MRI of Cardiovascular Malformations

Bruno Kastler

MRI of Cardiovascular Malformations

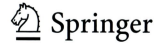 Springer

Author
Bruno Kastler
Professor of Radiology and Head of Radiology
Service de Radiologie A et C
Centre Hospitalier Universitaire Jean Minjoz
bd. Alexander Fleming
25000 Besançon
France
Director of Laboratoire I4S
(Health, Innovation, Intervention, Imaging, Engineering)
Université de Franche-Comté
Besançon
France
Associate Professor of Radiology
Department of Radiology
Centre Hospitalier Universitaire
Sherbrooke, Québec
Canada
kastler@ufc-chu.univ-fcomte.fr

ISBN 978-3-540-30701-3   e-ISBN 978-3-540-30702-0
DOI 10.1007/978-3-540-30702-0
Springer Heidelberg Dordrecht London New York

Library of Congress Control Number: 2010930082

Cover design: eStudioCalamar Figures/Berlin

Printed on acid-free paper

Springer is part of Springer Science+Business Media (www.springer.com)

This book is devoted to:

Children with congenital heart disease (with the hope that this book may modestly contribute to a better understanding and treatment of their disease).

My children, Tiphaine, Adrian and Florian (who patiently acted as dummies to prepare this atlas).

My nephews and nieces, Amandine, Hermance and Lysandre; Benjamin, Milena, Zelia and Aurelien.

My wife Blandine, already 35 years by my side.

Professor Wackenheim, who inspired me to illustrate pathological cases by diagrams.

Preface

For many years, the diagnosis of congenital cardiovascular anomalies was based on conventional radiography, catheterization and angiography. Non-invasive cardiac imaging was dramatically improved in the middle of the 1970s with the development of echocardiography, which considerably reduced the need for cardiac catheterization. This book summarizes years of "clinical collaborative work" to confirm the value of MRI, alongside echocardiography, in the management and follow-up of patients with congenital cardiovascular anomalies. This adventure began in 1987 in Strasbourg in close collaboration with Angelo Livolsi (hospital paediatric cardiologist), during examinations performed on Saturday afternoons and Sundays and often as an emergency at night, Philippe Germain (cardiologist) and Lionel Donato (hospital paediatrician). When I was appointed Professor of radiology at Besançon hospital, this adventure continued with the help of Yvette Bernard (Professor of cardiology) and her skills and competence in paediatric cardiac echocardiography.

MRI is a unique non-invasive imaging modality, a highly desirable feature in a paediatric population, which combines in one examination depicting complex cardiac anatomy measuring cardiac function and flow in one examination. The indications for MRI have been clearly established; it is perfectly complementary to echocardiography and has replaced diagnostic angiography. The primary indications are visualization of great vessels, especially coarctation of the aortic and aortic arch anomalies, right ventricular outflow tract anomalies, particularly to study the pulmonary artery and its branches, and anomalous systemic and pulmonary venous connections. MRI is also very useful for the diagnosis of complex forms and for postoperative follow-up after specific surgical procedures. Cardiac catheterization is now reserved for some types of congenital heart disease when obtaining hemodynamic information is mandatory.

The future of MRI is clearly ensured, as the spectacular progress in magnetic resonance have been accomplished these last years (imaging speed, flow analysis, angiography), will only reinforce contribution of this fundamental imaging modality and keep its indications essential.

Besancon, France

Bruno Kastler

Acknowledgement

I would like to thank:

Daniel Vetter for the excellent work of transcription of my diagrams in Illustrator® for Mac®.

Michel Gaudron who worked on the digital images.

Monique Dubois, Marie-Christine for updating the references.

Contents

Contributors

Sebastien Aubry Radiologie A & C, Centre Hospitalier Universitaire Jean-Minjoz, Boulevard Fleming, 25030 Besançon, France

Yvette Bernard Service de cardiologie, Centre Hospitalier Universitaire Jean-Minjoz, Boulevard Fleming, 25030 Besançon, France

Lionel Donato Service de pédiatrie, Hôpital de Hautepierre, Avenue Molière, 67098 Strasbourg, France

Philippe Germain Hospitaux Universitaires de Strasbourg, 1, rue de la 1re-Armée, 67000 Strasbourg, France

George Hadjidekov Radiologie A & C, Centre Hospitalier Universitaire Jean-Minjoz, Boulevard Fleming, 25030 Besançon, France

Jérome Jehl Radiologie A & C, Centre Hospitalier Universitaire Jean-Minjoz, Boulevard Fleming, 25030 Besançon, France

Bruno Kastler Professor of Radiology and Head of Radiology, Service de Radiologie A et C, Centre Hospitalier Universitaire Jean-Minjoz, bd. Alexander Fleming, 25000 Besançon, France
Director of Laboratoire I4S (Health, Innovation, Intervention, Imaging, Engineering), Université de Franche-Comté, Besançon, France
Associate Professor of Radiology, Department of Radiology, Centre Hospitalier Universitaire, Sherbrooke, Québec, Canada

Laurent Laborie Radiologie A & C, Centre Hospitalier Universitaire Jean-Minjoz, Avenue Molière, 67098 Strasbourg, France

Angelo Livolsi Service de pédiatrie, Hospitaux Universitaires de Strasbourg, Hôpital de Hautepierre, Avenue Molière, 67098 Strasbourg, France

Philippe Manzoni Radiologie A & C, Centre Hospitalier Universitaire Jean-Minjoz, Boulevard Fleming, 25030 Besançon, France

Armand Parsai Radiologie A & C, Centre Hospitalier Universitaire Jean-Minjoz, Boulevard Fleming, 25030 Besançon, France

Daniel Vetter Service IRM, Hospitaux Universitaires de Strasbourg, Hôpital de Hautepierre, Avenue Molière, 67098 Strasbourg, France

Patient Preparation: Magnetic Resonance Imaging Techniques

1

Magnetic resonance imaging plays a major role in the assessment of congenital heart disease [1–3]. The general principles of image acquisition are the same as in other clinical settings, but the assessment of congenital heart disease presents a number of specific features, which are described in this chapter by reviewing the main sequences used and their clinical value.

1.1 Examination Conditions

As in adults, cardiovascular MRI does not constitute an emergency examination for two essential reasons: the difficulties of patient surveillance during the examination and, especially, the very limited availability of MR machines that are already severely overbooked.

As an elective procedure, the major difficulty consists of ensuring good patient immobilization during the examination. Three main situations can be distinguished according to the child's age:

- In very young patients (especially below the age of 3–6 months), good immobilization is generally obtained quite easily during sleep following a feed.
- Similarly, when the examination can be explained to the child and when the parents are allowed to stay beside the MR apparatus, this examination can generally be performed in children older than 6 or 7 years without any particular medication for fairly short examination times.
- In contrast, the situation is much more difficult in children between the ages of 1 and 6 years. If sufficient time is available (at the end of the day's programme), MRI can be performed without anaesthesia, by lightly sedating the child with chloral hydrate solution administered after the baby's bottle or with intrarectal Hypnovel® (midazolam). This generally

ensures satisfactory immobilization within about 30 min, and repeated sequences can be launched during this interval. When this waiting time is not available, MRI must be performed in coordination with an anaesthetist. Some radiologists immobilize the child with Velpeau® bandages in plastic frames designed to be installed inside the coil.

In extreme cases, when anaesthesia must be avoided, good results can be obtained by letting an agitated child fall asleep on its mother's stomach (Fig. 1.1).

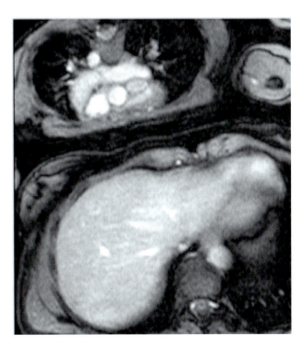

Fig. 1.1 A 4-year-old child, refractory to the usual sedatives, lying on his mother's stomach. Gating with the child's ECG allowed satisfactory imaging of the left ventricular walls (see Fig. 1.11). This last resort method can be effective when anaesthesia must be avoided, but the use of a whole body coil leads to a marked reduction of the signal-to-noise ratio for the analysis of small anatomical structures

B. Kastler, *MRI of Cardiovascular Malformations*,
DOI: 10.1007/978-3-540-30702-0_1, © Springer-Verlag Berlin Heidelberg 2011

A coil with a good apparent diffusion coefficient must be used, preferably a quadrature coil. A "head" coil or "knee" coil is generally used in young patients and a "chest" coil is used in older children. The region to be studied must be positioned in the centre of the coil. The child must be comfortably placed and well covered, and ventilation in the tunnel may need to be turned off. Baby vests must not have any metal clips or safety pins.

Small ECG electrodes with carbon contact clips and no metal parts must be arranged to obtain a good amplitude ECG recording with a clearly visible monophasic R wave to ensure reliable gating.

1.2 Sequences Used

The major difference in relation to adult imaging concerns the naturally high heart rate of infants (110–150 bpm). Gating of sequences with the R wave of the ECG therefore provides only a brief time window for signal acquisition, making it impossible to obtain 10–12 slices (on multislice spin-echo sequences) or 20–30 cardiac cycles (by cine-MRI) as in adults, but only about one quarter of these imaging rates. On the other hand, sequences are more rapidly completed in view of the rapid heart rate when cardiac gating is satisfactory (gating for each heart beat and not for every two or three heart beats). Only T1 weighting is possible due to the short TR related to the rapid heart rate (i.e. morphological imaging, without clearly defined tissue characterization). It should be noted that, in ECG-gated multislice imaging, each image is obtained at a distinct instant of the cardiac cycle, as shown in Fig. 1.2.

A 200-mm field of view with a 160 (anteroposterior) × 256 matrix is usually used to acquire images with a slice thickness of 3–5 mm and 2–4 accumulations, which corresponds to a resolution in the imaging plane of about 1 mm with an acquisition time of about 4 min. On modern machines, equipped with powerful gradients (fast imaging), the noise generated by gradient switching constitutes a considerable problem, as this noise can sometimes be very strident and intense and can wake or frighten the sleeping child, in which case, some sequences may need to be avoided (a "quiet" mode is available on some machines).

Four types of sequences are distinguished according to the desired type of information (Table 1.1).

Ultrafast or real-time imaging (for example, echoplanar imaging which produces an image in 100 ms)

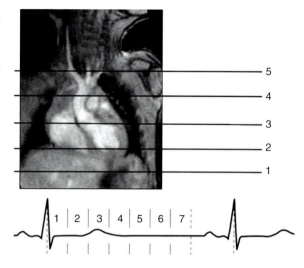

Fig. 1.2 In ECG-gated multislice imaging, each slice corresponds to a distinct instant of the cardiac cycle. Some images are therefore acquired in diastole, while others are acquired in systole; this acquisition mode is consequently unsuitable for precise measurements, which must be performed on cine images, on which diastole and systole are well defined

Table 1.1 Four types of sequences are used

Approach	Type of sequence	Application
Morphological	Black-blood: spin-echo and variants, double IR prepared	Anatomy of structures
Kinetic	Bright-blood: gradient-echo cine-MRI, balanced-SSFP	Wall motion and blood flow
Flowmetric	Velocity mapping	Flow quantification (especially shunts)
Angiographic	With or without gadolinium	Vascular imaging

does not have a satisfactory spatial resolution and contrast at the present time, but can be useful for localizing sequences.

1.3 Morphological Approach

The primary indication for MRI is generally morphological analysis, which is usually obtained by black blood techniques (low signal of flowing blood) and is based on spin-echo techniques.

Spin-echo-based sequences provide fairly good natural contrast between cardiac chambers (and/or

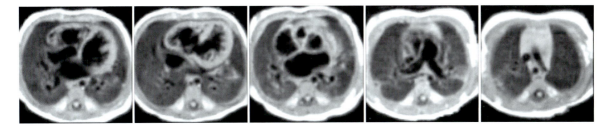

Fig. 1.3 Axial spin-echo sequence in a neonate with transposition of the great vessels. Several successive acquisitions were performed (0.5 T) (see Chaps. 3 and 7)

vessels lumen), in which mobile spins present a low signal intensity, in contrast to the walls, which present a higher signal intensity.

MR imaging sequence, including spin-echo-based techniques, has benefited from constant technical progress with the primary emphasis on speed.

It must, however, be outlined that bright-blood techniques (enhanced signal of inflow blood), particularly, the recently introduced balanced-SSFP, generate fast images with high spatial resolution, which offer highly detailed anatomical information.

1.3.1 Conventional Spin-Echo Sequence

Classically, the multislice spin-echo sequence is used with 2–4 imaging planes according to the child's heart rate. Several serial contiguous acquisitions can be used to acquire a larger volume (Fig. 1.3).

The spatial resolution of these T1-weighted images (short TR dictated by the rapid heart rate in infants) is satisfactory (about 1 mm in the plane of view). The acquisition time can be shortened by adopting asymmetrical matrices adjusted to the structures studied [4]. Several accumulations are necessary for thin slices (3 mm). A disadvantage of this sequence, that can sometimes be prohibitive, concerns the artefacts propagated in the direction of phase coding, which can become very important at high fields (Fig. 1.4). As these artefacts are essentially related to respiratory movements, swapping the direction of phase and frequency encoding can reduce them.

1.3.2 Variants

Variants of the spin-echo sequence have been proposed aiming at increasing imaging speed and optimizing image quality.

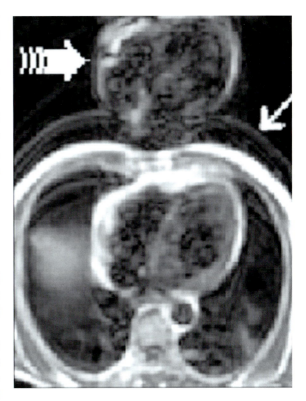

Fig. 1.4 Artefacts (classical spin-echo) obtained along the phase-encoding direction (in this case anteroposterior) related to respiratory (*long arrow*) and cardiac (*large arrow*) movements in a case of poor cardiac gating

1.3.3 Fast Spin-Echo or Turbo-Spin-Echo

On these sequences, 2–12 phase coding steps are obtained after each excitation (segmented imaging). The acquisition time is consequently divided by the corresponding turbo factor. The main purpose of these sequences is to provide identical spatial resolution to that of classical spin-echo sequences with a shorter acquisition time. Potential limitations of fast spin-echo sequences include blurring due to signal variation from one line of k space to the other and respiratory motion artefacts. Respiratory motion algorithm or navigator echo techniques using diaphragmatic motion have been proposed. Fast spin-echo acquisition time is compatible with breath-holding, which is essential to prevent motion artefacts. These sequences provide the best image quality when breath-holding (possible in elderly cooperative children or adults) is performed correctly. However in our experience, this type of sequence has proven useful in paediatric cardiology, despite respiratory movements.

1.3.4 Double IR Sequences

Another drawback of fast spin-echo sequences is incomplete blood signal, stagnant blood being mistaken as tissue. A double inversion pulse has been added at the beginning of the sequence for blood signal suppression and optimization of black blood imaging [5, 6]. First a non-selective 180° pulse occurs at the r wave trigger. A second selective 180° pulse restores the signal of section to be imaged (cardiac walls higher signal), whereas the nulled blood (black signal) flows in at a specific inversion time (TI). Single slice or better multislice double IR T2-weighted black blood sequences allowing excellent image quality during one breath-hold [7] are now becoming gold standard for black blood imaging and used routinely in replacement of fast spin-echo sequences. Double IR sequences can be combined with half Fourier acquisition.

1.3.5 Half Fourier Single Shot Fast Spin-Echo Sequences

An extreme version of Fast spin-echo imaging consists of completing, in a single passage, a half Fourier acquisition by means of echo signals generated by many refocusing RF impulses (typically 80) following the initial excitation at 90° (HASTE-Siemens, SSFSE-GEMS, SSTSE-Philips). These T2-weighted sequences present a major advantage in terms of speed, images being acquired within a heartbeat [8, 9], but the spatial resolution remains fairly poor and the use of a half Fourier acquisition makes the sequence very sensitive to spectral folding and motion artefacts (Fig. 1.5).

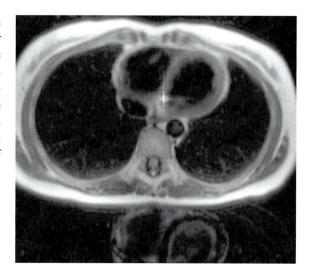

Fig. 1.5 Example of the results obtained with a Haste sequence (very rapid variant of spin-echo sequence), requiring only one heart beat. Spatial resolution is limited and several artefacts related to the use of a half Fourier acquisition are observed, but this type of sequence is very useful in practice due to its very short acquisition time, when breath-hold images cannot be obtained in young children

When available, half Fourier single shot FSE sequences, because they are very rapid, provide useful sets of localizing images and are a valuable alternative in patients unable to hold their breath. This type of sequence delivers a large number of 180° radiofrequency pulses, and can cause RF energy deposit and patient overheating (see: febrile patient), which is why limitation devices, taking the patient's weight into account, must be used (SAR). Black blood sequences should be performed before gadolinium injection as this latter impairs proper blood suppression by the specific unselective IR pulse.

1.4 Gradient-Echo Cine Imaging

Gradient-echo techniques offer two advantages for cardiovascular imaging: good visualization of the hyperintense blood pool, and cine imaging, which is very useful to assess contraction of the cardiac walls and blood flow.

The contrasts obtained on gradient-echo sequences are practically inverted compared to spin-echo sequences, as illustrated in Fig. 1.6. The dark colour of circulating blood, visible on spin-echo, is replaced by a

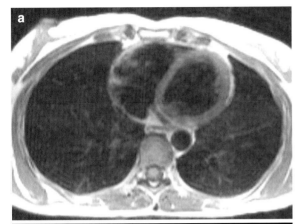

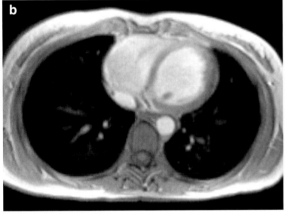

Fig. 1.6 (**a**) Spin-echo sequence (blood is black, walls have an intermediate signal intensity). (**b**) Gradient-echo sequence (blood is white, walls have an intermediate signal intensity)

gradient (Flash-Siemens, FFE-T1 Philips, SPGR-GE) and others restore transverse magnetization by steady-state (FISP-Siemens, FFE-T2 Philips, Grass-GE). The most useful techniques recently introduced in cardiovascular imaging now use balanced and symmetrical flow compensating gradients: Balanced-SSFP (Fiesta/GE, True-FISP/Siemens, Balanced-FFE/Philips). These sequences generate cine-MRI (with T2/T1 image weighting) [10] and furthermore excellent anatomical details. Advantages include faster imaging, better blood pool signal enhancement not relying on inflow effects and higher SNR. Drawbacks are sensitivity to field inhomogeneity (metallic artefacts, magnetic susceptibility), motion artefacts (respiration, pulsatile through plane flow under certain conditions), and most of all, significantly less sensitivity to abnormal flow patterns (flow void jets due to stenosis, regurgitation, ASD, VSD) in comparison to traditional GE cine-MRI. In view of the above-mentioned limitations, traditional GE cine-MRI is still performed. Unlike black blood techniques, it can be performed not only before but also after gadolinium administration.

1.4.1 Beating Heart Applications

The succession of diastolic and systolic images during the cardiac cycle allows assessment (and possibly quantification) of global and segmental wall contraction [11]. This application is less useful in children than in adults, but may be useful for assessment of cardiomyopathies (especially right ventricular dysplasia) or ischaemic disease (Fig. 1.10).

1.4.2 Qualitative Assessment of Blood Flow Applications

Another advantage of gradient-echo sequences concerns signal void, which occurs in the blood pool in the case of very rapid or turbulent flow (stenoses or regurgitating valves, flow jets in shunts), which cause flow void jets across the hyperintense blood pool corresponding to disturbances of flow [12, 13]. However, this pathological sign remains purely qualitative and not quantitative, as the dephasing effects are related to the TE time (the longer the TE, the more intense is the

high signal intensity of the blood pool on gradient-echo images. Muscle (and myocardial) tissue presents an intermediate signal intensity (grey) and adipose tissue has a high signal intensity on both types of sequences. The two examples shown in Figs. 1.7 and 1.8 illustrate the differences between spin-echo and gradient-echo sequences. One of the advantages of these differential contrasts is to facilitate identification of air and vascular structures, as shown in Figs. 1.8 and 1.9.

Gradient-echo therefore constitutes a useful complement to spin-echo for multislice anatomical imaging, but most importantly, these sequences allow repeated acquisition in the same plane at different successive instants of the cardiac cycle. Closed loop visualization of these images corresponds to the cine mode, which is very useful for cardiac applications. There are several types of gradient-echo sequences: some dephase transverse magnetization with a dephasing

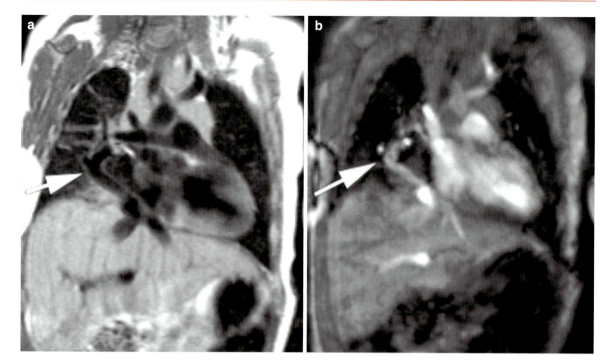

Fig. 1.7 Example of anomalous pulmonary venous connection of the right inferior pulmonary into the inferior vena cava (*arrow*); this child also presents azygos continuation of the inferior vena cava (see Chap. 4, Fig. 19). (**a**) Spin-echo sequence. (**b**) Gradient-echo sequence (cine-MRI). Tracheobronchial structures have low signal intensity on both sequences, while vessels have low signal intensity on spin-echo sequences and high signal intensity on gradient-echo sequences

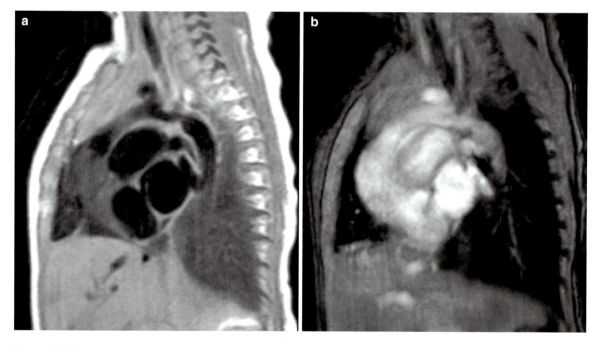

Fig. 1.8 Sagittal oblique images in an infant with D-transposition of the great vessels. (**a**) Spin-echo sequence. (**b**) Gradient-echo sequence. Pathognomonic "gun barrel" appearance of the aorta (anterior) and pulmonary artery (dilated, posterior). Inversion of vascular contrast between the two sequences

Fig. 1.9 Aortic arch anomaly (Neuhauser anomaly, see Chap. 5, Fig. 13) on two different axial slices. The advantage of gradient-echo (cine images on the *right*) compared to spin-echo (images on the *left*) is that it clearly demonstrates vascular structures

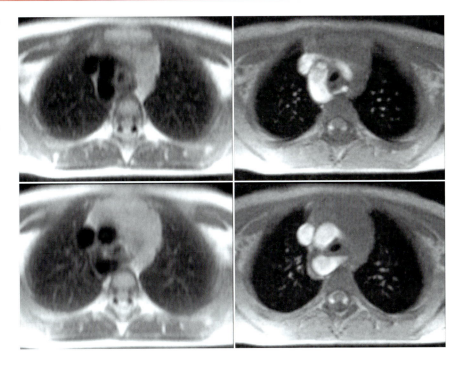

signal void). In practice, it is a very useful sign (as in colour-coded duplex echocardiography), for example, to estimate the extent of valvular regurgitation (Fig. 1.11) or to detect a left–right shunt (Fig. 1.12). As mentioned earlier, balanced-SSFP sequences are now used routinely in place of traditional GE cine-MRI. However, when abnormal flow pattern analysis is required, traditional GE cine-MR (with optimized long TE) should still be performed.

1.5 Phase Velocity Mapping for Flow Quantification

Phase velocity mapping sequences [14, 15] are based on phase encoding of the NMR signal proportionally to the velocity of spins in a given direction (generally perpendicular to the imaging plane). Phase velocity mapping sequences are gradient-echo cine sequences with slightly modified gradients.

The flow velocity curve during the cardiac cycle can be extracted from the phase images obtained for various arterial or venous regions of interest. Figure 1.13 illustrates the use of this sequence to measure aortic blood flow. The blood flow rate Q in this region during each cardiac cycle can be easily determined from the mean flow rate V and the surface area of the region of interest S: $Q_{mL/cycle} = V \times S$. It should be noted that, as for duplex echocardiography, velocity is more severely underestimated as the direction of flow shifts from the plane perpendicular to the imaging plane. This technique can therefore be used only when the imaging plane is perpendicular to the vessel studied. Finally, the range of velocities to be encoded must be carefully selected to avoid aliasing phenomena when the flow velocity exceeds the encoding range (as in Doppler). Prior definition of the direction of flow and its order of magnitude is therefore essential to obtain good measuring conditions.

1.5.1 Measurement of the QP/QS Shunt Ratio

The main application of this technique in congenital heart disease is non-invasive measurement of shunt ratios [16, 17] by comparison with pulmonary (QP, typically measured in the pulmonary artery trunk) and systemic blood flow (QS, typically measured in the ascending aorta). Figure 1.14 illustrates this concept in a case of ostium secundum ASD. Two separate acquisitions must be performed in this case due to the

Fig. 1.10 Diastolic and systolic images from cine-MRI sequences obtained in the child presented in Fig. 1.1. This 4-year-old boy suffered from Kawasaki disease inducing anterior myocardial infarction. An attempt to visualize the coronary arteries failed, but cine imaging clearly shows the large anterior akinetic area (*arrows*). The ejection fraction can be calculated by planimetry of the diastolic and systolic ventricular contours

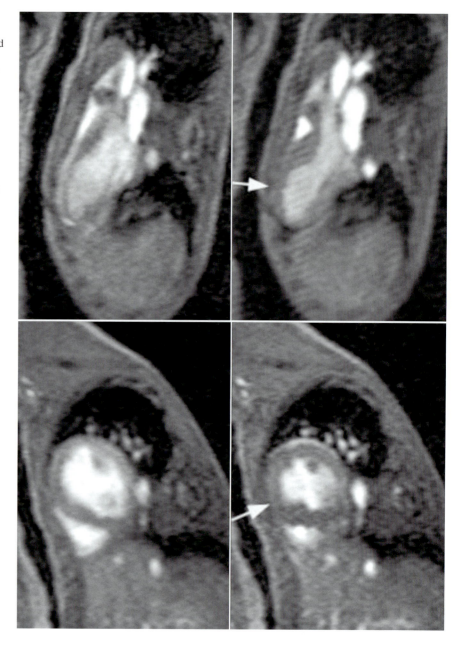

different orientations of the ascending aorta (vertical) and pulmonary artery trunk (inclined superiorly and posteriorly). Velocity measurements are usually corrected by a complementary measurement performed on a static region (muscle tissue) to correct for any systematic dephasing. As the flow rate measured is proportional to the surface area of the region of interest, vascular margins must be very carefully contoured, as the acceptable error is ± 10%.

1.5.2 Assessment of Direction of Flow

When velocity encoding gradients are applied in the imaging plane (and not perpendicular to this plane), phase images indicate the direction of flow in the imaging plane. One of the possible applications is analysis of the false channel in aortic dissection, to determine whether or not it is circulating (complication of Marfan syndrome, for example). Assessment

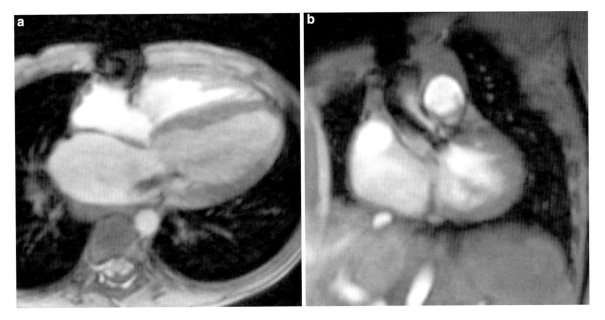

Fig. 1.11 Systolic gradient-echo cine images obtained in an infant with mitral regurgitation (**a**) and congenital aortic stenosis (**b**). Trails of signal void indicate the presence of rapid and turbulent jets related to valvular lesions

of flow lines is also useful to define the region with the highest velocity, to select the zone in which flow quantification can be used to calculate pressure gradients (Figs. 1.15 and 1.16).

1.5.3 Pressure Gradient Estimation

Like Doppler echocardiography, MRI can be used to estimate pressure gradients ΔP across stenotic segments, from the maximum velocity V, according to the simplified Bernouilli equation $\Delta P = 4 \times V^2$. An important application concerns coarctation of the aorta [18, 19]. An example of pressure gradient measurement in pulmonary stenosis is shown in Fig. 1.16. However, certain difficulties of this approach must be emphasized.

- Echo times (TE) must be very short to avoid intravoxel dephasing which would induce signal loss and therefore loss of information at the site of measurement.
- To avoid underestimating the gradient, the measurement must be performed precisely at the site of maximum stenosis. For these reasons, pressure gradient measurement is difficult to perform in practice.

These velocity mapping sequences therefore constitute a very useful complement to conventional anatomical imaging, as they provide a supplementary, functional dimension, particularly for comparative right–left flow quantification or to estimate flow in Blalock-Taussig shunts, for example.

1.5.4 MR Angiography

Gradient-echo sequences already provide a good "angiographic" approach, as shown in Figs. 1.7–1.9. MR angiography differs from standard sequences by a technique designed to achieve maximum contrast between stationary tissues and circulating blood, and also by projective rather than tomographic presentation of the data. The operation of transformation of raw data (stacks of parallel images) into projections oriented in any direction is called MIP (maximum intensity projection). Three main principles of MR angiography are currently used. The first two do not require injection of contrast agent [20–23] and are based on phase modulation of the spins or the time of flight (TOF) effect. The third method is the most effective and is based on enhancement of the intravascular signal following bolus injection of gadolinium (contrast-enhanced angiography) [22–25].

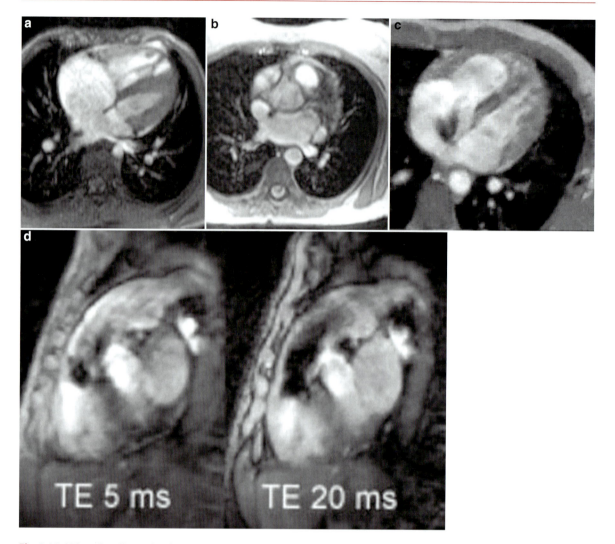

Fig. 1.12 Value of gradient-echo cine sequences for the analysis of shunts. In the presence of a large atrial septal defect, the flow velocities corresponding to the shunt can be low. In this case, there is no visible signal void, but the defect is often more clearly visualized than on spin-echo sequences (image (**a**) with large ostium secundum ASD and (**b**) high sinus venosus ASD). When flow velocities in the defect are higher ((**c**) ASD and (**d**) high VSD), the jet has a signal void appearance (*black*). Image (**d**) shows that the infundibular signal void is more marked with a long TE (20 ms) than with a short TE (5 ms). The MR signs of pathological jet must therefore be interpreted cautiously in the light of the results obtained with a sequence with which the radiologist is more familiar

1.5.5 Non-enhanced MR Angiography

Phase-contrast angiography is well adapted to the study of slow flows, but is not suitable for infants or children, who present fairly high and very pulsatile circulatory velocities. The TOF technique is more appropriate for these situations, but blood flow must be perpendicular to the imaging plane. The entry of fully magnetized, unsaturated spins into the imaged slice, in contrast with the already saturated spins of the surrounding tissues,

Fig. 1.13 Flow measurement in the ascending aorta during the cardiac cycle. The image is acquired perpendicular to the ascending aorta. The phase image corresponds to the velocity mapping perpendicular to the imaging plane (systolic image). The graph on the *right* shows the mean velocity measured at each instant of the cardiac cycle in the region of interest corresponding to the ascending aorta. The integral of the velocities in this zone of interest corresponds to aortic systolic flow (ejection flow)

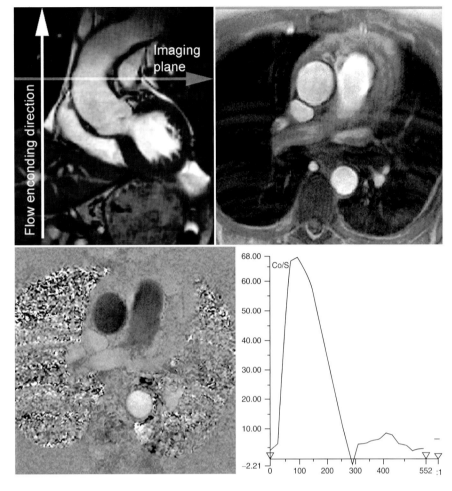

induces excellent vascular contrast. In addition, saturation pulses can be applied above or below the imaged slice to selectively suppress venous or arterial flow, as shown in Fig. 1.17.

TOF sequences can be acquired in 2DFT (successive acquisitions of thin separate images) or 3DFT (global acquisition of a volume composed of elementary partitions) modes. The 2DFT mode provides optimal vascular contrast, but a poor signal-to-noise ratio. In 3DFT mode, the signal-to-noise ratio is better, but saturation effects are observed as blood travels in the imaged volume, which decreases vascular contrast. Forty to sixty 2 mm thick images are usually acquired in about 6–8 min.

1.5.6 Contrast-Enhanced MR Angiography

The best results at the present time are obtained with fast 3DFT sequences, acquired during first passage of a T1 contrast agent. These gradient-echo sequences (TR about 5 ms and TE about 2 ms) allow about thirty 1–2 mm thick images to be obtained in about 10 s for a limited resolution (1.5 mm pixels, for example) and about 20 s for a higher resolution (pixels measuring about 1 mm) (Fig. 1.18).

Apart from rapid acquisition, compatible with one breath-hold in older children and adults, the decisive advantages are:

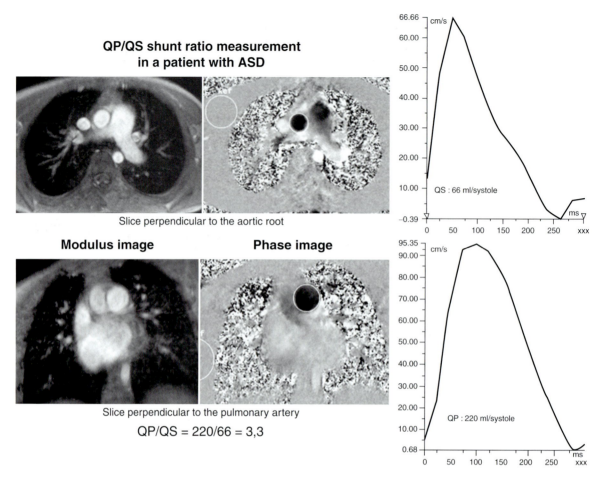

QP/QS shunt ratio measurement in a patient with ASD

Slice perpendicular to the aortic root

Modulus image   **Phase image**

Slice perpendicular to the pulmonary artery

QP/QS = 220/66 = 3,3

QS : 66 ml/systole

QP : 220 ml/systole

Fig. 1.14 Example of measurement of a shunt ratio in a 6-year-old boy with ostium secundum ASD. On the *top part* of the figure, the measurement is performed perpendicularly to the ascending aorta. The "modulus" image is on the *left* and the corresponding "phase" image (systole) is in the *middle*. Velocity curves in the cardiac cycle are shown on the *right*. The *bottom* images show measurement in another imaging plane, perpendicular to the pulmonary artery trunk. In this case, the shunt ratio is high (QP/QS = 220/66 = 3.3). This measuring modality is relatively easy and appears to be reliable

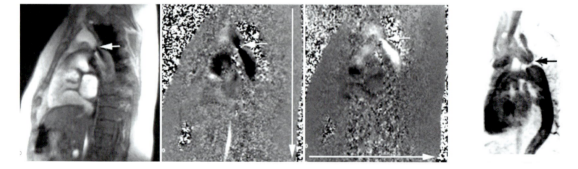

Fig. 1.15 Sagittal oblique images obtained in a young girl with coarctation of the aorta. The image on the *left* corresponds to a systolic gradient-echo "module" image through the isthmic coarctation (*arrow*). The *middle* images correspond to velocity mapping images obtained after velocity coding in the imaging plane in the craniocaudal (*vertical long arrow*) and anteroposterior (*horizontal long arrow*) directions. The highest velocities are observed in the zone of maximum strangulation of the coarctation. The image on the *right* corresponds to gadolinium-enhanced MR angiography (Dota-Gd, Guerbet, France)

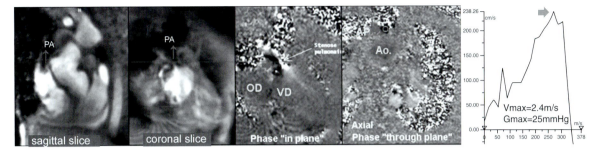

Fig. 1.16 Example of pulmonary valve stenosis. The two images on the *left* correspond to systolic "module" images obtained in the coronal and sagittal planes. The *middle* image is a coronal image showing the axial plane used to measure veloci-ties. The maximum velocity measured in the pulmonary artery (*arrows*) was 2.4 m/s, which corresponds to a pulmonary gradient of about 25 mmHg

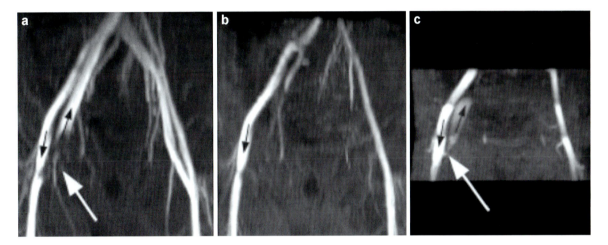

Fig. 1.17 TOF MR angiography (without injection of contrast agent) obtained in a 12-month-old infant with right femoral arteriovenous fistula. (**a, b**) Correspond to 2DFT acquisitions (stacks of serial thin axial slices). No presaturation is applied in image (**a**). The venous signal void over the fistula is related to turbulence in the shunt (*white arrow*). More distally, the right iliac vein is dilated compared to the contralateral vein. In (**b**), venous presaturation (inferior) is applied to each slab suppressing all venous signals (including distal to the fistula), leaving only the arteriogram. The image on the *right* (**c**) corresponds to a 3DFT acquisition in three slabs with underlying venous presaturation of each slab. A venous signal related to the shunt is visible in the central image

- Large field of view with no constraints related to the direction of flow compared to the imaging plane as in the case of the TOF technique.
- Excellent vascular contrast due to the marked reduction of T1 induced by passage of gadolinium bolus.
- 3D MIP reconstruction and time-resolved dynamic sequences [26] allowing evaluation of small vacular structure patency and separation of the venous and arterial phases and of pulmonary and systemic circulation (see Fig. 1.14 E, F Chap. 7).

However, this technique presents certain limitations. A good quality venous line must be set up to allow a sufficient bolus injection rate. The choice of imaging volume is critical, as it must be sufficiently large to include all of the vascular structures of interest, but must be sufficiently small to allow an acceptable acquisition time. Finally, the interval between injection and launching of the sequence must be precisely adjusted so that the time of acquisition of the central line of the Fourier plan (start or middle of the sequence) exactly corresponds to the time of passage of the gadolinium

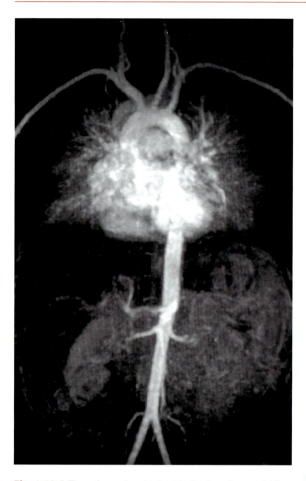

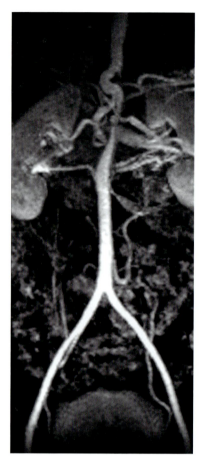

Fig. 1.18 MR angiography obtained in 8 s in a 6-year-old boy with injection of 4 mL of gadolinium (0.2 mL/kg). A large field of view can be obtained in this small child with an adult chest coil extending from the origin of supra-aortic vessels to the iliac vessels

Fig. 1.19 Examples of abdominal coarctation of the aorta in an adolescent, visualized by gadolinium-enhanced MR angiography (Dota-Gd, Guerbet, France), with a brief breath-hold of 10–20 s (see Chap. 6). MIP projections comprise bothersome superimposition effects, poor distinction between the stenotic abdominal aorta and the origin of the coeliac trunk, which is why, analysis of elementary images or multiplanar reconstructions in other planes is essential to ensure correct interpretation of the examination

bolus. This factor makes MR angiography of the right ventricular outflow tract and pulmonary branches particularly difficult due to the very rapid transit in these structures. Figure 1.19 provide several examples of the results obtained with this technique which, in the future, should considerably limit the indications for conventional angiography (except for coronary vessels).

1.6 Conclusion

Multiple sequences can be used in paediatric cardiovascular MRI. The examination must not be limited to purely morphological imaging, but must also take advantage of the possibilities of functional imaging provided by cine-MRI techniques, velocity mapping and MR angiography.

References

1. Higgins CB, editor. MRI of congenital heart disease. In: Essentials of cardiac radiology and imaging. New York: J.B. Lippincott; 1992. p. 283–331.
2. Ho VB, Kinney JB, Sahn DJ. Contributions of newer MR imaging strategies for congenital heart disease. Radiographics. 1996;16:43–60.

3. Bank ER. Magnetic resonance of congenital cardiovascular disease. An update [review]. Radiol Clin North Am. 1993;31:553–72.

4. Kastler B, Livolsi A, Germain P. Strip scanning a method to improve pediatric cardiovascular MRI. In: SMRI, Ninth Annual Meeting, Chicago; 3–6 April 1991.

5. Edelman RR, Chien D, Kim D. Fast selective black blood MR imaging. Radiology. 1991;181(3):655–60.

6. Simonetti OP, Finn JP, White RD, Laub G, Henry DA. "Black blood" T2- weighted inversion-recovery MR imaging of the heart. Radiology. 1996;199(1):49–57.

7. Boiselle PM, White CS. New techniques in cardiothoracic imaging. New York: Informa Healthcare USA; 2007. p. 81–2.

8. Stehling MK, Holzknecht NG, Laub G, Böhm D, von Smekal A, Reiser M. Single-shot T1- and T2-weighted magnetic resonance imaging of the heart with black blood: preliminary experience. MAGMA. 1996;4(3–4):231–40.

9. Winterer JT, Lehnhardt S, Schneider B, Neumann K, Allmann KH, Laubenberger J, et al. MRI of heart morphology. Comparison of nongradient echo sequences with single- and multislice acquisition. Invest Radiol. 1999;34(8):516–22.

10. Carr JC, Simonetti O, Bundy J, Li D, Pereles S, Finn JP. Cine MR angiography of the heart with segmented true fast imaging with steady-state precession. Radiology. 2001;219(3):828–34.

11. Graham TP Jr. Ventricular performance in congenital heart disease. Circulation. 1991;84:2259–74.

12. Mohiaddin RH, Longmore DB. Functional aspects of cardiovascular nuclear magnetic resonance imaging. Techniques and application [review]. Circulation. 1993;88:264–81.

13. Weber OM, Higgins CB. MR evaluation of cardiovascular physiology in congenital heart disease: flow and function. J Cardiovasc Magn reson. 2006;8(4):607–17.

14. Rees S, Firmin D, Mohiaddîn R, Underwood R, Longmore D. Application of flow measurements by magnetic resonance velocity mapping to congenital heart disease. Am J Cardiol. 1989;64:953–6.

15. Rebergen SA, Niezen RA, Helbing WA, van der Wall EE, de Roos A. Cine gradient-echo MR imaging and MR velocity mapping in the evaluation of congenital heart disease. Radiographics. 1996;16(3):467–81.

16. Brenner LD, Caputo GR, Mostbeck G, et al. Quantification of left to right atrial shunts with velocity-encoded cine nuclear magnetic resonance imaging. J Am Coll Cardiol. 1992;20:1246–50.

17. Boehrer JD, Lange RA, Willard JE, Grayburn PA, Hillis LD. Advantages and limitations of methods to detect, localize, and quantitate intracardiac left- to-right shunting [review]. Am Heart J. 1992;124:448–55.

18. Oshinski JN, Parks WJ, Markou CP, et al. Improved measurements of pressure gradients in aortic coarctation by magnetic resonance imaging. J Am Col Cardiol. 1996;28:1818–26.

19. Simpson IA, Chung KJ, Glass RF, Sahn DJ, Sherman FS, Hesselink J. Cine magnetic resonance imaging for evaluation of anatomy and flow relations in infants and children with coarctation of the aorta. Circulation. 1988;78:142–8.

20. Bradley WG. Flow phenomena in MR imaging. AJR Am J Roentgenol. 1988;150:983–94.

21. Edelmann RR. Basic principles of magnetic resonance angiography. Cardiovasc Intervent Radiol. 1992;15:3.

22. Kastler B, Patay Z, Vetter D. Imagerie du flux. in Comprendre l'IRM. Paris: Masson; 2006 (6th edition). P. 189–214.

23. Kastler B. Principles of MR angiography. In: Patay Z, Kastler B, Anzalone N, editors. Applied neuroMR angiography CD-ROM. Antwerpen: Lasion; 1996.

24. Holmqvist C, Larsson EM, Stahlberg F, Laurin S. Contrast-enhanced thoracic 3D-MR angiography in infants and children. Acta Radiol. 2001;42:50–8.

25. Lohan DG, Krishnam M, Saleh R, Tomasian A, Finn JP. MR imaging of the thoracic Aorta. Magn Reson Imaging Clin N Am. 2008;16(2):213–34.

26. Lohan DG, Krishnam M, Saleh R, Tomasian A, Finn JP. Time- resolved MR angiography of the thorax. Magn Reson Imaging Clin N Am. 2008;16(2):235–48.

Cardiovascular Anatomy and Atlas of MR Normal Anatomy

MRI with its large field of view, excellent spontaneous vessel-tissue contrast, good spatial resolution, and functional approach to blood flow is very well adapted to visualization of cardiac as well as mediastinal structures, in contrast with echocardiography, which is limited by bone or air artifacts [1–15]. However, as for any "tomographic" technique, multiplanar MRI requires mental 3D reconstruction of cardiovascular anatomy from a series of sequential images 3–10 mm thick, obtained after processing.[1]

A good knowledge of normal cardiac anatomy in the "useful" imaging planes usually performed (axial, coronal, sagittal, and guided according to the anatomical axis of the heart) is therefore an essential prerequisite. This approach allows segmental cardiovascular analysis[2] [16–20] by identifying the various cardiac chambers and great vessels, their location, and their mode of connection.

Healthy subjects with usual connections (SVC and IVC → RA → RV → PA and PV → LA → LV → Ao[3]) present a right–left arrangement of cardiac chambers which is correlated with the thoracic and abdominal arrangement. Due to the orientation of the anatomical axis of the heart, the "right" chambers are actually in a "right anterior" position compared to the "left" chambers, which are situated in a "left posterior" position (Figs. 2.1–2.3). Furthermore, due to crossover (twisting) of the great vessels at their origin, the pulmonary artery and aorta do not comply with this right–left symmetry. At its origin, the ascending aorta ("left-sided" structure) is situated centrally and posteriorly (and to the right) of the pulmonary artery ("right-sided" structure), which is situated anteriorly (and to the left) (Figs. 2.1 and 2.4).

Many variants of position and cardiac and vascular connection (inversion) can be observed in congenital malformations. The various chambers (atria/ventricles) are therefore identified by morphological criteria as "morphologically right" (mRA, mRV) or "morphologically left" (mLA, mLV) regardless of their actual position ("right" or "left").

After a general review of the principles of cardiovascular imaging and a few basic concepts, this chapter describes cardiovascular anatomy, illustrated by an atlas of normal imaging, which is completed by segmental sequential analysis (see Chap. 3).

2.1 General Principles

MRI examination, particularly in children, requires perfect sedation (or possibly even general anesthesia), as the slightest movement can significantly alter the image quality (see Chap. 1).

After a localizing sequence, the examination starts with axial spin-echo sequences, providing a precise and reliable three dimensional tomographic visualization of cardiovascular anatomy. On T1-weighted spin-echo-based sequences, the blood, circulating rapidly in vessels and cardiac chambers, usually generates spontaneous contrast ("low signal intensity" – black) compared to mediastinal fat ("high signal intensity" – white) and soft tissues (vessel walls and myocardium, "isosignal" – gray). Chambers and airways (lungs, trachea, etc.),

---

[1]Real-time imaging is possible on more recent machines, which allows selection, on a beating heart image, of the most appropriate imaging plane to visualize the structure of interest.

[2]In the same way as for echocardiography, angiography or autopsy.

[3]SVC and IVC = superior vena cava and inferior vena cava, RA and LA = right and left atrium, RV and LV = right and left ventricle, PA = pulmonary artery and Ao = aorta.

B. Kastler, *MRI of Cardiovascular Malformations*,
DOI: 10.1007/978-3-540-30702-0_2, © Springer-Verlag Berlin Heidelberg 2011

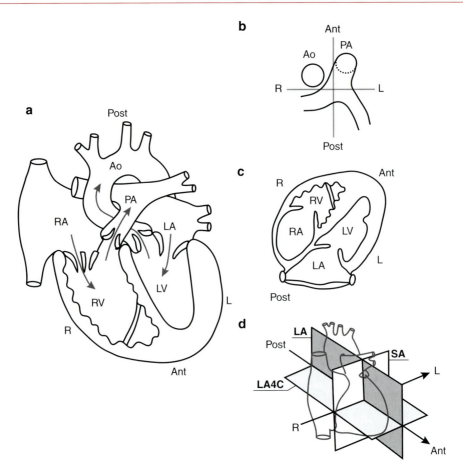

Fig. 2.1 Normal arrangement of cardiac chambers and great vessels. (**a**) Anatomical diagram, (**b**) Section through the origin of the aorta (Ao) and pulmonary artery (PA), (**c**) "Four-chamber" axial image. (**d**) Diagram of the arrangement of the cardiac chambers in the thorax. (**a**) The aorta (Ao) emerges from the (morphologically) left ventricle (LV-mLV), and the pulmonary artery (PA) emerges from the (morphologically) right ventricle (RV-mRV). (**b**) At its origin, the ascending aorta is in a central position, posteriorly and to the right of the pulmonary artery, which is situated anteriorly and to the left. (**c**, **d**) "Right" chambers are "right anterior" and "left" chambers are "left posterior" (also see Figs. 2.2 (anatomical axis) and 2.4 (short-axis and long-axis images) and Figs. 2.4, 2.6, and 2.7 ("four-chamber" axial images). Right atrium (RA) and left atrium (LA). Note that the loop rule indicating that both the Ao and mRV are situated on the same side applies here (*see below*)

bone and calcifications also appear black (see Chap. 1). The field of view is adapted to the child's thorax including the heart, mediastinum, lungs, and extends into the neck or even the abdomen to analyze the position of abdominal viscera.

2.2   Choice of Imaging Planes

Although acquisition of a first series of axial images is essential, the choice of the other imaging planes (the most appropriate: other axial series, coronal, sagittal, and/or oblique series) cannot be standardized. The examination protocol is adapted to each individual case by referring to the clinical file and the problems not resolved by echocardiography, and also the information gradually obtained during acquisition of MR sequences. The use of oblique slices containing vascular structures (situated away from the heart) is sometimes very useful, as these structures are not always clearly visualized on echocardiography. The limiting factor when elaborating this examination protocol (as is often the case in imaging) is the duration of the examination. The use of rectangular fields of view with asymmetrical matrices (e.g., 96×256) and several

Fig. 2.2 Anatomical axis of
the heart. The anatomical
axis of the heart or long-axis
(base-apex) is usually
directed anteriorly, inferiorly,
and to the left. Consequently,
the atria are situated
posteriorly and superiorly,
and the ventricles are situated
anteriorly and inferiorly (see
text and Figs. 2.1c and 2.5c)

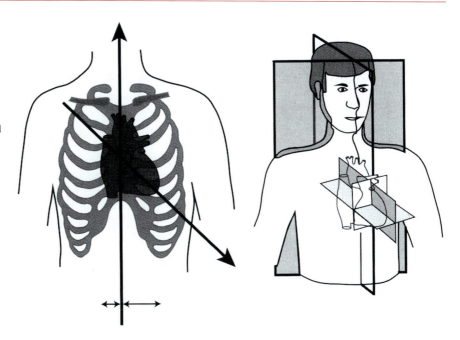

excitations (at least 4) reduces the examination time
and movement artifacts [21, 22]. Under these conditions, the acquisition time of a conventional spin-echo
(SE) sequence is in the range of 2–4 min (series of 5
images in a given imaging plane). Fast imaging
sequences have strongly reduced imaging time down
to a few seconds allowing breath-hold acquisition.4
However, the total examination time for a thorough
examination comprising a series of 6–10 sequences is
around 30–45 min. This procedure is well tolerated
even by very young, sick, or premature patients.

To improve visualization of small vessels, we rec-
ommend two series of thin (3–5 mm), intertwined, and
overlapping (2–3 mm) slices in each plane of interest.

2.3 Study of Blood Flow

MR study of blood flow is based on two techniques:
black-blood imaging and bright-blood imaging (see
Chap. 1).

2.3.1 Black-Blood Imaging

The spin-echo sequence (historically, the first imaging
sequence to be developed) is currently the most com-
monly used black-blood technique for cardiac imaging. Due to long acquisition times, black blood fast
spin-echo sequences have replaced traditional spin-
echo sequences. In black blood fast spin-echo
sequences circulating blood is generally black (as
blood flows out of the slice and due to spin dephasing
[23–30]). The images obtained are excellent for anatomical delineation generating "spontaneous" contrast
between circulating blood which is black and soft tissues (and thrombus) which are gray (fat appears white).
However, when blood circulates slowly (venous flow
or end-diastole arterial flow as, for example, in aortic
aneurysm or false lumen), flow effects may be confus-
ing. An intermediate intravascular signal or even a
high signal intensity due to inflowing unsaturated
blood can be observed and may be mistaken for
obstruction or thrombus [31]. This situation can be
clarified by using sequences with saturation bands outside the Fov of interest [24, 30] (which restore the
usual contrast between black circulating blood and
gray thrombus) or bright-blood imaging (circulating
blood is white and thrombus is gray), which is briefly
discussed later [25–36].

---

4 Not always possible in practice in very young patients – feasible
in elderly cooperative children and adults.

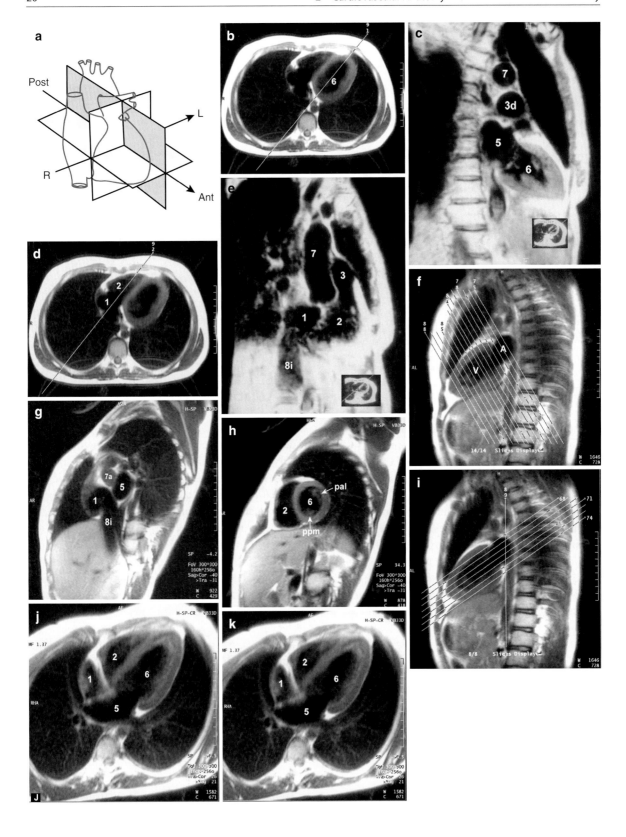

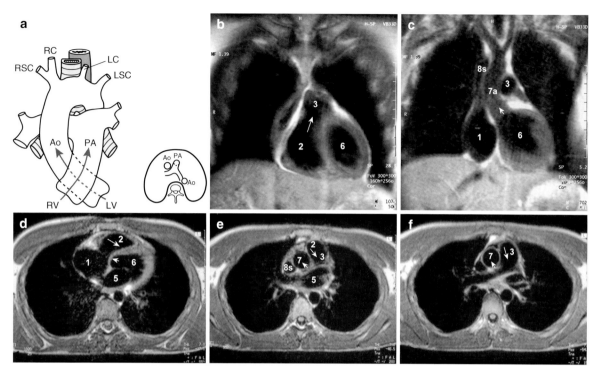

Fig. 2.4 *Crossover* (Twisting) of the aorta (Ao) and pulmonary artery trunk (PA) at their origin. Schematic diagram (**a**) and coronal *fast spin-echo* images through the origin of the pulmonary artery (*long arrow, 3* – **b**) and the aorta (*short arrow, 7* – **c**). Axial *fast spin-echo* images through the origin of the aorta (**d**) and pulmonary artery (**e, f**). The ascending aorta (Ao-7) at its origin is in a central position, posteriorly and to the right of the pulmonary artery (PA-3) which is situated anteriorly and to the left. The vessels cross over at their origin (*short* and *long arrows*): the *pulmonary artery* emerges from the right ventricle (*2*) and the *aorta* emerges from the left ventricle (*6*); right atrium (*1*), superior vena cava (*8s*)

Incomplete blood signal suppression and respiratory motion artifacts are also potential limitations of fast spin-echo sequences. Respiratory motion algorithm or navigator echo techniques using diaphragmatic motion have hence been proposed. A double inversion pulse can be added at the beginning of the sequence for blood pool signal suppression and optimization of black blood imaging [37]. Single slice or better multislice double IR T2 weighted sequences allowing excellent image quality during one breath-hold[4] [38]) are now becoming the gold standard for black blood imaging and are used routinely, replacing fast spin-echo sequences. Black blood sequences should be performed before gadolinium injection as the latter impairs proper blood suppression by the IR pulse.

Fig. 2.3 Images in the anatomical axis of the heart. (**a**) Schematic diagram. (**b–g**) Long-axis *two-chamber (vertical dark gray plane)* and *four-chamber (true four-chamber image* – horizontal light gray plane) and short-axis *two-chamber* images. The "left chamber" long-axis images (**c**) and "right chamber" long-axis images (**e**) were obtained from the axial image ("four-chamber"), by placing the imaging planes in the anatomical axis of the heart on the left (**b**) and right (**d**) chambers, respectively. Short-axis images (double oblique *true short-axis*) are obtained from the long-axis image (**f**), by placing the imaging planes perpendicular to the anatomical axis of the heart: posterior images through the atria (**g**) and anterior images through the ventricles (**h**). (**j, k**) Four-chamber axial images in the anatomical axis of the heart (*true four-chamber image*), obtained from the long-axis image (**f**) by placing imaging planes parallel to the anatomical axis of the heart; right atrium (*1*), right ventricle (*2*), left atrium (*5*), left ventricle (*6*), ascending aorta (*7*), inferior vena cava (*8i*), anterolateral papillary muscles (pal), and posteromedian papillary muscles (ppm)

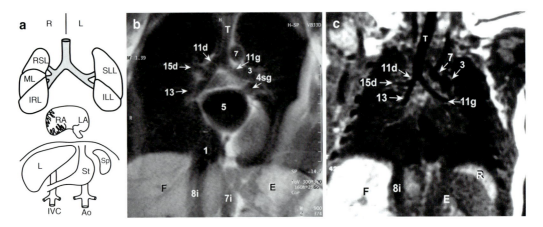

Fig. 2.5 Correlation between the atrial, thoracic, and abdominal arrangements in situs solitus (normal atrial position). (**a**) Schematic diagram. (**b, c**) Coronal spin-echo images in a child (**b**) and an infant (**c**). Right-left pulmonary asymmetry: right main bronchus (11d) on the right and left main bronchus (11g) on the left correlated with the atrial positions; right atrium (RA-1) on the right and left atrium on the left (LA-5). The same applies to the position of abdominal organs: Liver (L) on the right and spleen (Sp) and stomach (St) on the left, inferior vena cava (IVC-8i) on the right and abdominal aorta (Ao-7i) on the left. Right upper lobe (RUL), left upper lobe (LUL), middle lobe (ML), right lower lobe (RLL), left lower lobe (LLL); pulmonary artery (left-3), left superior pulmonary vein (*4sg*), ascending aorta (*7a*), left main bronchus (*11g*), *bronchus intermedius* (*13*), right upper lobe bronchus (*15d*) (also see Chap. 3, Figs 3.2 and 3.19b and Chap. 5, Fig. 5.23)

Fig. 2.6 "Morphologically" right atrium (mRA) and "morphologically" left atrium (mLA). (**a**) Schematic diagram. (**b**) Axial images in an infant. (**c, d**) Axial images in a young adult. The "morphologically" right atrial appendage (*1d*) has a triangular shape with a broad implantation on the right atrium (*1*) (situated on the right) which is connected to the superior vena cava (*1*). The "morphologically" left atrial appendage (*5g*) has a finger-like shape with a narrow implantation on the left atrium (*5*) (situated on the left); pulmonary infundibulum (*2i*) below the pulmonary artery, right superior (*4sd*), right inferior (*4id*), and left inferior (*4ig*) pulmonary veins, ascending and descending aorta (*7* and *7d*), superior vena cava (*8s*); note the origin of the right coronary artery (*20*) (also see Chap. 3, Fig. 3.19b)

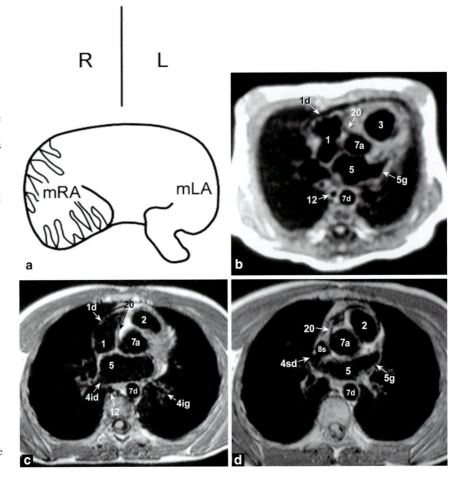

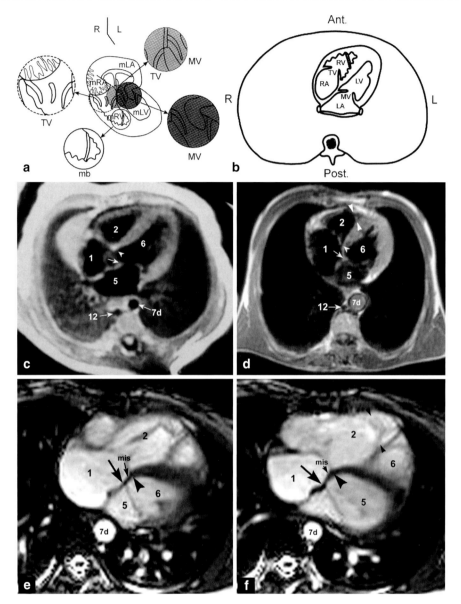

Fig. 2.7 "Morphologically" right ventricle (mRV) and "morphologically" left ventricle (mLV). (**a**) Schematic diagram. (**b**) "Four-chamber" axial spin-echo images through the ventricular chambers in an (**c**) and an adolescent (**d**). Gradient-echo cine-MR axial images (**e** and **f**). Morphologically right atrium (mRA) and left atrium (mLA). Identification of mRV and mLV is based on the insertion of the atrioventricular valve leaflets in relation to the interventricular septum: the tricuspid valve (TV– *arrowhead* - not VM) which always opens into an mRV, is always situated more anteriorly (and inferiorly to the apex of the heart) compared to the mitral valve (MV– *arrow*), which always opens into an mLV and which is situated more posteriorly. This offset of the valves delineates the membranous interventricular septum (mis). The mRV is also identified (second criterion) by the presence of trabeculations and the moderator band (between *arrow heads*); right atrium (*1*) and left atrium (*5*), right ventricle (*2*) and left ventricle (*6*), descending aorta (*7d*), azygos vein (*12*) (also see Chap. 3, Figs. 3.17c and d, 3.19c, 3.20e, 3.21b, and 3.24d and Chap. 7, Fig. 7.14 and Chap. 8, Figs. 8.14 and 8.22)

2.3.2 Bright-Bood Imaging

Bright-blood imaging techniques give physiologic information on blood flow. Bright-blood imaging uses gradient-echo (GE) sequences with flow compensation (circulating flow-white and soft tissues-dark gray). The acquisition time is sufficiently short to allow breath-hold images[4] [25–27]. They provide dynamic ECG-gated cine-MRI images [25–27, 33–36, 39, 40], or MR angiography images [28–31] on which soft tissues are almost completely suppressed by saturation and/or by special algorithms such as Maximum Intensity Projection (MIP). This imaging therefore allows a dynamic approach to normal flow (bright-blood) and a semiquantitative approach to abnormal flow (black flow void *jets* in stenoses, shunts, and regurgitations) [33–36] (see Chap. 1).

It is also possible to obtain flow quantification (velocity mapping) by using specific sequences (phase-contrast MR angiography) (see Chap. 1) [40–48].

Recently introduced Balanced-SSFP (Fiesta/GE, True-FISP/Siemens, Balanced-FFE/Philips) [49] sequences generate excellent, strongly flow-enhanced cine-MR images not relying on inflow effects. They are now used routinely in place of traditional GE cine-MRI and for anatomical cardiovascular analysis, as a complement to black-blood images, whenever the latter are inconclusive. Contrary to black-blood sequences, they can be performed not only before but also after gadolinium administration (see Chap. 1).

Contrast-enhanced gradient-echo images (CE-MR angiography) using intravascular Gadolinium administration can also be obtained displaying 3D luminal information on a large Fov (see Chap. 1).

2.4 Segmental Analysis of Cardiac Anatomy

Segmental analysis of cardiac anatomy (see Figs. 2.4–2.7; atlas and Chap. 3, Fig. 3.17) [16] and vascular connections is performed by carefully selecting the orientation of slices on axial, coronal, or sagittal planes, as well as oblique planes, according to the anatomical axes of the heart or vessels studied (aorta, pulmonary artery, vena cava, or pulmonary vein, surgical procedures, etc.).

Axial images (generally performed first) (atlas Figs. A) define the position of the ascending aorta, which is "normally" in a "central" situation posteriorly and to the right of the pulmonary artery (which is situated anteriorly and to the left) (A6), identify the "morphologically" right and left atria and ventricles (A10–12), evaluate the caliber of branches of the pulmonary artery (A4–6), and identify pulmonary veins "normally" converging onto the left atrium (A7, 8, and F10).

Coronal images (atlas Figs. F) more clearly visualize the superior vena cava and inferior vena cava normally draining into the right atrium (F7, 10), the left ventricle and its outflow tract giving rise to the ascending aorta, and the trachea and the main bronchi (bronchial arrangement, Fig. 2.5 and atlas F11). Posterior images show the left atrium (F10, 11) and descending aorta, and anterior images show the right ventricle with the origin of the pulmonary artery.

Sagittal images (Atlas Fig. S) are well adapted to the study of all of the right ventricular outflow tract (ventricle, infundibulum and pulmonary artery trunk) (S3–5), as well as the trachea (S2).

"Short-axis" two-chamber and "long-axis" two-chamber and four-chamber images (Fig. 2.3) respecting the right–left symmetry clearly distinguish the right chambers from the left chambers [50] (the right atrium is identified by drainage of the venae cavae). They can be used to confirm transposition of the great vessels or a ventricular or atrial septal defect.

Sagittal oblique images (equivalent to "LAO") (Fig. 2.8) are essential to study the aortic arch.

2.5 Normal Cardiovascular Anatomy

Identification of the numerous pathological variants, particularly in the context of congenital heart disease, requires a perfect knowledge of normal anatomy. Although some paired organs have a "symmetrical" arrangement (cerebral hemispheres, kidneys, etc), other paired organs are not symmetrical (lungs, bronchial tree, branches of the pulmonary artery, atria, and ventricles). Some "asymmetrical" viscera and vessels are also clearly lateralized to the right (liver, inferior vena cava), while others are lateralized to the left (stomach, spleen, abdominal aorta, and heart) (Fig. 2.5). Determination of the disposition or situs of asymmetrical atrial, pulmonary [18], and abdominal structures [19] (normal position: situs solitus – Figs. 2.5, 2.6, 2.7, and 2.9) is important in congenital heart disease, as some malformations are associated with situs anomalies.

The anatomical axis of the heart (base-apex long-axis) is usually directed anteriorly, inferiorly, and to the left, and not according to one of the conventional orthogonal axes (right-left, superior-inferior, anterior-posterior) (Fig. 2.2 and see Chap. 3,

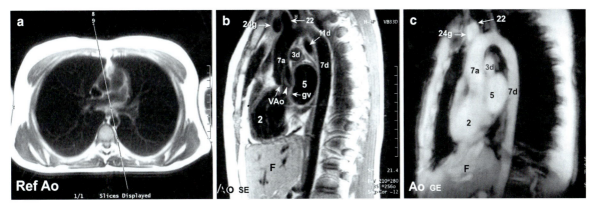

Fig. 2.8 Imaging plane (**a**) to obtain a LAO image containing the aortic arch. Spin-echo black-blood image (**b**) and gradient-echo bright-blood (**c**) images. The aortic valve (AoV) is clearly visualized (the posterior leaflet is continuous with the anterior leaflet of the mitral valve) (Fig 2.8 and see Chap. 2 3, Fig. 6.22c). Ascending and descending thoracic aorta (*7a* and *7d*), right pulmonary artery (*3d*), left atrium (*5*), right ventricle (*2*), left brachiocephalic vein (*24g*), right main bronchus (*11d*)

Sect. 3.2.4.1.7).[5] Consequently, the atria are situated posteriorly and superiorly, and the ventricles are situated anteriorly and inferiorly (the right chambers are actually right anterior and the left chambers are left anterior); hence, the value of so-called "long-axis" two-chamber and four-chamber images is parallel to the anatomical axis of the heart, and "short-axis" two-chamber images are perpendicular to this axis [50] (Fig. 2.5).

Compared to conventional orthogonal planes,[6] the cardiac mass is therefore not arranged symmetrically: the left atrium is the posteriormost chamber (anterior to the spine), the right ventricle is the anteriormost chamber (posterior to the sternum), the right atrium is the chamber situated mostly to the right and the left ventricle is the chamber situated mostly to the left. This particular arrangement is clearly visualized on axial images (particularly on the so-called "four-chamber" image – Fig. 2.1 and atlas A10–12) and is also observed on coronal (right atrium to the right and left ventricle to the left) (atlas F4–7) and sagittal images (right ventricle anteriorly and left atrium posteriorly) (atlas S2–5).

Cardiac chambers also have specific morphological features corresponding to well-defined criteria. In Chap. 3, we shall see that a chamber considered to be strictly normal anatomically can occupy an abnormal situation; the same applies to the great vessels.

The differentiation of "right-sided" structures from "left-sided" structures is further complicated by twisting of the great vessels at their origin: the aorta, which emerges from the left ventricle, belongs to the systemic or "left" circuit, but is actually situated on the right and posteriorly to the pulmonary artery which belongs to the pulmonary or "right" circuit ("right-sided" structure situated on the left and anteriorly) – Figs. 2.1 and 2.4; atlas A6).

After a brief description of the anatomy of each structure, the MR criteria for recognition of "morphologically" right and left chambers and the distinction between aorta and pulmonary artery are described.

2.6 MR Segmental Cardiovascular Anatomy

2.6.1 "Morphologically" Right Atrium (mRA)

The right atrium, normally situated to the right and posteriorly, is divided into a venous component, vestibule, septum, and atrial appendage. The venous component normally receives the superior vena cava superiorly (into which merge the right and left brachiocephalic veins) and the inferior vena cava

---

[5] It is more "horizontal" in newborn infants compared to adults, where it is more vertical.

[6] Axial, coronal, and sagittal.

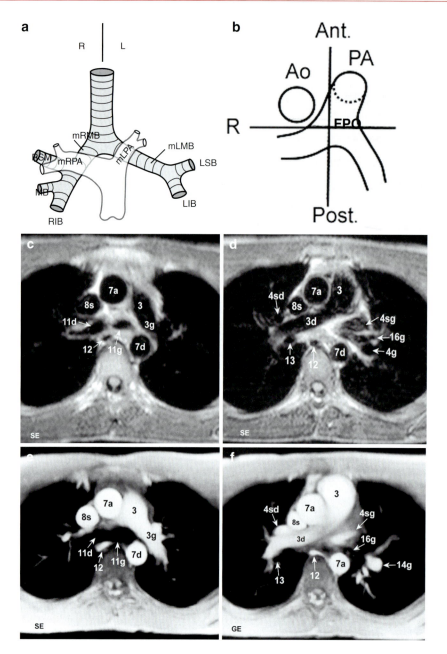

Fig. 2.9 Right and left pulmonary artery and bronchial arrangement. Schematic diagram (**a**) and section (**b**). The right (mRPA) and left (mLPA) pulmonary arteries, right (mRMB) and left (mLMB) main bronchus, right (RULB) and left (LULB) upper lobe bronchus, right middle lobe bronchus (RMLB), right (RLLB) and left (LLLB) lower lobe bronchus, aorta (Ao), and pulmonary artery (PA). MR axial images through the right (**d** and **f**) and left pulmonary arteries (**c** and **e**). (**c, d**) Anatomical spin-echo black-blood images. (**e, f**) Gradient-echo bright-blood images. At its origin, the aorta (7) is situated anteriorly and to the right of the pulmonary artery (3). The pulmonary artery divides into a long, large right branch situated in a "coronal" (oblique) plane (**a, b** and 3d **d, f**, atlas F8) and a shorter left branch continuous with the trunk situated in a "sagittal" (oblique) plane (**a, b** and 3g, **c, e**, atlas S4). Vascular structures appear white on gradient-echo sequences, allowing

vessels to be distinguished from bronchial structures in the hila (atlas A4, A6). This right–left pulmonary artery arrangement is correlated with the tracheobronchial arrangement, i.e., short, vertical, and eparterial right main bronchus (tri-lobed lung) and long, horizontal, and hyparterial left main bronchus (bilobed lung) (diagram). As described in Chap. 3, the thoracic arrangement is used to establish the atrial arrangement or atrial situs (Fig. 2.5b, c, atlas F11 and see Chap. 3, Figs. 3.1, 3.2, 3.4 and 3.7 and Chap. 5, Figs. 5.23 and 5.24). Pulmonary artery (3), right branch (3d) and left branch (3g), ascending and descending thoracic aorta (7a and 7d), left and right superior pulmonary veins (4sd and 4sg), superior vena cava (8s), left and right main bronchus (11d and 11g), bronchus intermedius (13), left lower lobe artery (14), left lower lobe bronchus (16g).*Eparterial: parallel and posterior to the pulmonary artery **Hyparterial: crossing underneath the pulmonary artery inferiorly (which receives the hepatic veins) and the coronary sinus (close to the septum). The inferior vena cava has a valve (Eustachian valve of the inferior vena cava). The coronary sinus also has a valve (Thebesian valve of the coronary sinus). The crista terminalis is a vertical structure in the prolongation of the Eustachian valve, which separates the venous component from the appendage (Fig. 2.11a, c). All of the pectinate muscles, arising from the crista terminalis, converge onto the right atrial appendage. Filamentous structures attached to the crista terminalis are consistent with a Chiari's network reseau (arrows), embryological remains of no pathological significance (Fig. 2.10).

The triangular right atrial appendage has a large implantation base superiorly, laterally, and anteriorly

to the venous component (Fig. 2.6, atlas A7 and see Chap. 3, Figs. 3.19b et 3.24d).

The criteria for identification of the right atrium are:

- Broad triangular shape of the atrial appendage (Fig. 2.6, atlas A7 and see Chap. 3, Figs. 3.19b and 3.24c)
- Connection to the superior vena cava and especially the inferior vena cava (more reliable criterion) (Atlas F7, 10, S1, and Fig. 2.3 short-axis);
- The presence of a crista terminalis on axial MR images (arrows, Fig. 2.11a and c) is a feature that is of particular value to identify the mRA in anomalies of position of the heart such as Dextrocardia (Chap. 3, Fig. 3.28).

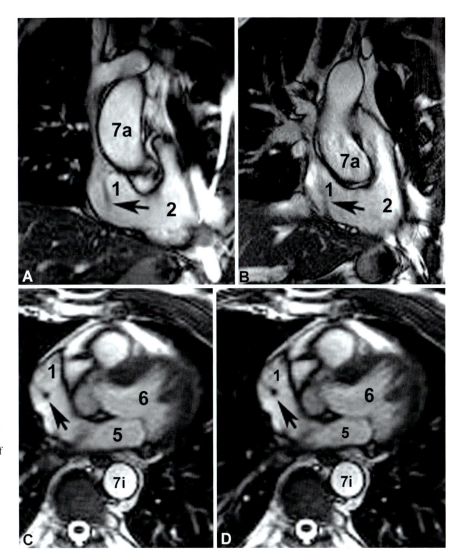

Fig. 2.10 Coronal (**a** and **b**), and axial (**c** and **d**) gradient-echo images. The presence of posterior filamentous structures attached to the crista terminalis is consistent with a Chiari's network, (*arrows*), embryological remains of no pathological significance

Fig. 2.11 Axial gradient-echo (**a** and **c**), spin-echo (**b**), and CT (**d**) images. Small heart anatomical and physiological structures to be remembered: The moderator band (mb A) which extends anteriorly from the main papillary muscle on the anterior wall to the interventricular septum; the vertical structure of the crista terminalis (CT ct, on images **a** and **c**) in the prolongation of the Eustachian valve, separating the venous component from the appendage of the right atrium (the presence of the crista terminalis is also a feature which is of particular value to identify the mRA in anomalies of position of the heart (see Chap. 3, Fig. 3.28)); the fibrous spur (*arrow* **b**) separating the left appendage and the abutting superior left pulmonary vein (4sg); the offset of the mitral (*arrowhead*) and tricuspid (*arrow*) valves, which delineates the membranous interventricular septum, (mis) is also visible (**a**); pectinate muscles within the left atrial appendage (5g) which are well seen on this CT image with an excellent spatial resolution (**d**). Right atrium (*1*), left atrium (*5*), right ventricle (*2*), left ventricle (*6*), descending aorta (*7d*)

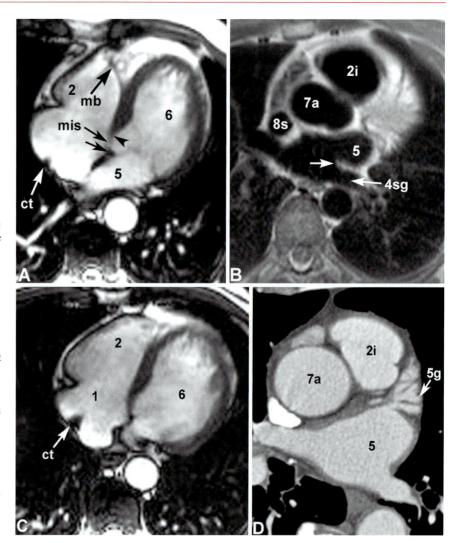

2.6.2 "Morphologically" Left Atrium (mLA)

The left atrium, *normally situated posteriorly and to the left,* is also divided into a venous component, vestibule, septum, and atrial appendage. The smooth-walled venous component normally receives the four (*or more*) pulmonary veins. The valve of fossa ovalis largely covers the superior part of the septum secundum, even ensuring, in the absence of fusion of these two structures, a watertight shunt-free seal between the atria, provided the pressure in the left atrium exceeds that in the right atrium, as a patent foramen ovale is detected in one-third of the general population [17]. The pectinate muscles, less well developed than on the right, are almost exclusively situated in the atrial appendage (Fig. 2.11d). The morphology of the

left atrial appendage is also very different from that of the right atrial appendage. It has a hooked finger-like shape with a narrow connection to the atrium (Fig. 2.6, atlas A7 and F6, 7 and see Chap. 3, Fig. 3.16).

The criteria for identification of the left atrium are therefore:

- Narrow finger-like atrial appendage (Fig. 2.6, atlas A7 and see Chap. 3, Fig. 3.16)
- Connection to the pulmonary vein (less reliable criterion) (atlas F8–10, A7 and 8).

N.B.: the criteria for identification of the atria based on morphological differences between the right atrial appendage and left atrial appendage are not always obvious on MR or echocardiographic imaging. The venous connections are also not an absolute criterion. Chapter 3 describes in more detail other more reliable criteria that are more readily accessible on MRI for determination of atrial situs (bronchial arrangement, see Fig. 2.5, Chap. 3).

2.6.3 "Morphologically" Right Ventricle (mRV)

The right ventricle (Fig. 2.7), normally situated anteriorly and to the right, has a triangular pyramid shape, composed of three walls: anterior (sternocostal), inferior (diaphragmatic), and medial, convex towards the right ventricle (interventricular septum). The base of the right ventricle corresponds to the tricuspid valve and, more anteriorly to the left, the pulmonary valve, which covers the subpulmonary conus arteriosus or infundibulum (myocardial tube separating the semilunar and atrioventricular valves). It comprises an entry chamber (compartment), an apex (containing many coarse trabeculations), and an ejection chamber (arterial compartment corresponding to the muscular infundibulum). The tricuspid valve[7] opens into the right ventricle. It is composed of three triangular leaflets: anterior, inferior, and medial or septal, corresponding to the three walls. The insertion of one of the leaflets in relation to the interventricular septum is characteristic of the tricuspid valve. The tricuspid valve is always situated more anteriorly (and inferiorly towards the apex of the heart) compared to the mitral valve (which is situated more posteriorly, offset of the valves) (Fig. 2.7 and atlas A9, 10 – also see Chap. 3, Figs. 3.17c and d, 3.19c, 3.20e, 3.21b and 3.24d).

This offset of the valves delineates the membranous interventricular septum[8] (mis) Fig. 2.7 and atlas A10). The right ventricle presents many trabeculations corresponding to papillary muscles; the moderator band (septomarginal trabecula) extends from the main papillary muscle on the anterior wall to the interventricular septum, anteriorly and below the infundibulum (Atlas A9, 10).

Criteria for identification of the right ventricle are therefore:

- The tricuspid valve which always opens into a right ventricle; it is identified by its more anterior septal insertion compared to that of the mitral valve (offset of the valves depicted on "four-chamber long-axis" image and axial images (Fig. 2.7 and Atlas A9, 10)).
- The presence of a muscular subpulmonary infundibulum (conus) (atlas, sagittal images – long-axis images Fig. 2.3e), situated between the pulmonary valve and the tricuspid valve (space between the tricuspid and pulmonary rings) (see axial image, atlas A8, 9 through the pulmonary infundibulum).
- The presence of coarse trabeculations and the moderator band, generally clearly visible on axial images (atlas A9, 10).

2.6.4 "Morphologically" Left Ventricle" (mLV)

The left ventricle (Fig. 2.7), normally situated to the left and anteriorly, has a truncated conical ellipsoid shape (bullet shape) and its myocardium is normally much thicker than that of the right ventricle.[9] It has two externally convex walls, the right septal wall (the posterior two-thirds correspond to the smooth interventricular septum) and the free left wall, which is less trabeculated than the right endocardial surface. The base is entirely occupied by the mitral and aortic rings, which are continuous. Like the right ventricle, the left ventricle comprises an entry chamber (atrial compartment), an apex (containing fine trabeculations), and an ejection chamber. The mitral valve,[10] opens into the left ventricle. Also known as the bicuspid valve, it is composed of two quadrilateral leaflets (or cups), the anterior leaflet and the posterior leaflet, with no insertion on the interventricular septum. There is a "mitro-aortic" continuity between the posterior part of the aortic root (posterior aortic leaflet) and the anterior leaflet of the mitral valve (Fig. 2.8 and see Chap. 2, Fig. 22c). The absence of insertion of the mitral valve onto the septum and the presence of two papillary muscles (anterolateral and posteromedian) on the free wall are characteristic of the left ventricle. The mitral valve is always situated posteriorly compared to the tricuspid valve (offset of the valves) (Fig. 2.7 and atlas A9 and 10).

---

[7]Strictly speaking, according to the new nomenclature, we should use the term "right atrioventricular valve", but we deliberately continue to use the term "tricuspid valve".

[8]A septal defect situated in this posterior part of the membranous septum or interatrioventricular portion is responsible for a left ventricle-right atrium communication.

[9]This difference of thickness (and size), less marked at birth due to the fetal "balanced" right-left circulation, gradually increases, so that the heart progressively takes on the appearance of an "adult" heart with a dominant "systemic" left ventricle.

[10]Here again, according to the new nomenclature, we should use the term "left atrioventricular valve", but we deliberately continue to use the term "mitral valve".

Criteria for identification of the left ventricle are therefore:

- The mitral valve always opens into the left ventricle; it is identified by its more posterior position compared to the septal insertion of the tricuspid valve (offset of the valves depicted in "four-chamber long-axis" images and axial images (Fig. 2.7 and atlas A9, 10)).
- The presence of "mitro-aortic" continuity between the aortic and mitral rings (Fig. 2.8, atlas A8, S2).
- The presence of two papillary muscles (anterolateral and posteromedian) inserted onto the free wall (short-axis image (Fig. 2.3h)).

2.6.5 Pulmonary Artery

The pulmonary artery trunk[11] normally arises from the right ventricle, at the pulmonary orifice (comprising three semilunar cusps) at the summit of the infundibulum (conus), situated to the left and anteriorly to the aorta (atlas A6): it travels posteriorly, to the left and slightly superiorly and rolls around the left anterior surface of the ascending aorta forming a curve with a right posterior concavity (Figs. 2.4 and 2.9). Behind the left margin of the aorta, it divides into the left pulmonary artery continuous with the trunk, situated in an almost sagittal plane (atlas A4 and S4) crossing the left main bronchus almost perpendicularly by forming an arch with a superolateral convexity over the bronchus (Figs. 2.4 and 2.9), and thet right pulmonary artery (larger and longer than the left pulmonary artery), situated in a coronal plane (atlas A6 and F8) in front of the right main bronchus. The ligamentum arteriosum (remnant of the fetal circulation) arises from the superior edge of the pulmonary artery and joins the descending aorta close to its origin (normally, the ductus arteriosus rapidly involutes at birth).

The criteria for identification of the pulmonary artery are:

- Bifurcation into left and right pulmonary arteries (Fig. 2.9 and atlas A4–6, F8, 9).
- Discontinuity between the tricuspid and pulmonary rings, in the normal configuration, due to the presence of the subpulmonary conus arteriosus (see morphologically right ventricle).

---

[11]The diameter of the PA at its origin in adults is normally equal to 0.85 times that of the aorta.

2.6.6 Aorta

The aorta normally emerges from the left ventricle in a "central," posterior and right position (compared to the pulmonary artery). It has an ascending portion first, and then a horizontal portion, usually describing a left-sided arch over the pulmonary artery trunk (Fig. 2.4). It is situated in a vertical plane, oblique anteroposteriorly and from right to left (LAO, Fig. 2.8). The ascending portion, almost entirely intrapericardial, contains the aortic orifice with three semilunar valves: one posterior (noncoronary), and the other two right and left anterolateral giving rise to coronary arteries. The horizontal segment gives rise to three arteries: brachiocephalic trunk anterior to the trachea, left common carotid artery lateral to the trachea, and left subclavian artery lateral to the esophagus. The isthmus of the aorta, situated at the origin of the descending aorta, is located between the origin of the left subclavian artery and the insertion of the ligamentum arteriosum.

The criteria for identification of the aorta are:

- Absence of division and the origin of supra-aortic vessels (Fig. 2.8).
- Origin of the coronary artery (both coronary sinuses are always situated over the pulmonary artery regardless of the aorta/pulmonary artery arrangement).
- "Mitro-aortic" continuity between the posterior part of the aortic root (posterior semilunar cusp) and the anterior leaflet of the mitral valve[11].

2.7 Atlas of Normal MR Anatomy of the Heart and Mediastinum

The following atlas is numbered in the direction of blood flow for cardiac chambers and great vessels. Numbering arbitrarily starts at the right atrium (1). The right ventricle is therefore number 2, the pulmonary artery is number 3, the pulmonary veins are number 4 etc. Names in bold type correspond to the new nomenclature (the old nomenclature is sometimes indicated in parentheses). Names with capital letters correspond to abbreviations used in the diagrams and some of the figures in this book.

Images were acquired by various spin-echo or fast spin-echo black-blood techniques.

- A1–15: Craniocaudal series of axial images (fast spin-echo segmented with cardiac gating, slice thickness: 5 mm).

- F1–14: Anteroposterior series of coronal images (ECG-gated spin-echo, slice thickness: 7 mm).
- S1–7: Sagittal images from right to left (half-Fourier ECG-gated fast spin-echo, slice thickness: 7 mm).

1	right atrium RA
1'	morphologically right atrium situated on the left
1d	right atrial appendage RAa
2	right ventricle RV
2'	morphologically right ventricle RV situated on the left
pp	main papillary muscle
mb	moderator band (septomarginal trabecula)
2i	pulmonary infundibulum
3	pulmonary artery trunk PA, pulmonary valve PuV
3d	right pulmonary artery RPA
3g	left pulmonary artery LPA
4	pulmonary vein PV
4sd	right superior pulmonary vein
4sg	left superior pulmonary vein
4id	right inferior pulmonary vein
4ig	left inferior pulmonary vein
5	left atrium LA
5'	morphologically left atrium situated on the right
5g	left atrial appendage LAa
6	left ventricle LV
6'	morphologically left ventricle situated on the right
pal	anterolateral papillary muscle
ppm	posteromedian papillary muscle
7	aorta Ao
7a	ascending aorta AAo
7d	descending thoracic aorta Dao
7i	abdominal aorta AbdAo
8 s	superior vena cava SVC
8sd	right superior vena cava RSVC
8sg	left superior vena cava LSVC
8i	inferior vena cava IVC
T 9	Trachea
10	Esophagus
Th	Thymus

11d	right main bronchus R
11g	left main bronchus L
12, 12d	azygos vein AzV
12g	(left) hemiazygos vein (superior or inferior)
13	Bronchus intermedius
14	lower lobe artery (14d-right, 14g-left)
15	lobar bronchus (right upper lobe-15d, middle lobe-15m, left upper lobe-15g)
16	lower lobe bronchus (right-16d, left-16g)
17	superior pericardial recess
18	circumflex artery
19	left anterior descending artery
20	right coronary artery RCo
Tc	left coronary artery trunk
21	left coronary artery LCo
cs	coronary sinus
VM or M	left atrioventricular valve (mitral -bicuspid-valve) (arrow), Gv
MV or M	anterior leaflet,
TV or T	pv posterior leaflet
VT or T	right atrioventricular valve (tricuspid valve) (arrowhead)
VAo	aortic valve
PuV	pulmonary valve
22	brachiocephalic trunk (innominate artery)
23d	right common carotid artery RC
23g	left common carotid artery LC
24d	right brachiocephalic vein (right innominate vein) RBCV
24g	left brachiocephalic vein (left innominate vein) LBCV
Mi	internal mammary artery (internal thoracic artery)
25d	right subclavian artery RSC
25g	left subclavian artery LSC
26i	posterior mitral papillary muscle (inferior papillary muscle of left ventricle)
27	mediastinal trunk (s) (right superior mediastinal artery)
ct	crista terminalis
Lin	lingular bronchus
HV	hepatic veins
VR	renal veins
PV	portal vein

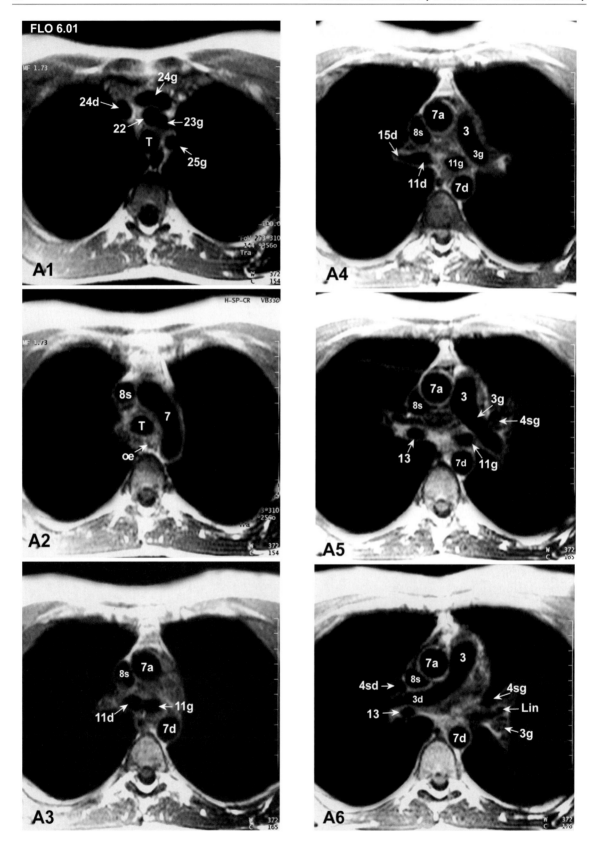

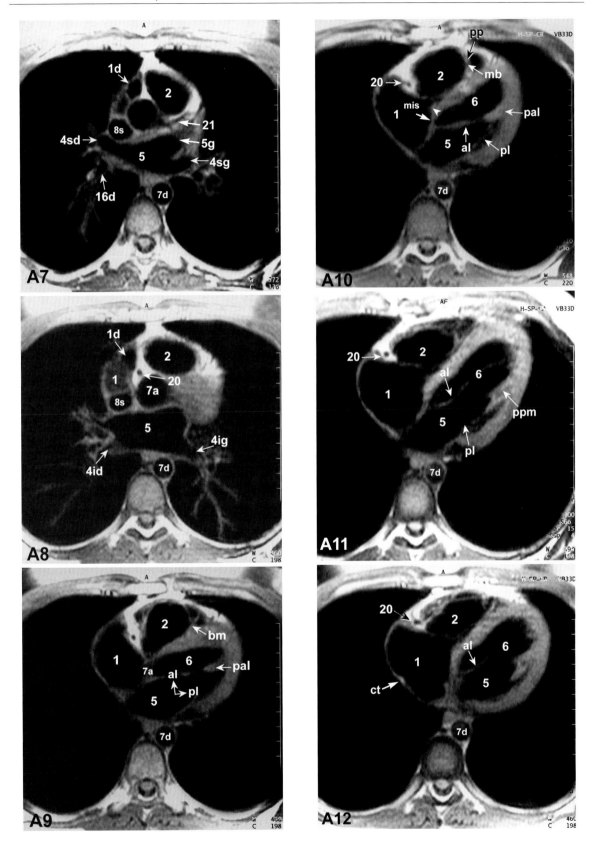

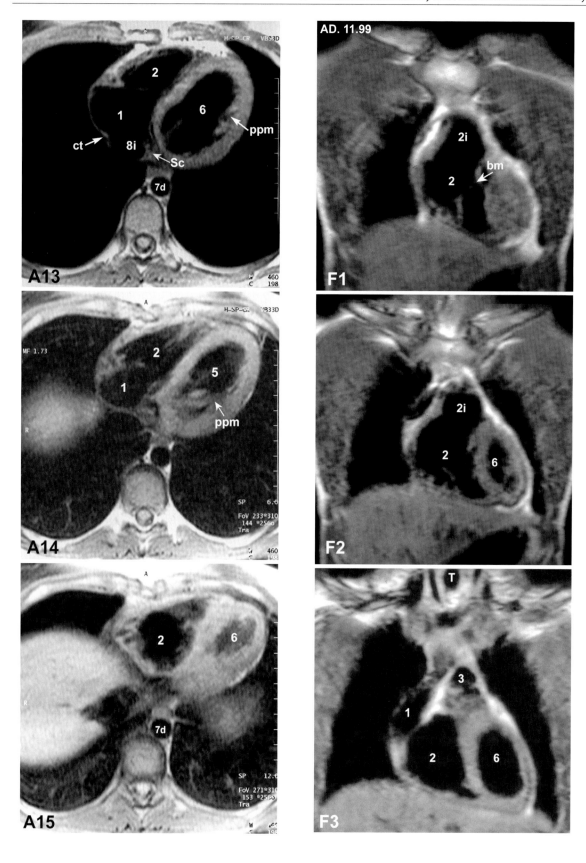

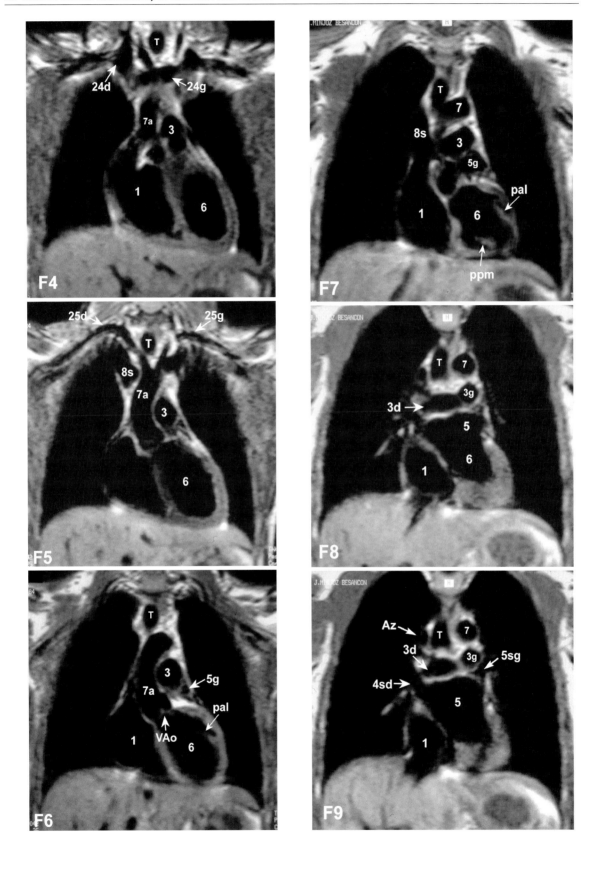

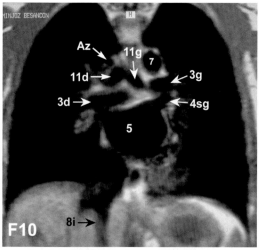

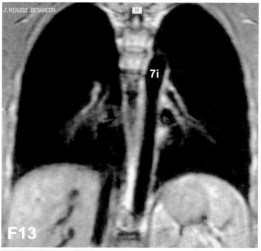

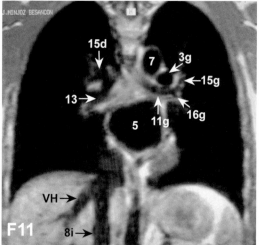

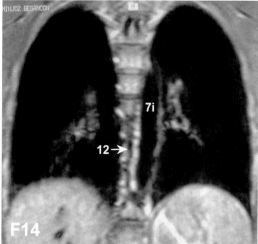

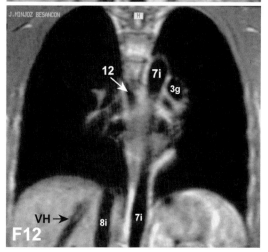

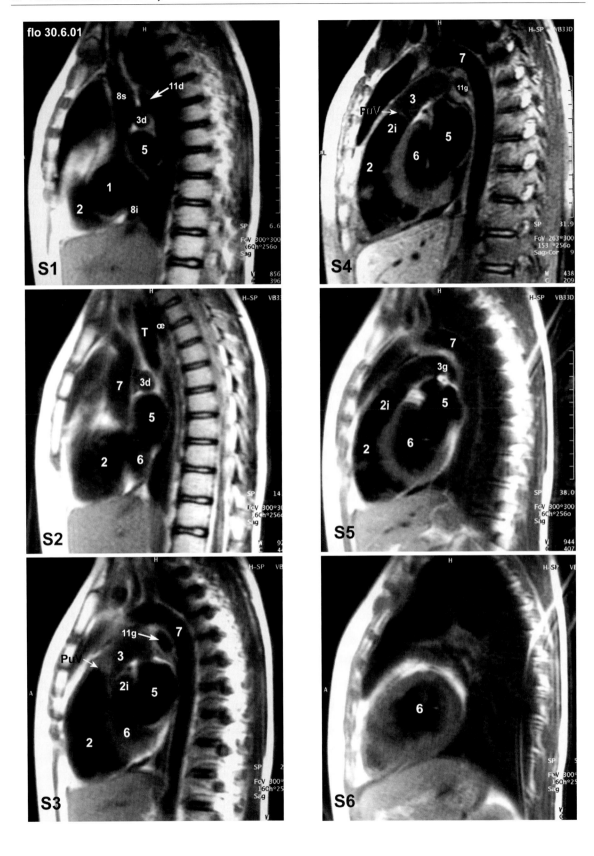

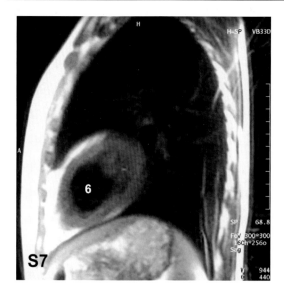

References

1. Fletcher BD, Jacobstein MD, Nelson AD, et al. Gated MRI of congenital cardiac malformation. Radiology. 1984;150:137–40.
2. Higgins CB, Byrd BF, Farmer DW, et al. MRI in patients with congenital heart disease. Circulation. 1984;70: 851–60.
3. Jacobstein MD, Fletcher BD, Nelson AD, Goldstein S, Alfidi RJ, Riemenschneider TA. ECG-gated nuclear magnetic resonance imaging: appearance of the congenitally malformed heart. Am Heart J. 1984;107:1014–20.
4. Higgins CB, Byrd BF, McNamara MT, et al. Magnetic resonance imaging of the heart: a review of the experience in 172 subjects. Radiology. 1985;155:671–9.
5. Fletcher BD, Jacobstein MD. MRI of congenital abnormalities of the great vessels. AJR. 1986;146:941–8.
6. Didier D, Higgins CB, Fisher MR, et al. GatedMRI in congenital heart disease: initial experience in 72 patients. Radiology. 1986;158:227–35.
7. Boxer RA, Singh S, La Corte MA, et al. Cardiac MRI in children with congenital heart disease. J Pediatr. 1986;109:460–4.
8. Gomes AS, Lois JF, George B, Alpan G, Williams RG. Congenital abnormalities of the aortic arch. Radiology. 1987;165:691–5.
9. Chung KJ, Simpson IA, Newman R, et al. Cine-MRI for evaluation of congenital heart disease: role in pediatric cardiology compared with echocardiography and angiography. J Pediatr. 1988;113:1028–35.
10. Sieverding L, Klose U, Apitz J. Morphological diagnosis of congenital and acquired heart disease by MRI. Pediatr Radiol. 1990;20:311–9.
11. Parson JM, Baker EJ, Hayes A, et al. MRI of the great arteries in infants. Int J Cardiol. 1990;28:73–85.
12. Bank ER. Magnetic resonance of congenital cardiovascular disease: an update. Radiol Clin North Am. 1993;31: 553–72.
13. Kastler B, Livolsi A, Germain P, et al. MRI in congenital heart disease of newborns. Preliminary results in 23 patients. Eur J Radiol 1990;10:109–17.
14. Livolsi A, Kastler B, Germain P, et al. Indication de l'imagerie par résonance magnétique dans les cardiopathies congénitales en période néonatale. Ann Cardiol Angéiol. 1991;40:129–33.
15. Kastler B, Livolsi A, Germain P, et al. MRI in the management of congenital heart disease in newborn and s. Hospimedica. 1991;9:31–41.
16. Guilt Gl, et al. Levotransposition of the aorta: identification of segmental cardiac anatomy using MR imaging. Radiology 1986;161:673–9.
17. Hagen PT, Schoz DG, Edward WD. Incidence and size of patent foramen ovale during the first 10 decades of live: an autopsy study of 965 normal hearts. Proc Staff Meet Mayo Clin. 1984;59:1489–94.
18. Soto B et al. Identification of thoracic isomerism from the plain chest radiograph. AJR Am J Roentgenol. 1978;131: 995–1002.
19. Tonkin IL, Tonkin AK. Visceroatrial situs abnormalities: sonographic and computed tomographic appearence. AJR Am J Roentgenol. 1982;138:509–15.
20. Stanger P, Rudolph AM, Edwards JE. Cardiac malpositions: an overview based on a study of 65 necropsy specimens. Circulation. 1977;56:159–72.
21. Kastler B, Livolsi A, Germain P. Strip scanning a method to improve pediatric cardiovascular MRI. SMRI, 9th Annual Meeting, Chicago, April 3–6, 1991. (JMRI).
22. Kastler B, et al. MRI Artifacts a comprehensive approach. RSNA, 81th Assembly and Annual Meeting, Chicago, November 26–December 3, 1996. Artefacts en IRM. Feuillets de Radiologie 1994;34(6):493–514.
23. von Schulthess GK, Higgins CB. Blood flow imaging with MR: spin-phase phenomena. Radiology. 1985;157:687–95.
24. Felmlee JP, Ehman RL. Spatial presaturation: a method for suppressing flow artifacts and improving depiction of vascular anatomy in MR imaging. Radiology. 1987;164:559–64.
25. Link KM, Lesko NM. Magnetic resonance imaging in the evaluation of congenital heart disease. Magn Reson Q. 1991;7:173–90.
26. Higgins CB, editor. MRI of congenital heart disease. Essentials of cardiac radiology and imaging. Philadelphia: Lippincott; 1992. p. 283–331.
27. Wehrli FW, Haacke EM. Principles of MR imaging. In: Potchen EJ, Haacke EM, Siebert JE, Gottschalk A, editors. Magnetic resonance angiography: concepts and applications. St Louis: Mosby-Year Book; 1993. p. 9–34.
28. Listerud J. First principles of magnetic resonance angiography. Magn Reson Q. 1991;7:136–70.
29. Kastler B, editor. Dans: Comprendre l'IRM: Imagerie du flux. 6th ed. Paris: Masson; 2006. p. 189–213.
30. Atkinson D, Teresi L. Magnetic resonance angiography. Magn Reson Q 1994;10:149–72.
31. von Schulthess GK, Fisher S, Crooks LE, et al. Gated MR imaging of the heart: intracardiac signals in patients and healthy subjects cardiac. Radiology. 1985;156(1):125–32.

32. Kastler B. Principles of MR angiography. In: Patay Z, Kastler B, Anzalone N, editors. Applied neuroMR angiography CD-ROM. Antwerpen: Lasion; 1996.

33. Sechtem U, Pflugfelder PW, White RD, et al. Cine MR imaging: potential for the evaluation of cardiovascular function. AJR Am J Roentgenol. 1987;148:239–46.

34. Sechtem U, Pflugfelder P, Cassidy MC, Holt W, Wolfe C, Higgins CB. Ventricular septal defect: visualization of shunt flow and determination of shunt size by cine MR imaging. AJR Am J Roentgenol. 1987;149:689–92.

35. Baker EJ, Ayton V, Smith MA, et al. Magnetic resonance imaging at a high field strength of ventricular septal defects in infants. Br Heart J. 1989;62:305–10.

36. Simpson IA, Chung KJ, Glass RF, Sahn DJ, Sherman FS, Hesselink J. Cine magnetic resonance imaging for evaluation of anatomy and flow relations in s and children with coarctation of the aorta. Circulation. 1988;78:142–8.

37. Edelman RR, Chien D, Kim D. Fast selective black blood MR imaging. Radiology. 1991;181(3):655–60.

38. Boiselle PM, White CS. New techniques in cardiothoracic imaging. New York: Informa Healthcare; 2007. p. 81–2.

39. Weber OM, Higgins CB. MR evaluation of cardiovascular physiology in congenital heart disease: flow and function. J Cardiovasc Magn Reson. 2006;8(4):607–17.

40. Rebergen SA, Niezen RA, Helbing WA, van der Wall EE, de Roos A. Cine gradient-echo MR imaging and MR velocity mapping in the evaluation of congenital heart disease. Radiographics. 1996;16(3):467–81.

41. Mostbeck GH, Caputo GR, Higgins CB. MR measurement of blood flow in the cardiovascular system. AJR Am J Roentgenol. 1992;159:453–61.

42. Nayler GL, Firmin DN, Longmore DB. Blood flow imaging by cine magnetic resonance. J Comput Assist Tomogr. 1986; 10:715–22.

43. Bogren HG, Klipstein RH, Firmin DN, et al. Quantification of antegrade and retrograde blood flow in the human aorta by magnetic resonance velocity mapping. Am Heart J. 1989;117:1214–22.

44. Rees S, Firmin D, Mohiaddin R, Underwood R, Longmore D. Application of flow measurements by magnetic resonance velocity mapping to congenital heart disease. Am J Cardiol. 1989;64:953–6.

45. Pelc NJ, Herfkens RJ, Shimakawa A, Enzmann DR. Phase contrast cine magnetic resonance imaging. Magn Reson Q. 1991;7:229–54.

46. Kilner PJ, Firmin DN, Rees RSO, et al. Valve and great vessel stenosis: assessment with MR jet velocity mapping. Radiology. 1991;178:229–35.

47. Rebergen SA, Van Der Wall EE, Doornbos J, De Roos A. Magnetic resonance measurement of velocity and flow: technique, validation, and cardiovascular applications. Am Heart J. 1993;126:1439–56.

48. Pelc NJ, Sommer G, Li KCP, Brosnan TJ, Herfkens RJ, Enzmann DR. Quantitative magnetic resonance flow imaging. Magn Reson Q. 1994;10:125–47.

49. Carr JC, Simonetti O, Bundy J, Li D, Pereles S, Finn JP. Cine MR angiography of the heart with segmented true fast imaging with steady-state precession. Radiology. 2001;219(3):828–34.

50. Dinsmore RE, Wismer GL, Levine RA, Okada RD, Brady TJ. Magnetic resonance imaging of the heart: positioning and gradient angle selection for optimal imaging planes. AJR Am J Roentgenol. 1984;143:1135–42.

Sequential segmental analysis is based on the identification of the cardiac chambers, great vessels, and their mode of connection. Following a preliminary echocardiographic assessment of the cardiac anomalies (1–3), MRI must systematically visualize each of the three cardiac compartments (atrial, ventricular and arterial) which, in the normal heart, are connected concordantly on the right (RA→RV→PA[1]) or on the left (LA→LV→Ao). In congenital heart disease, each of these segments may occupy an abnormal position. This chapter reviews exhaustively a large number of anomalies. In some cases, MRI completes echocardiographic assessment, while in other cases it is not essential. However, this chapter presents several typical examples which are not discussed in subsequent chapters.

Identification of each compartment (atrial, ventricular and arterial) is considered separately.

3.1 Identification of Visceroatrial Situs

Identification of the visceroatrial situs is based on analysis of three groups of anatomical structures: the atria, tracheobronchial and pulmonary artery system (most reliable criterion) [1–4], and, in the abdomen, the positions of the inferior vena cava (IVC) and abdominal aorta in relation to the spine, and the positions of abdominal viscera [5–9].

Atrial situs can be determined by analysis of the morphology of the atria on axial images (Fig. 3.2a).

Criteria for "morphological" identification of the right and left atria were described in the previous chapter. The most reliable criterion is based on the very distinct appearance of the left and right atrial appendages (visualized on axial images): the right atrial appendage has a broad-based triangular shape, while the left atrial appendage has a hooked finger-like appearance with a narrow connection to the atrium (see Chap. 2, Fig. 2.6).

However, when this distinction cannot be formally established (differentiation of the atrial appendages on MRI images or transthoracic echocardiography[2] [11], is sometimes difficult in the case of complex anomalies), other structures must be analysed.

First of all, the venous connections are determined, although they are less discriminant than analysis of the atrial appendages. Coronal and short-axis images (see Chap. 2, atlas F7, F10 and Fig. 2.4g) clearly show the superior vena cava (SVC) and IVC normally draining into the right atrium. The site of insertion of the IVC is a more reliable[3] criterion than that of the SVC, which can abnormally drain into the left atrium (Fig. 3.6 and see Chap. 4, Figs. 4.3 and 4.4). Analysis of axial and coronal image (in several planes, see Chap. 2, atlas A7, A8 and F10) can show whether the pulmonary veins converge normally onto the left atrium, bearing in mind that anomalies of pulmonary return may also be observed (the most frequent being return of the superior pulmonary vein into the IVC – see Chap. 4, Figs. 4.18 and 4.19).

Fortunately, determination of atrial situs is based on other criteria: the anatomical arrangement of thoracic

---

[1]Due to crossover (twisting) of the great vessels at their origin, the PA which is part of the pulmonary or 'right' circuit at its emergence is situated anteriorly and to the left of the aorta, while the aorta, at its emergence, is situated posteriorly and to the right, although it is part of the systemic or 'left' circuit. *See loop rule below.*

[2]This R/L atrium distinction is easier on transoesophageal echocardiography [10], but cannot be performed in young infants.
[3]Except when the retrohepatic IVC is absent and is continuous with the azygos vein (see Fig. 3.7 left isomerism and Chap. 4, Figs. 4.6 and 4.7).

B. Kastler, *MRI of Cardiovascular Malformations,*
DOI: 10.1007/978-3-540-30702-0_3, © Springer-Verlag Berlin Heidelberg 2011

viscera (reliable and well demonstrated by MRI in contrast with echocardiography) and the situs of abdominal viscera (less discriminant)[4] (Figs. 3.1 and 3.2).

There are four types of situs (Fig. 3.1):

- Situs solitus (normal atrial situs)
- Situs inversus (mirror image)
- Right isomerism (two morphologically right atria)
- Left isomerism (two morphologically left atria) which are grouped under the term situs ambiguus, indeterminate situs or heterotaxy

3.1.1 Situs Solitus: Normal Atrial Situs

In the normal heart – normal atrial situs ("morphologically" right atrium on the right and "morphologically" left atrium on the left) or situs solitus (Figs. 3.1a and 3.2 and see Chap. 2, Figs. 2.2 and 2.6).

- The "morphologically" right lung (tri-lobed) and its bronchial divisions (short, vertical, eparterial[5] right main bronchus with trifurcation[6]) and pulmonary artery divisions (right pulmonary artery coursing in a coronal (slighty right oblique) plane in front of the right main bronchus) are normally situated on the right (Figs. 3.1a, 3.2b and 3.3a).
- The "morphologically" left lung (bilobed) and its bronchial divisions (long, horizontal, hyparterial[7] left main bronchus with bifurcation[8]) and pulmonary artery divisions (left pulmonary artery with an anteroposterior course in a sagittal (slighty left

oblique) plane forming an arch above the left main bronchus) are normally situated on the left (Figs. 3.1a, 3.2b and 3.3a).
- The liver is on the right, the stomach and spleen are on the left, the IVC is situated on the right, and the abdominal aorta is on the left (Figs. 3.2a, b and 3.3a).

3.1.2 Situs Inversus

In situs inversus (Figs. 3.1b, 3.3b, 3.4, 3.5 and 3.15b), the "morphologically" left atrium is on the right and the "morphologically" right atrium is on the left. All the other viscera are also inverted (including the IVC on the left and the aorta on the right – Fig. 3.3b) (mirror image). Situs inversus is very rare.

3.1.3 Other Types of Situs: Situs Ambiguus

Other types of situs are classified under the term heterotaxy or cardiosplenic syndrome, which can be subdivided into right isomerism and left isomerism (Table 3.1).

3.1.3.1 Right Isomerism

Right isomerism (Figs. 3.1c, 3.3c and 3.6) comprises two "morphologically" right atria, thoracic right–right symmetry and usually juxtaposition of the IVC and aorta, which are situated on the same side of the spine (either on the right, or on the left), together with asplenia with a midline liver, and a right or midline stomach (or less frequently in a normal position) (Fig. 3.6) [12–18]. Right isomerism is usually associated with an atrial septal defect (Fig. 3.6), often a ventricular septal defect, and sometimes a double SVC (50% of cases) (Fig. 3.6) (also see Chap. 4, Figs. 4.2, 4.4 and 4.5), a right aortic arch, an anomalous pulmonary venous connection, and more rarely a double IVC (Fig. 3.6) (each vena cava is connected separately to its respective atrium). Anomalies of the atrioventricular junction are also frequently observed (atrioventricular septal defect, AVSD, Fig. 3.6), or less

---

[4]The concordance between anomalies of atrial and bronchopulmonary situs is excellent, but the same is not true for anomalies of abdominal situs. For example: (a) right–left bronchopulmonary inversion→right–left atrial inversion (situs inversus), (b) bronchopulmonary D-isomerism (or L-isomerism)→atrial D-isomerism (or L-isomerism), (c) asplenia is usually, but not always, accompanied by atrial D-isomerism and polysplenia is usually, but not always, accompanied by atrial L-isomerism.

[5]Eparterial: parallel and posterior to the pulmonary artery.

[6]After a short vertical course, bifurcation into the right upper lobe bronchus and bronchus intermedius, which then divides into the right middle lobe bronchus and right lower lobe bronchus.

[7]Hyparterial: crossing underneath the pulmonary artery.

[8]After a long horizontal course, bifurcation into the left upper lobe and left lower lobe bronchi.

Fig. 3.1 Correlation between atrial and thoracic arrangement: four types of combinations are possible. (**a**) situs solitus (normal atrial arrangement), (**b**) situs inversus (mirror image), (**c**): right isomerism (two morphologically right atria) and (**d**) left isomerism (two morphologically left atria). Morphologically right atrium (mRA), morphologically left atrium (mLA)

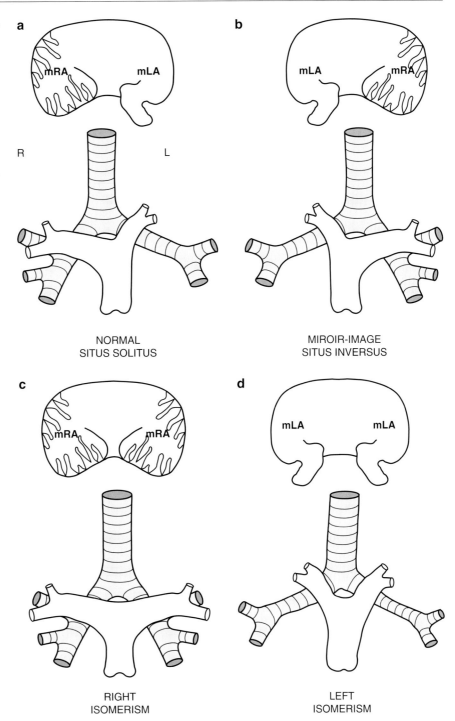

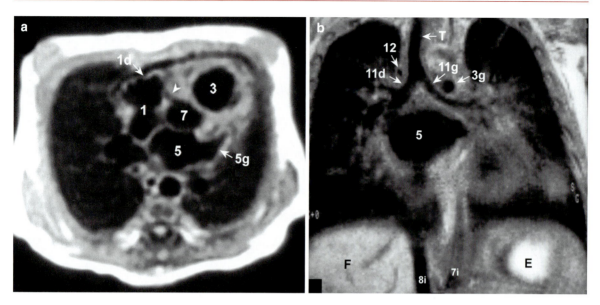

Fig. 3.2 Correlation between atrial, thoracic and abdominal arrangement in situs solitus (normal atrial arrangement): (**a**) axial image through the atria. *1* Identification of the 'morphologically' right atrium (mRA-1) situated on the right: the 'morphologically' right atrial appendage, situated on the right (*1d*) has a triangular shape with a broad implantation on the mRA anterior to the superior vena cava connection. *2* Identification of the 'morphologically' left atrium (mLA-5) situated on the left: the 'morphologically' left atrial appendage situated on the left (*5g*) has a finger-like shape with a narrow implantation on the mLA; pulmonary infundibulum (*2i*) below the pulmonary artery, aorta (*7*); note the origin of the right coronary artery (*arrowhead*) (also see Fig. 3.19b, and Chap. 2, Figs. 2.2 and 2.7; Chap. 5, Figs. 5.23 and 5.24). (**b**) Coronal image of the bronchial bifurca-tion and the abdomen. *1* Right–left pulmonary asymmetry: short, vertical, eparterial right main bronchus (*11d*) (which divides into the right upper lobe bronchus and right middle lobe bronchus) and long, horizontal, hyparterial left main bronchus (*11g*) (which divides into left upper lobe and left lower lobe bronchi). The left pulmonary artery (*3g*) has an anteroposterior course (in a slightly left oblique plane) and is seen on this image passing above the left main bronchus (also see Chap. 2, Fig. 2.8). The azygos vein (*12*) passes above the right main bronchus. The liver (Li) is in a normal position on the right and the stomach (St) is on the left. The inferior vena cava (*8i*) is on the right and drains into the right atrium (situated on the right). The abdominal aorta (*7i*) is on the left; morphologically left atrium (*5*) (also see Fig. 3.19b and Chap. 2, Fig. 2.2)

frequently a single ventricle (Fig. 3.6), and/or a single coronary artery. Finally, anomalies of the ventriculoarterial connection (transposition of the great vessels, double outlet right ventricle, right ventricular outflow anomaly (stenosis and obstruction), or even pulmonary atresia) (Fig. 3.6).

3.1.3.2 Left Isomerism

Left isomerism (Figs. 3.1d, 3.3d and 3.7) comprises two "morphologically" left atria, thoracic left–left symmetry, often, but not always, accompanied by polysplenia and, in 70% of cases, interruption of the retrohepatic IVC with azygos continuation [7, 12, 15, 19–24] (Fig. 3.7 and see Chap. 4, Fig. 4.4). It is also sometimes associated with ventricular septal defect and anomalies of the atrioventricular junction (AVSD). Unlike right

isomerism, a single ventricle is uncommon. Anomalies of the ventriculoarterial connection (left ventricular outflow tract obstruction, coarctation or hypoplasia of the aorta) may also be observed. Ventriculoarterial discordances corresponding to transposition (particularly simple D-transposition that will be discussed below) and pulmonary stenosis are observed less frequently than in right isomerism. Abdominal anomalies are frequently associated (intestinal malrotation, extrahepatic biliary atresia).

Right isomerism and left isomerism are also classically, but less appropriately, described as asplenia (Ivemark syndrome) and polysplenia (as splenic anomalies are not always concordant with anomalies of atrial situs) (see Table 3.1).

In the light of this description, MRI clearly plays an important role (complementary to that of echocardiography) in the determination of visceroatrial situs, particularly in the case of complex anomalies. This assessment is essentially based on analysis of the thorax on coronal images of the bronchial arrangement and, in the abdomen, examination of the position of the IVC in relation to the aorta and their positions in relation to the spine. Visualization of the tracheobronchial tree (most reliable criterion)[9] [1–3] is one of the major advantages of MRI. This also constitutes a major advantage for the assessment of other extracardiac anomalies, in which MRI is an essential complement to echocardiography.

After establishing atrial situs (first step in segmental analysis), the atrioventricular connections and ventriculoarterial connections must be defined on the basis of the criteria of identification of the "morphologically" right and "morphologically" left ventricles and their connexion to the great vessels (aorta and pulmonary artery), as they can be concordant or discordant in situs solitus and situs inversus (Fig. 3.9). This analysis is more difficult in the case of right or left isomerism, which may be associated with numerous additional anomalies (especially involving the atrioventricular connections).

Fig. 3.3 Correlation between the atrial, thoracic and abdominal arrangement. (**a**) Situs solitus (normal atrial arrangement). (**b**) Situs inversus (mirror image) (also see Fig. 3.15b). (**c**) Right isomerism (two right atria). (**d**) Left isomerism (two left atria). Right (R), left (L), morphologically right (mR) and morphologically left (mL), liver (Li), stomach (St), spleen (R), Sp (splenules), aorta (Ao), left (L) and right (R) superior vena cava (SVC) and inferior vena cava (IVC), azygos vein (AzV), hemiazygos vein (hAz)

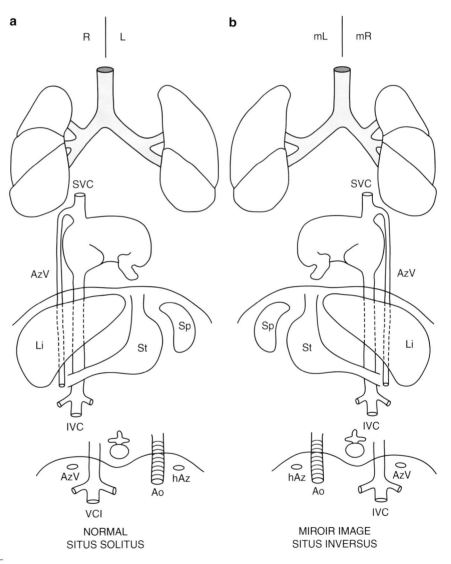

Fig. 3.3 (continued)

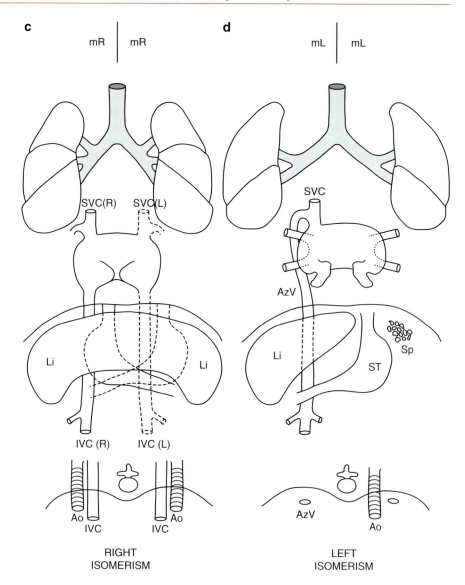

3.2 Atrioventricular and Ventriculoarterial Variants and Identification of Intersegmental Connections

Before analysing the atrioventricular and ventriculoarterial connections, the radiologist must first determine whether there are two ventricles or only one, and two systemic great vessels (aorta and pulmonary artery) or only one single outlet arterial connection. In the presence of bi-ventricular and bi-arterial connections, the criteria of identification of "morphologically" right and left ventricles and the great vessels are used to determine the type of atrioventricular and ventriculoarterial connections, which can be either concordant or discordant.

This assessment must also integrate the possibility of atrial isomerism (frequently associated with ASD) and univentricular (Fig. 3.6) and/or uni-arterial connection, which highlights the very large number of possible combinations and variants. Most of these possibilities are described and illustrated by diagrams and clinical cases, although this review cannot be completely exhaustive.

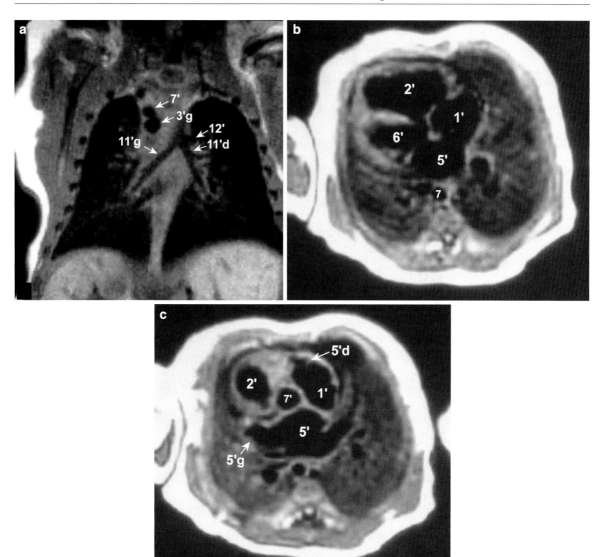

Fig. 3.4 Complete situs inversus with mirror image at all levels: thoracic and abdominal (**a**), ventricular (**b**) and atrial (**c**) (To facilitate identification of anomalies, turn the film over or swap right and left on your computer display screen, leading to R–L inversion = normal). Morphologically right atrium (*1′*) and left atrium (*5′*), right atrial appendage (*1d′*) and left atrial appendage (*1g′*), morphologically right ventricle (*2′*) and left ventricle (*6′*), aorta (*7′*) and pulmonary artery (left-*3g′*) (situated on the right!), eparterial right main bronchus (*11′d* situated on the left!) and hyparterial left main bronchus (*11′g* situated on the right!), azygos vein (*12′*) (also see Fig. 3.15b)

3.2.1 Atrioventricular Variants and Identification of Connections

Primarily, atrioventricular variants depend not only on the type of univentricular or bi-ventricular connections, but also on the situs. In situs solitus and situs inversus, these connections can be either concordant or discordant (Fig. 3.8). Right or left isomerism can be associated with many other anomalies of atrioventricular connections (Figs. 3.6 and 3.10), making analysis even more complicated.

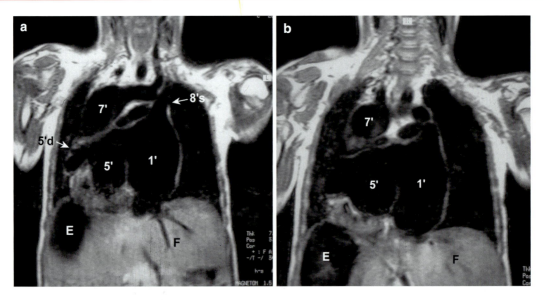

Fig. 3.5 Situs inversus in a 13-year-old child with pulmonary atresia, VSD and transposition of the great vessels (**a, b**). The morphologically right atrium (*1′*) is on the left, the superior vena cava (*8′s*) drains into the morphologically right atrium and the morphologically left atrium (*5′*) is on the right identified by its left finger-like atrial appendage (*5′g*), the gastric air bubble (E) on the right and the liver (F) on the left

Table 3.1 Right and left isomerism

		Right isomerism	Left isomerism
Clinical	Age	Neonate/child	Child/adult
	Gender	Male	Female
	Cyanosis	Severe	Usually absent
	Heart disease	Severe	Moderate
	Spleen	Absent	Multiple small spleens
	ECG	/	Abnormal P wave
	Prognosis	Severe	Good
	Mortality	High	Low
Anomalies	Aortic arch	R/L	R/L – coarctation/hypoplasia
	Great vessels	D/L-transposition	Transposition is rare
	Pulmonary stenosis	(70%)	Less frequent
	SVC	Always	Double (33%)
	IVC	Double (50%)	Retrocaval IVC absent
	Azygos	Normal (double)	Azygos continuation of IVC
	IVC/AbdAo	Juxtaposed to R or L of spine	(70%)
	Bronchus/lung	Two R types	Two L types
	Stomach	Central/R/L	R/L
	Liver	Central/R/L	Variable position
	Malrotation of intestinal loops	Microgastria	Yes
	Cardiac apex	R/L/central	R/L
	Pulmonary veins	TAPVC	PAPVC
	Atrial septum	Single atrium	ASD (85%)
	AV valve	Atresia-single valve	Normal-mitral valve anomaly
	Single ventricle	20%	/
	Ventricular septal defect	Yes	Frequent

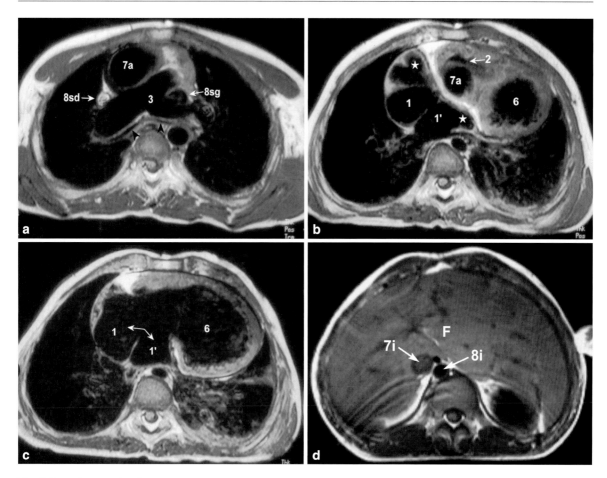

Fig. 3.6 A 13-year-old child with complex cyanotic heart disease in the context of right isomerism with left single ventricle and tight pulmonary stenosis. A left Blalock-Taussig shunt was performed first to revascularize the pulmonary artery, followed by a complete cavopulmonary shunt (see same patient Chap. 7, Fig. 7.22 and post-operative image Chap. 8, Fig. 8.9). Segmental analysis of the thoracic and visceroatrial situs clearly reveals the features of right isomerism. (**a–d**) Craniocaudad series of axial images: the dilated pulmonary trunk is clearly visualized (*3*) together with its division into left and right branches. Note the left–left symmetry of pulmonary and atrial structures with: two right pulmonary arteries (right–right symmetry) running in a 'slightly oblique' coronal plane anteriorly and parallel to the respective main bronchi; two main bronchi presenting a right symmetry (eparterial) and which are also hypoplastic (*arrowheads*); the atrium situated on the right (*1*) and the atrium situated on the left (*1′*) both present a broad triangular atrial appendage (*asterisk*), corresponding to a morphologically right atrium (these structures clearly correspond to two morphologically right atria (right isomerism)). There is a large atrial septal defect (*double arrow*). Also note the presence of two superior vena cavae, one on the right (*8sd*) and one on the left (*8sg*). The large single morphologically left ventricle (*6*) contrasts with the

rudimentary small right ventricular chamber (almost absent-2) usually situated anterosuperiorly, as in this case; ascending aorta (*7a*). (**e–h**) Anteroposterior series of coronal images, confirming and completing the findings of the previous images. The dilated pulmonary trunk (*3*) and branch left (*3g*) and right (*3d*) pulmonary arteries are clearly visualized (*3*). Note the right superior vena cava (*8sd*) which drains into the atrium situated on the right (*1*) and the left superior vena cava (*8sg*) which drains into the atrium situated on the left (*1′*); the same applies to the left inferior vena cava (IVC) stump, which receives an hepatic vein (Vh) (see Chap. 8, Figs. 8.9a, c). A palliative Blalock-Taussig shunt (*arrows*) was performed between the left subclavian artery (superiorly) and the left pulmonary artery (*3g* inferiorly); aorta (*7*). The liver (F, *black*) is in a midline position and the right IVC (*8i*) and abdominal aorta (*7i*) are juxtaposed and situated to the right of the spine (right isomerism) (**d–f**). The aorta (*7d*), initially situated on the left in the thorax crosses the midline as it passes through the diaphragm and is situated infradiaphragmatically (*7i*) next to the right IVC (*8i*) (F), both vessels are thus located to the right of the spine (**d–h**). The trachea (T) and main bronchi are hypoplastic. Note that the left bronchial division has a right morphology with division into an upper lobe bronchus – left – and middle lobe bronchus (bronchus intermedius)

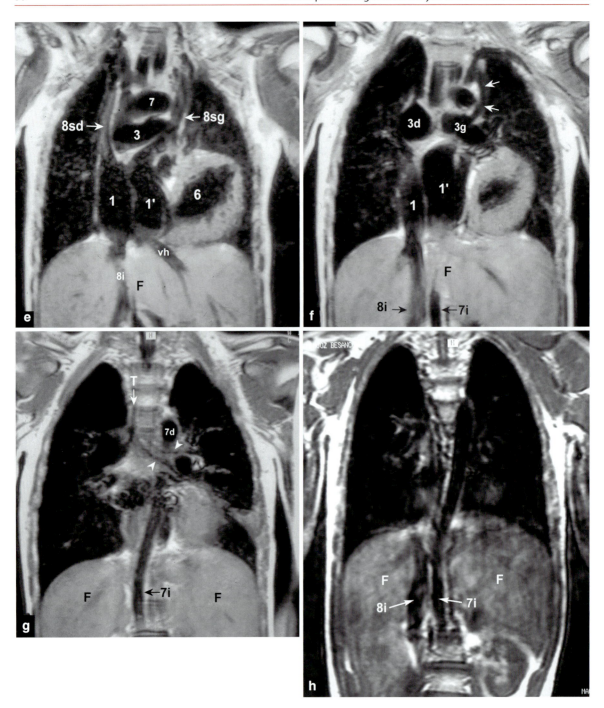

Fig. 3.6 (continued)

3.2.1.1 Bi-ventricular Connections

Situs solitus or inversus

In the usual arrangement (situs solitus) or in situs inversus, identification of each ventricle is essentially based on identification of the atrioventricular valve (the tricuspid valve opens into the mRV and the mitral valve opens into the mLV), that is the offset of the atrioventricular valves: the tricuspid valve is situated more anteriorly than the mitral valve (identification of the septal insertion of the tricuspid valve on axial and/or long-axis four-chamber images – Figs. 3.8b, d and 3.17 and see Chap. 2, Fig. 2.7 and atlas A9 and A10).

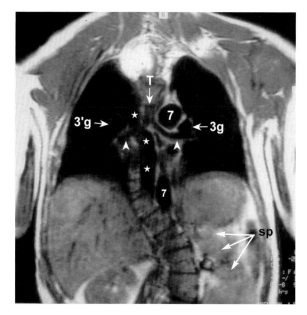

Fig. 3.7 Young girl with interruption of the retrohepatic IVC and azygos continuation in a context of left isomerism. Coronal spin-echo image through the tracheal bifurcation. Note the presence of left–left pulmonary symmetry with: two symmetrical, long and horizontal (hyparterial) left main bronchi (*arrowheads*); symmetrical left pulmonary arteries with an anteroposterior course forming an arch over the respective main bronchi (*3g* and *3'g*). The dilated azygos vein (*asterisks*) is situated posteriorly to the right hilum and drains into the superior vena cava (azygos continuation of the IVC); note the polysplenias (*splenules-sp*); aorta (*7*), trachea (*T*) (also see Chap. 4, Fig. 4.4)

The term *ventricular loop* is used to determine the position occupied by the ventricles (Figs. 3.8 and 3.17):

- In a right ventricular loop (RVL), the ventricles are situated in a normal position: the mRV is to the right of the mLV (which is on the left!).
- In a left ventricular loop (LVL), the ventricles are inverted: the mRV is to the left of the mLV (which is on the right!).

This concept of RVL or LVL corresponds to the more anatomical description of right-hand and left-hand arrangements (Fig. 3.8 [1, 3]).

Connections may be either concordant (mRA→mRV and mLA→mLV) or discordant (mRA→mLV and mLA→mRV), consequently resulting in four possibilities related to situs (see Fig. 3.9).

1. Concordance of the ventricular loop in relation to atrioventricular situs:
   - Situs solitus and RVL (mRA→mRV situated on the right).
   - Situs inversus and LVL (mirror image of the above: mRA→mRV situated on the left).
2. Discordance of the ventricular loop in relation to atrioventricular situs:
   - Situs solitus and left loop (mRA→mLV: situated on the right).
   - Situs inversus and right loop (mLA→mRV: situated on the right).

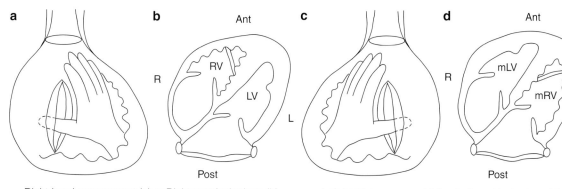

Right-hand arrangement (a) or Right ventricular loop (b)   Left-hand arrangement (c) or Left ventricular loop (d)

Fig. 3.8 Ventricular loop concept. In a right ventricular loop (RVL), the mRV is on the right of the mLV (**b**), and in a left ventricular loop (LVL) the mRV is on the left of the mLV (**d**). The ventricular loop is determined on axial images by identification of the mRV: the tricuspid valve always opens into a morphologically right ventricle and is identified by its septal insertion, which is situated more anteriorly than that of the mitral valve ('valve offset' seen on axial and long-axis four-chamber images, see morphologically

right and left ventricles, Chap. 2, Figs. 2.7, 2.9 and atlas A9, A10). This case does not present any anomaly of atrial situs. Right (R), left (L), anterior (A), posterior (P). This loop concept corresponds to the concept of right-hand (**a**) or left-hand (**c**) arrangement, based on the fact that a right hand (right loop B), or a left hand (left loop D), respectively, could be placed on the septal wall of the mRV with the thumb in the inlet chamber and the fingers in the ejection chamber (adapted and modified from Anderson [1, 3])

Fig. 3.9 Concordant or discordant atrioventricular connections in situs solitus and situs inversus (four possible combinations, see text). 'Morphologically' right atrium (mRA) and left atrium (mLA), 'morphologically' right ventricle (mRV) and left ventricle (mLV), right and left ventricular loops (RVL and LVL)

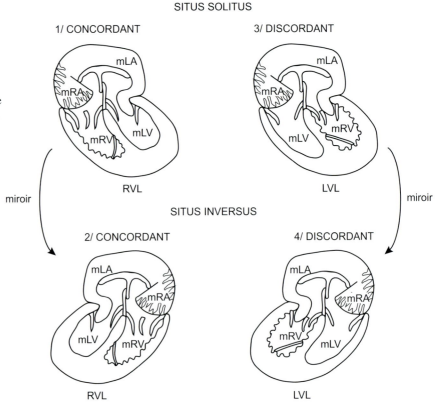

Atrial Isomerism and Differentiated "Morphologically" Right and Left Ventricles

In the presence of atrial isomerism (two atria of the same type) and two differentiated "morphologically" right and left ventricles, the atrioventricular connections can no longer be described as concordant or discordant, as they are, by definition, ambiguous. Determination of the ventricular loop is of prime importance (right-hand or left-hand arrangement, see Figs. 3.8 and 3.10), as it defines which type of "morphologically" right or left ventricle (mRV or mLV) is connected to the atrium situated on the right and the atrium situated on the left, respectively.

3.2.1.2 Univentricular Connections (or with a Dominant Ventricle)

In univentricular connections, the atria are connected to a single ventricle or a left or right dominant ventricle (the other ventricle is rudimentary or incomplete). The rudimentary right ventricle is generally situated antero-superiorly (Fig. 3.6, and see Chap. 4, Fig. 4.22 and

Chap. 5, Fig. 5.23) and the rudimentary left ventricle is situated posteroinferiorly. One or two "double-inlet" valves may also be present. When two valves are present, one may be stenotic, atresic (Figs. 3.11 and 3.12), incompetent, partly overriding[10] one of the ventricles or may present straddling.[11] When a single common valve is present, it can also be stenotic, atresic, incompetent, partially imperforate or may present "straddling". Figure 3.13 summarises the possible combinations integrating the atrial variants.

3.2.1.3 Atrioventricular Septal Defect

Fast spin-echo sequences completed by gradient-echo sequences clearly demonstrate ventricular and atrial septal defects, especially when they are multiple. A particular form of AVSD is situated at the junction of the interventricular and interatrial septa. These defects,

---

[10]When a valve overrides both ventricles, it is attributed to the ventricle that it covers by more than 50%.

[11]A valve presents 'straddling' when it is partly inserted (papillary muscles, tendinous cords) onto the contralateral ventricle.

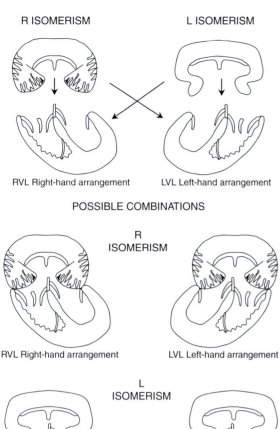

POSSIBLE COMBINATIONS

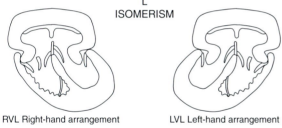

Fig. 3.10 Atrioventricular connections in right and left atrial isomerism. As in Fig. 3.9, there are four possible combinations: right or left ventricular loop (RVL–LVL) (right-hand arrangement and left-hand arrangement, respectively) for right isomerism and for left isomerism. 'Morphologically' right atrium (mRA) and left atrium (mLA) and 'morphologically' right ventricle (mRV) and left ventricle (mLV)

associating varying degrees of anomalies of atrioventricular valves, atrial and/or ventricular septal defects, are called AVSD.[12] There are many variants of AVSD, ranging from incomplete forms, such as ostium primum ASD or AVSD VSD and/or valve anomalies (tricuspid or mitral cleft, abnormal insertions, straddling, etc.) to complete forms: ASD, VSD, common valves, or even single atrium (Fig. 3.14).

---

[12]The septal defect situated on the posterior part of the membranous septum or interatrioventricular portion, responsible for left ventricle-right atrium communication, is a distinct entity that must be distinguished from AVSD.

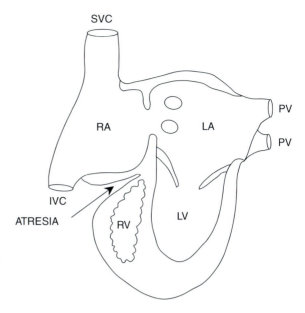

Fig. 3.11 Diagram of tricuspid atresia resulting in absence of communication between the right atrium (A) and right ventricle (RV), which is usually smaller than normal. A right–left shunt is mandatory for the patient's survival, generally via a ventricular or atrial septal defect (also see Chap. 7, Fig. 7.24). Left Atrium (LA), left ventricle (LV) superior vena cava (SVC) and inferior vena cava (IVC)

3.2.2 Ventriculoarterial Variants and Identification of Connections

3.2.2.1 Bi-Arterial Connections

In the presence of two trunci arteriosi (and two ventricles[13]), the connections can be concordant, discordant or may present a double outlet.

Ventriculoarterial Concordance

Ventriculoarterial concordance is observed in the usual arrangement in which the aorta emerges from the left ventricle situated on the left, and the pulmonary artery emerges from the right ventricle situated on the right (Fig. 3.15). At its origin, the aorta is in a "central" position, posterior and to the right of the pulmonary artery. Ventriculoarterial concordance is also present in situs inversus with mirror image.

---

[13]The terms ventriculoarterial concordance and discordance only apply when there are two differentiated ventricles, leading, in the presence of ventriculoarterial discordance, to the concept of transposition of the great vessels. In the case of a single or dominant left or right ventricle or double-outlet ventricle, the terms ventriculoarterial concordance and discordance no longer apply, leading to the more general concept of malposition of the great vessels (see below).

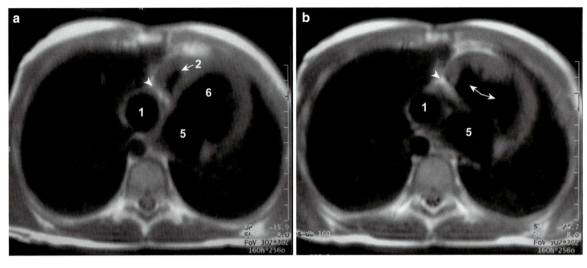

Fig. 3.12 An 11-year-old child with tricuspid atresia (Type 1b). Axial fast spin-echo images (**a, b**): the right atrioventricular groove (*arrow*) is continued by a white fat signal (in the place of the absent tricuspid valve), which completely separates the dilated right atrium (*1*) from the rudimentary right ventricular chamber (*2*); left atrium (*5*), left ventricle (*6*). This patient was treated by bidirectional cavopulmonary shunt ('hemi-Fontan') (see Chap. 7, Fig. 7.25 and 7.26 and Chap. 8, post-operative MRI, Fig. 8.10)

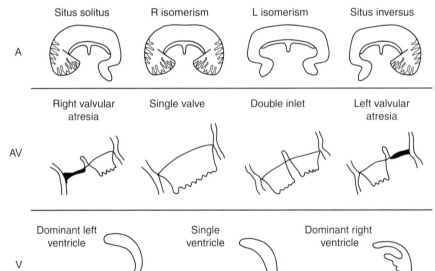

Fig. 3.13 Atrio-univentricular connections: possible combinations integrating the atrial (level A), ventricular (level V) and atrioventricular valve (level AV) variants. All combinations are possible between the three levels

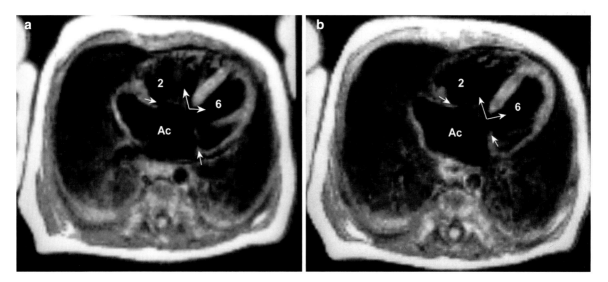

Fig. 3.14 Complete atrioventricular septal defect infant. Aial images (**a, b**) showing the common atrioventricular valve (*arrows*) extending to the right (*2*) and left (*6*) ventricles, a VSD (*double arrow*) and a complete septal defect with a single or common atrium (Ac)

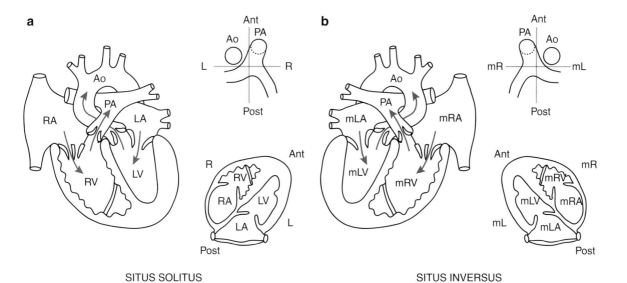

SITUS SOLITUS   SITUS INVERSUS

Fig. 3.15 Ventriculoarterial concordance. In the case of ventriculoarterial concordance, the aorta (Ao) emerges from the morphologically left ventricle (mLV) and the pulmonary artery (PA) emerges from the morphologically right ventricle (mRV). Ventriculoarterial concordance is observed in the normal arrangement with situs solitus (**a**) and in complete situs inversus (**b**) (also see Figs. 3.3 and 3.4). The opposite case corresponds to ventriculoarterial discordance (Fig. 3.16). In the normal arrangement, the aorta is in a 'central' position at its origin, posteriorly and to the right of the pulmonary artery. The right ventricle is to the right of the left ventricle; right atrium (RA) and left atrium (LA). Note that the rule of the Ao and mRV loop situated on the same side applies here (see below)

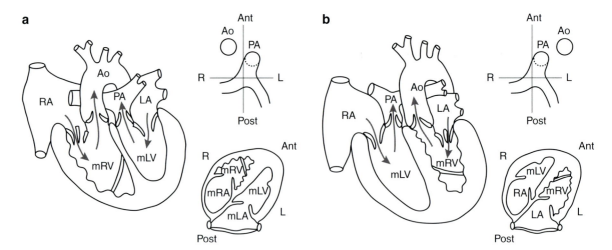

Fig. 3.16 Complete transposition (D-transposition) and corrected transposition (L-transposition) of the great vessels. (**a**) Ventriculoarterial discordance with atrioventricular concordance in complete transposition of the great vessels: the aorta (Ao), situated anteriorly and to the right of the pulmonary artery (PA) (D-transposition), emerges from a morphologically right ventricle (mRV) situated on the right (R ventricular loop); morphologically right atrium (mRA), left atrium (mLA) and left ventricle (mLV); right ventricular loop (RVL). (**b**) Double ventriculoarterial and atrioventricular discordance in corrected transposition: the aorta (Ao), situated anteriorly and to the left of the pulmonary artery (PA) (L-transposition), emerges from a morphologically right ventricle (mRV), which is situated on the left (L ventricular loop). A mirror image is possible in the two types of transposition (also see Chap. 7, Fig. 7.13). Note that the rule of the Ao and mRV loop situated on the same side applies here (see below); left ventricular loop (LVL)

Fig. 3.17 Segmental analysis at the arterial level (Ao images: axial images through the origin of the aorta and pulmonary artery) and at the ventricular level (V images: axial images through the ventricular chambers), to determine the type of anomaly (for diagram, see Fig. 3.15a and 3.16a, b). Note that the rule of the Ao and mRV loop situated on the same side (95% of cases) applies here (see below). (**a, b**) *Normal subject* (**c, d**) *Complete transposition* (**e, f**) *Corrected transposition*. (**a, b**) *Normal subject* (AoN VN): at the arterial level AoN, normal relations of the great vessels: at its origin, the ascending aorta (*7a*) is in a central position, situated posteriorly and to the right of the pulmonary artery (*3*), which is situated anteriorly and to the left; at the ventricular level VN, normal position of the ventricles: the morphologically right ventricle (*2*) is on the right (right loop), and is identified by the tricuspid valve (*arrowhead*) localized on the right and situated more anteriorly (and inferiorly towards the apex of the heart) compared to the mitral valve (*arrow*), which is more posterior and to the left, which identifies the morphologically left ventricle (*6*); descending aorta (*7d*), right atrium (*1*) and left atrium (*5*). (**c, d**) *Complete transposition* (D-transposition) (AoD VD): at the arterial level AoD, the great vessels are transposed: the ascending aorta (*7a*) is situated anteriorly and to the right (D-transposition) and the pulmonary artery (*3*) is situated posteriorly and to the left in a 'central position'; at the ventricular level VD, normal position of the ventricles: the morphologically right ventricle (*2*) is on the right (right loop), and is identified by the tricuspid valve (*arrowhead*) localized on the right and situated more anteriorly (and inferiorly towards the apex of the heart) compared to the mitral valve (*arrow*), which is more posterior and to the left, which identifies the morphologically left ventricle (*6*). Note the presence of a moderator band (between *white arrowheads*), another criterion for identification of the morphologically right ventricle; right atrium (*1*), left atrium (*5*). Overall: the ascending aorta (*7a*), situated anteriorly and on the right (D-transposition), emerges from the morphologically right ventricle (situated on the right: right loop) and the pulmonary artery (*3*), situated posteriorly and on the left, emerges from the morphologically left ventricle. There is ventriculoarterial discordance but atrioventricular concordance. (**e, f**) *Corrected transposition* (L-transposition) (AoL VL): at the arterial level AoL, the great vessels are transposed: the ascending aorta (*7a*) is situated anteriorly and to the left (L-transposition) of the pulmonary artery (*3*); at the ventricular level VL: there is ventricular inversion, the morphologically right ventricle (*2′*) is situated on the left (left loop) and is identified by the tricuspid valve (*white arrowhead*) localized on the left and situated more anteriorly (and inferiorly towards the apex of the heart) compared to the mitral valve (*white arrow*), which is more posterior and on the right, which identifies the morphologically left ventricle (*6′*). The right ventricle (trabeculated) is hypertrophied because it is connected to the aorta and the systemic circulation (the right ventricle is the systemic ventricle). Also note the presence of a moderator band (*black arrowhead*); right atrium (*1*) and left atrium (*5*). Overall: the ascending aorta (*7a*), situated anteriorly and on the left (L-transposition), emerges from the morphologically right ventricle (situated on the left: left loop) and the pulmonary artery (*3*), situated posteriorly and on the right, emerges from the morphologically left ventricle (situated on the right). There is ventriculoarterial and atrioventricular discordance

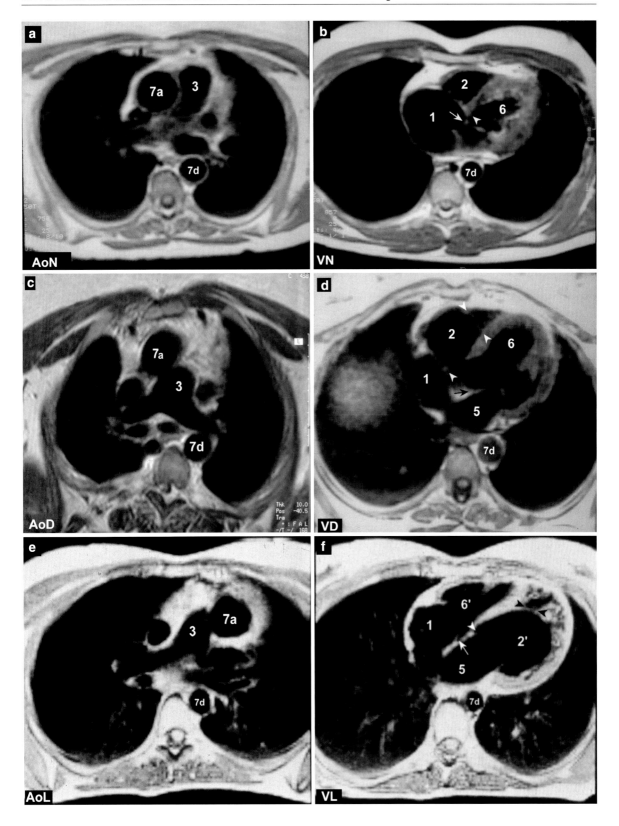

Ventriculoarterial Discordance

Ventriculoarterial discordance is observed in transposition of the great vessels: the aorta emerges from an mRV and the pulmonary artery emerges from an mLV (Fig. 3.16). There are two variants (Figs. 3.16a, b and 3.17): simple complete transposition (D-transposition) and corrected transposition of the great vessels (L-transposition).

• Simple complete transposition (D-transposition)

This anomaly (Table 3.2 and Figs. 3.16–3.20) consists of atrioventricular concordance[14] (situs solitus or situs inversus) with ventriculoarterial discordance[15]: the aorta (situated anteriorly and on the right – D-transposition) emerges from an mRV and the pulmonary artery (situated posteriorly and on the left) emerges from an mLV. These features are clearly visualized on axial and/or short-axis images, on which the two vessels initially have a parallel course instead of crossing over ("gun barrel" appearance) (Fig. 3.18). The mRV is to the right of the mLV resulting in a RVL (D loop) (Figs. 3.17, 3.19, 3.20). The aortic valve is higher than normal due to the presence of a subaortic conus, inducing tricuspid-aortic discontinuity (while the absence of subpulmonary conus on the left results in mitro-pulmonary continuity). Transposition of the great vessels can also be associated with other anomalies (ventricular septal defect, pulmonary valve stenosis, patent ductus arteriosus, etc.). Haemodynamically, there are two, parallel closed circuit pulmonary and systemic circulations (Fig. 3.16a). In this type of anomaly, mixing of the two circulations (to supply the pulmonary outflow tract) is exclusively ensured by the ductus arteriosus for as long as it remains patent (functional) and/or by a ventricular septal defect. Surgical correction is rapidly required

---

[14]The concept of atrioventricular concordance implies that, strictly speaking, the term complete transposition cannot be used in atrial isomerism where atrioventricular connections are ambiguous.

[15]The term ventriculoarterial discordance (which does not describe the atrioventricular connections) is obviously not synonymous with complete transposition of the great vessels (D-transposition) (there is also a corrected variant of transposition of the great vessels [L-transposition] associated with ventriculoarterial discordance together with atrioventricular discordance).

Table 3.2 Atrioventricular and ventriculoarterial connections in the complete transposition (D-transposition) and corrected transposition (L-transposition)

Normal		Complete transposition (D)		Corrected transposition (L)	
RA	LA	RA	LA	RA	LA
↓	↓	↓	↓	↓	↓
RV	LV	RV	LV	LV	RV
↓	↓	↓	↓	↓	↓
PA	Ao	Ao	PA	PA	Ao

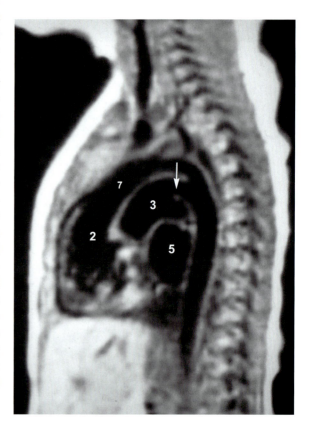

Fig. 3.18 Complete transposition (D-transposition) of the great vessels in a newborn. Sagittal oblique image in the pulmonary artery-aorta axis: the ascending aorta (*7*) situated anteriorly and on the left, and the pulmonary artery (*3*), situated posteriorly and on the right, have a parallel course without crossing over ('gun barrel image'). The aorta emerges from the right ventricle (*2*) and the pulmonary artery emerges from the left ventricle. The patent ductus arteriosus (*arrow*) is clearly visualized; left atrium (*5*) (also see Chap. 1, Fig. 1.8, Chap. 7, Fig. 7.14 and Chap. 8, Fig. 8.14)

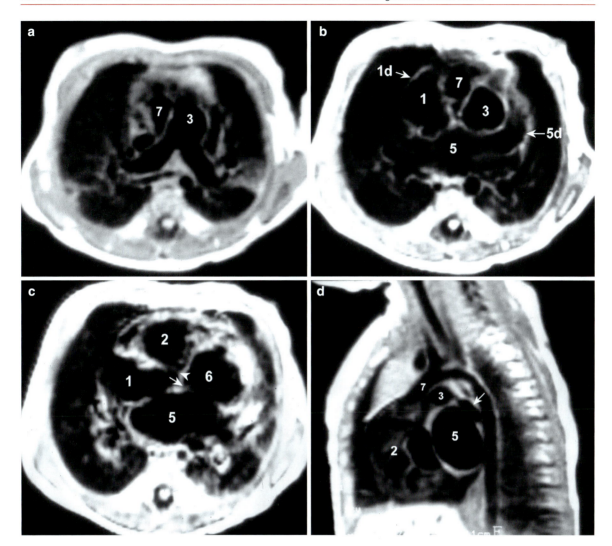

Fig. 3.19 Complete transposition (D-transposition) of the great vessels in a newborn. (**a, b**) Axial spin-echo image (through the origin of the aorta and pulmonary artery): the ascending aorta (*7*), situated anteriorly and on the right (D-transposition), emerges from the morphologically right ventricle (*2*) and the pulmonary artery (*3*), situated posteriorly and on the left (in a *central position*) emerges from the morphologically left ventricle (*6*). Note that the 'morphologically' right atrial appendage (*1d*) which has a triangular shape and a broad connection to the right atrium (*1*) is situated on the right and the 'morphologically' left atrial appendage (*5d*) which has a finger-like shape with a narrow connection to the left atrium is situated on the left (*5*). (**c**) Axial spin-echo image (through the ventricular chambers): the morphologically right ventricle (*2*) is on the right (right loop); it is identified by the tricuspid valve (*arrowhead*) situated on the right and more anteriorly (and inferiorly towards the apex of the heart). The mitral valve (*arrow*) is situated more posteriorly and to the left, identifying the morphologically left ventricle (*6*). (**d–f**) Sagittal images from right to left: ascending aorta (*7*), situated anteriorly and on the left, and pulmonary artery (*3*), situated posteriorly and on the right, have a parallel course without crossing over ('gun barrel image'). The aorta emerges from the right ventricle (*2*) and the left ventricular pulmonary artery. Patent ductus arteriosus (*arrow*); left atrium (*5*); This patient presented a ventricular septal defect: between 2 and 6 in (**f**); also see Chap. 7, Fig. 7.14 and Chap. 8, Fig. 8.1, 8.4, 8.21 and 8.22 for postoperative features)

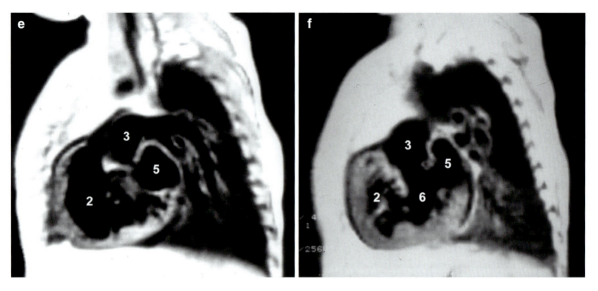

Fig. 3.19 (continued)

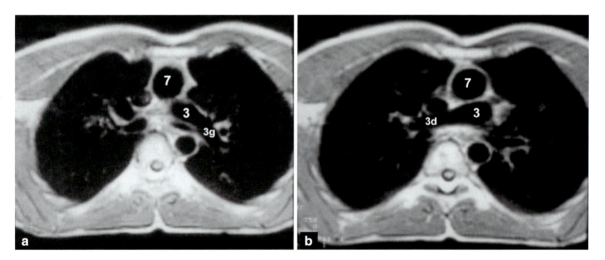

Fig. 3.20 Complete transposition (D-transposition) of the great vessels in an adolescent. (**a**, **b**) Axial spin-echo images through the origin of the aorta and pulmonary artery: the ascending aorta (*7*), situated anteriorly and on the right (D-transposition), emerges from the morphologically right ventricle and the pulmonary artery (*3*), situated posteriorly and on the left (in a central position), emerges from the morphologically left ventricle. (**c**) Short-axis oblique image: the aorta (*7*), situated anteriorly and on the right and the pulmonary artery (*3*), situated posteriorly and on the left, have a parallel course ('gun barrel image'). The aorta emerges from the right ventricle (*2*) and the pulmonary artery emerges from the left ventricle (*6*). This patient was treated by a Mustard atrial switch procedure (also see Chap. 7, Figs. 7.14 and 7.15 and Chap. 8, Fig. 8.14, 8.15, 8.21, 8.22 for post-operative features). (**d**) Axial spin-echo image through the ventricular chambers: the morphologically right ventricle (*2*) is on the right (right loop), it is identified by the tricuspid valve (*arrowhead*) situated on the right and more anteriorly (and inferiorly towards the apex of the heart) compared to the mitral valve (*arrow*), which is more posterior and to the left (which identifies the morphologically left ventricle – *6*). Also note the presence of a moderator band (between the two *black arrowheads*). (**e–h**) Anteroposterior series of coronal images: the aorta (*7*), situated anteriorly clearly emerges from the morphologically right ventricle (*2* – trabeculated) and the pulmonary artery, situated posteriorly (*3*) emerges from the morphologically left ventricle (*6* – smooth wall); right pulmonary artery (*3d*), left pulmonary artery (*3g*), right atrium (*1*)

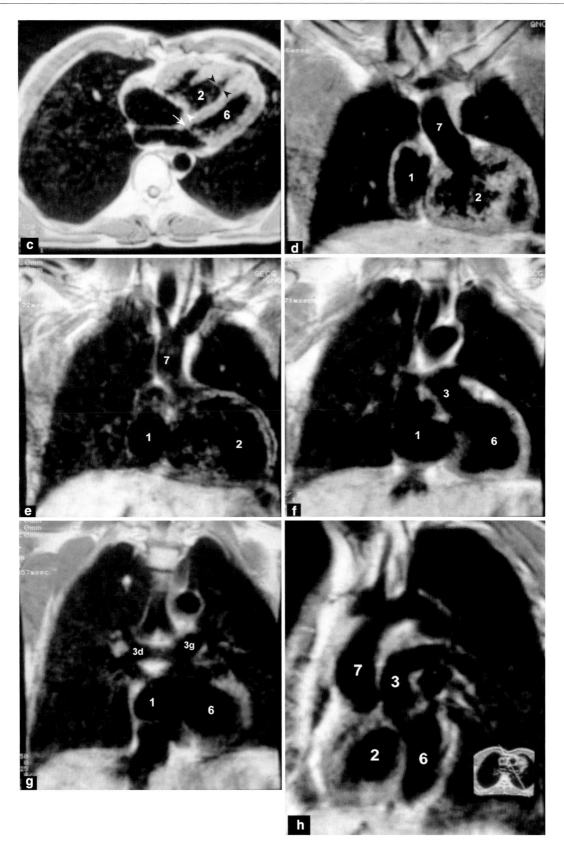

Fig. 3.20 (continued)

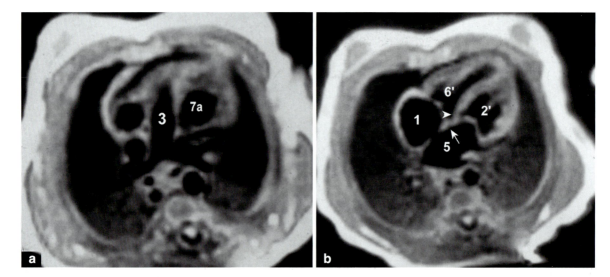

Fig. 3.21 Corrected transposition (L-transposition) of the great vessels in a newborn. (**a**) Axial spin-echo image through the origin of the aorta and pulmonary artery: the great vessels are transposed: the aorta (*7a*) is situated anteriorly and to the left (L transposition) of the pulmonary artery (*3*). (**b**) Axial spin-echo image through the ventricular chambers: the morphologically right ventricle (*2′*) is on the left (left loop) and is identified by the tricuspid valve (*arrow*) situated on the left and more anteriorly (and inferiorly towards the apex of the heart) compared to the mitral valve (*arrowhead*), which is more posterior and to the right, which identifies the morphologically left ventricle (*6′*). The right ventricle is similar in size or even larger than the left ventricle because it is connected to the aorta and systemic circulation (the right ventricle is the systemic ventricle) (also see Chap. 7, Fig. 7.17)

after performing emergency balloon atrial septotomy (Rashkind procedure [25], Fig. 3.19c) allowing circulatory mixing in the atrium. Surgical correction can be performed by two techniques: arterial switch or atrial switch (see detailed description in Chap. 8).

• Corrected transposition of the great vessels (L-transposition)

This is a distinct entity with double atrioventricular[16] and ventriculoarterial discordance and, therefore, normal blood circulation (Table 3.2 and Figs. 3.16b, 3.17, 3.21, 3.22). The aorta (situated anteriorly and on the left, L-transposition) emerges from an mRV which is connected to an mLA and the pulmonary artery (situated posteriorly and on the right) emerges from an mLV which is connected to an mRA. The mRV is to the left of the mLV resulting in a LVL (L-loop). The mRV is the systemic ventricle, as it is trabeculated, thickened and dilated. The tricuspid valve opens into a right ventricle situated on the left and the valve

offset is therefore inverted: the septal insertion of the tricuspid valve (on the left of the septum) is situated anteriorly compared to the mitral valve (these anomalies are clearly visible on multislice short-axis and axial images, Figs. 3.17, 3.21, 3.22). L-transposition is also associated with aorto-tricuspid discontinuity and a common fibrous mitropulmonary valve. Congenitally corrected transposition is often associated with other anomalies: ventricular septal defect, pulmonary stenosis, or Ebstein anomaly (of the left-sided tricuspid valve).

Mirror arrangements of simple transposition and corrected transposition are also possible.

Transposition and Malposition of the Great Vessels

The terms malposition and transposition, concerning the respective positions of the great vessels in relation to their origin, must be clearly defined. The great vessels may differ from normal while maintaining normal anteroposterior relations: in situs solitus (normal arrangement), the origin of the aorta is situated posteriorly and to the right of the origin of the pulmonary artery; in situs inversus, the origin of the aorta is

---

[16]Once again, in the presence of atrial isomerism with ambiguous atrioventricular connections, the term corrected transposition is, strictly speaking, inappropriate.

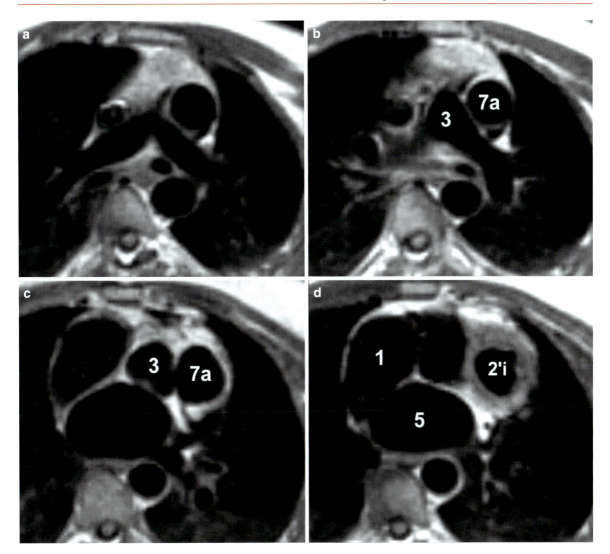

Fig. 3.22 Corrected transposition (L-transposition) (L loop) of the great vessels in an adolescent. Craniocaudad axial spin-echo images. (**a**, **b**) Axial images through the origin of the aorta and pulmonary artery: the great vessels are transposed: the ascending aorta (*7a*) is situated anteriorly and to the left (L-transposition) of the pulmonary artery (*3*). (**c–f**) Axial images through the ventricular chambers: the morphologically right ventricle (*2'*) is on the left (left loop) and is identified by the presence of a moderator band (between *arrowheads*) and by the fact that it is trabeculated, and has an infundibulum (*2'i* here subaortic). It is also hypertrophied because it is connected to the aorta and the systemic circulation (the right ventricle is the systemic ventricle). The offset of the atrioventricular leaflets is also clearly identified: the tricuspid valve (*arrowhead*) situated on the left and more anteriorly (and inferiorly towards the apex of the heart) compared to the mitral valve (*arrow*), which is more posterior and on the right; right atrium (*1*) and left atrium (*5*). (also see Chap. 7, Fig. 7.17). In this case, the atrioventricular valves were not clearly visualized and the mRV could not be identified by the offset criterion. Other criteria must therefore be used to identify the mRV

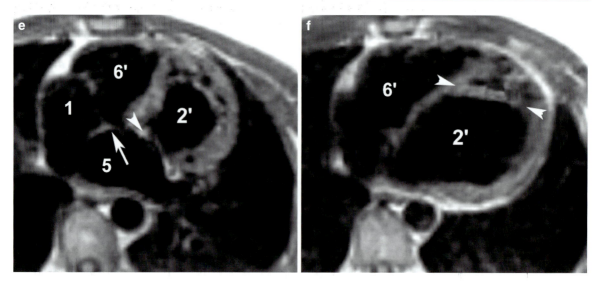

Fig. 3.22 (continued)

situated to the left of the pulmonary artery, but the anteroposterior relations are not modified. The great vessels are normally connected to their respective ventricles (Ao-mLV and PA-mRV). There is a simple right–left mirror inversion of the cardiovascular arrangement.

In transposition of the great vessels, the aorta arises from the right ventricle and the pulmonary artery arises from the left ventricle. The origin of the aorta is generally situated more anteriorly than that of the pulmonary artery (loss of anteroposterior relations). When the transposed aorta arises to the right of the pulmonary artery, it corresponds to complete transposition or D-transposition, and when it arises to the left of the pulmonary artery, it corresponds to corrected transposition or L-transposition.

In malposition, the great vessels present abnormal anatomical relations at their origin but are not necessarily associated with ventriculoarterial discordance. In the same way as for transpositions, when the origin of the transposed aorta is situated to the right of the pulmonary artery, the anomaly is described as D-malposition and when the aorta is situated to the left of the pulmonary artery, it is described as L-malposition. The two types of D- and L-transpositions can be considered to be particular forms of malposition. In the absence of transposition (no ventriculoarterial discordance), two particular types of malpositions are described. Appropriate origin of a great vessel from its

ventricle and inappropriate origin of the other vessel from the same ventricle corresponds to double outlet right ventricle and double outlet left ventricle (*see below*). The vessels are usually arranged side by side. The aorta is usually to the right of the pulmonary artery in DORV (D-malposition), but can be on the right or the left in DOLV (D- or L-malposition). Figure 3.27 summarizes the various possible positions of the aorta in relation to the pulmonary artery.

Double Outlet Arterial Connections

In this type of anomaly, the two great vessels (aorta and pulmonary artery) emerge from the same morphologically right or left ventricle: double outlet left or right ventricle or single or indeterminate[17] ventricle (Figs. 3.6, 3.23 and 3.24).

In double outlet right ventricle, the only possible left ventricular outflow tract is via a ventricular septal defect, which can be situated at various levels (underneath the

---

[17]When there is an anomaly of the relations between the aorta and the pulmonary artery, the term malposition of the great vessels can no longer be used, as the two vessels arise from the same cavity (right, left or single ventricle) and are therefore not transposed from one cavity to the other: transposition of the great vessels is therefore a particular form of a more general anomaly of malposition of the great vessels (see Fig. 3.2).

Fig. 3.23 Diagrams of arterial connections. (**a**) In double outlet right ventricle (DORV). (**b**) In double outlet left ventricle (DOLV). (**c**) In single or indeterminate ventricle (ID) (also see Chap. 7, Fig. 7.18 and 7.20). The aorta (Ao) and pulmonary artery (PA) emerge from the right ventricle (RV) in DORV and the left ventricle (LV) in DOLV and from the same ventricle in the case of a single ventricle. Right atrium (RA), left atrium (LA), left ventricle (LV)

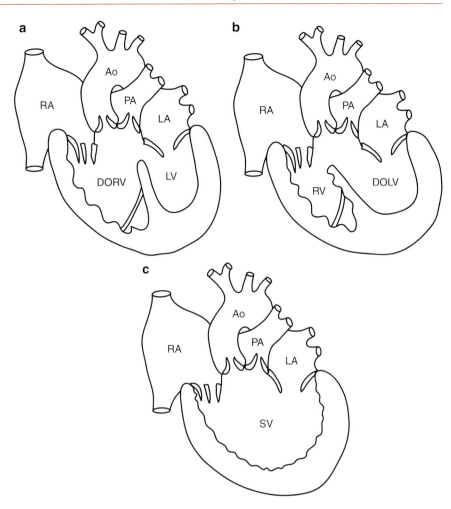

aorta, underneath the pulmonary artery or underneath both arteries). The site of the VSD is important, as it determines the direction of flow: in subaortic VSD, blood circulation is relatively normal, while in subpulmonary VSD, the circulation is comparable to that of transposition of the great vessels. Subaortic VSD is also frequently associated with pulmonary stenosis (resulting in cyanotic heart disease similar to tetralogy of Fallot). The two vessels are generally side by side, with the aorta on the right with a double subaortic and subpulmonary conus (these characteristics are clearly visualized on the coronal images on Fig. 3.24).

3.2.2.2 Bi-Ateraial connections

Single Outlet Connections

In single ventriculoarterial connections, the ventricles are connected with:
- A truncus arteriosus (Figs. 3.25 and 3.26b and see Chap. 7, Figs. 7.3–7.5), which presents several variants.
- Only one of the two vessels (solitary trunk), while the other is hypoplastic or atresic (pulmonary or aortic atresia).

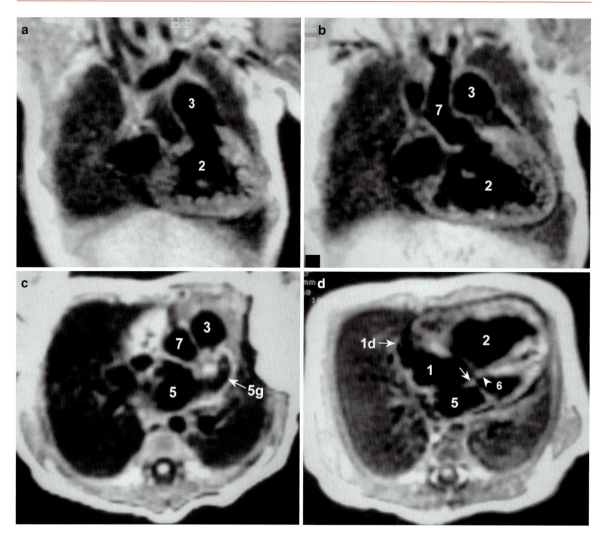

Fig. 3.24 Double outlet right ventricle: the pulmonary artery and aorta both emerge from the right ventricle. (**a, b**) Coronal spin-echo images through the origin of the pulmonary artery and the aorta: the pulmonary artery (3) and aorta (7) both emerge from the trabeculated right ventricle (2). (**c**) Axial spin-echo image through the origin of the great vessels which travel side by side with the aorta, as here, usually to the right with double subaortic and subpulmonary conus; note that the left atrial appendage (5g) has a finger-like shape with a narrow connection to the left atrium (5). (**d**) "Four-chamber" axial spin-echo image. The right ventricle (2) is in a normal position to the right (right loop) of the left ventricle (6): it is identified by the tricuspid valve (*arrowhead*) situated on the right and more anteriorly (and inferiorly towards the apex of the heart) compared to the mitral valve (*arrow*), which is more posterior and on the left. Also note that the right atrial appendage (1d) has a triangular shape and a broad connection to the right atrium (1) (see post-operative MRI appearance, Chap. 8, Fig. 8.31)

3.2.3 Loop Rule

The loop rule proposed by Van Praagh [26, 27] can be used to indirectly predict the ventricular loop from the respective positions of the great vessels (and vice versa). According to this rule, in 95% of normal or abnormal hearts, a RVL corresponds to an aorta situated on the right of the pulmonary artery and vice versa (the aorta and mRV are generally situated on the same side).

However, this very useful rule is not infallible (and can sometimes be misleading). For example, in complete transposition of the great vessels with situs solitus, the aorta is situated on the right and in front of the

Fig. 3.25 Normal arrangement (**a**) and variants of single outlet ventriculoarterial connections: type I truncus arteriosus (TA) (**b**), solitary trunk with hypoplasia or pulmonary atresia (**c**) or aortic atresia (**d**). Aorta (Ao), pulmonary artery (PA), right (R) and left (L) branches (also see Chap. 7, Fig. 7.3)

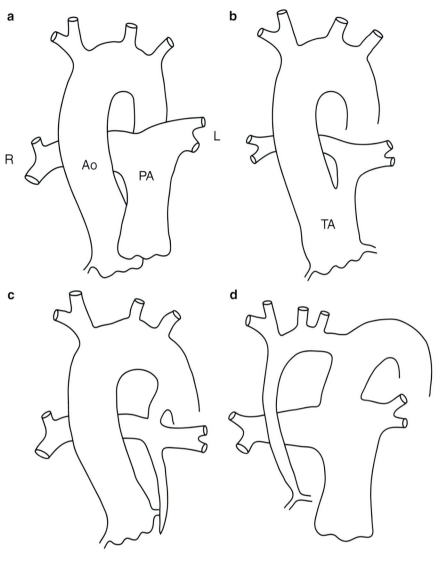

pulmonary artery in only 60% of cases. A second criterion for identification of the mRV must always be used (offset atrioventricular valves or moderator band). Figure 3.27 summarizes the various possible positions of the aorta in relation to the pulmonary artery.

3.2.4 Cardiac Position

So far, we have only considered anomalies of position and/or connection of the cardiac chambers without discussing anomalies of cardiac position. In fact, an anomaly of cardiac position is only rarely accompanied by a true morphological anomaly and anomalies of cardiac position must therefore be considered separately. The heart generally occupies a predominantly left-sided position in the thorax (levocardia), but it can be predominantly situated on the right (dextrocardia – see Chap. 2 Fig. 2.6e, f) or, more rarely, in a central position (mesocardia). This cardiac position is independent of the position of the apex, which can also be left-sided, right-sided(Fig. 3.28) or central.

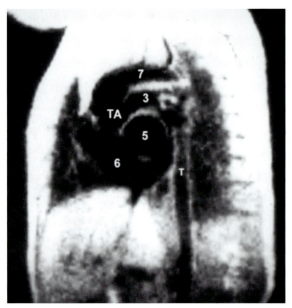

Fig. 3.26 Type I truncus arteriosus in a neonate: sagittal image through the truncus arteriosus (TA) which emerges above the left ventricle (*6*) and gives rise to both the aorta (*7*) and the pulmonary artery (*3*); left atrium (*5*)

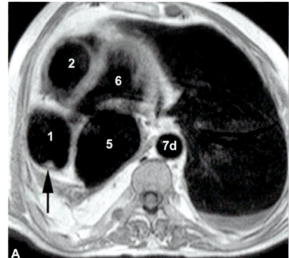

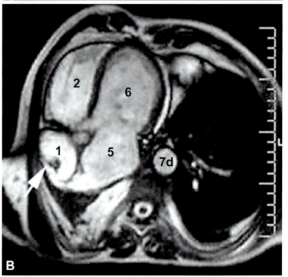

Fig. 3.28 Dextrocardia in a young adult patient. Axial fast spin-echo and cine-MR images. Note the presence of a crista terminalis (*arrow*), which is here a feature of particular value to identify the mRA in anomalies of position of the heart. Right atrium (*1*), left atrium (*5*), right ventricle (*2*), left ventricle (*6*), descending aorta (*7d*) (for dextrocardia see Chap. 7 Fig. 7.7, for crista terminalis also see Chap. 2, Fig. 2.10)

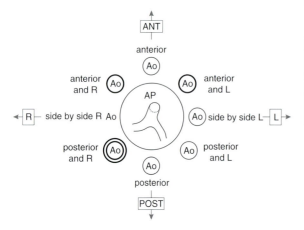

Fig. 3.27 Respective positions of the aorta (*outer circle*) in relation to the pulmonary artery (PA in the *centre*). Aorta situated posteriorly and to the right: normal, anteriorly and to the *right*: D-transposition, anteriorly and to the *left*: L-transposition, side by side: double outlet right ventricle

References

1. Anderson RH, Becker AE, Freedom RM, Macartney FJ, Quero-Jimenez M, Shinebourne EA, et al. Sequential segmental analysis of congenital heart disease. Pediatr Cardiol. 1984;5:281–8.
2. Soto B et al. Identification of thoracic isomerism from the plain chest radiograph. AJR. 1978;131:995–1002.
3. Anderson RH, Ho SY. Sequential segmental analysis of congenitally malformed hearts: advances for the 1990's. Austral Assoc J Cardiac Thorac Surg. 1993;2:10–7.
4. Anderson C, Devine WA, Anderson RH, Debich DE, Zuberbuhler JR. Abnormalities of the spleen in relation to congenital malformations of the heart: a survey of necropsy findings in children. Br Heart J. 1990;63:122–8.
5. Shinebourne EA, Macartney FJ, Anderson RH. Sequential chamber localization-logical approach to diagnosis in congenital heart disease. Br Heart J. 1976;38:327–40.
6. Guilt GL et al. Levotransposition of the aorta: identification of segmental cardiac anatomy using MR imaging. Radiology. 1986;161:673–9.
7. Stanger P, Rudolph AM, Edwards JE. Cardiac malpositions: an overview based on a study of 65 necropsy specimens. Circulation. 1977;56:159–72.
8. Tonkin IL, Tonkin AK. Visceroatrial situs abnormalities: sonographic and computed tomographic appearance. AJR. 1982;138:509–15.
9. Sharma S, Devine W, Anderson RH, Zuberbuhler JR. The Determination of atrial arrangement by examination of appendage morphology in 1842 heart specimens. Br Heart J. 1988;60:227–31.
10. Stumper OFW, Sreeram N, Elzenga NJ, Sutherland GR. Diagnosis of atrial sirus by transesophageal echocardiography. J Am Coll Cardiol. 1990;16:442–6.
11. Sapire DW, Ho SY, Anderson RH, Righy ML. Diagnosis and significance of atrial isomerism. Am J Cardiol. 1986;58:342–6.
12. Anderson RH, Becker AE, Freedom RM, et al. Sequential segmental analysis of congenital heart disease. Pediatr Cardiol. 1984;5:281–7.
13. van Mierop LHS, Gessner IH, Schiebler GL. Asplenia and polysplenia syndromes. Birth Defects. 1972;8:74–82.
14. Rose V, Izukawa T, Moes CAF. Syndromes of asplenia and polysplenia. A review of cardiac and non-cardiac malformations in 60 cases with special reference to diagnosis and prognosis. Br Heart J. 1975;37:840–52.
15. Ruttenberg HD, Neufeld HN, Lucas Jr RV, et al. Syndromes of congenital heart disease with asplenia. Distinction from other forms of congenital cyanotic cardiac disease. Am J Cardiol. 1964;13:387–406.
16. Caruso G, Becker AE. How to determine atrial situs? Considerations initiated by 3 cases of absent spleen with a discordant anatomy between bronchi and atria. Br Heart J. 1979;41:559–67.
17. Freedom RM, editor. Asplenia and polysplenia (a consideration of syndromes characterized by right or left atrial isomerism). In: Angiocardiography of congenital heart disease. New York: Macmillan; 1984:643.
18. Macartney FJ, Zuberbuhler JR, Anderson RH. Morphological considerations pertaining to recognition of atrial isomerism. Consequences for sequential chamber localization. Br Heart J. 1980;44:657–67.
19. Liberthson RR, Hastreiter AR, Sinha SM, et al. Levocardia with visceral heterotaxy-isolated levocardia: pathologic anatomy and its clinical implications. Am Heart J. 1973;85:40–54.
20. Becker AE, Anderson RH. Pathology of congenital heart disease. London: Butterwoths; 1981.
21. Jelinek JS, Stuan PL, Done SL, Ghaed N, Rudd SA. MRI of polysplenia syndrome. Magn Reson Imaging. 1989;7:681–6.
22. Pernot C, Hoeffel JC, Worms AM, Auguste JP. La continuation azygos de la veine cave inférieure. Ann Radiol. 1978;21:525–30.
23. Schultz CL, Morrison S, Brian PJ. Azygos continuation of the inferior vena cava: demonstration by NMR. J Comput Assist Tomogr. 1984;8:774–6.
24. Coulomb M, Rose-Pittet L, Dalsoglio S, Lebas JF, Paillasson F, Gros Ch, et al. Continuation azygos droite de la veine cave inférieure. A propos de 3 observations avec étude IRM. J Radiol. 1987;68:45–50.
25. Waldhausen JA, Boruchow I, Miller WW, Rashkind WJ. Transposition of the great arteries with ventricular septal defect. Palliation by atrial septostomy and pulmonary artery banding. Circulation. 1969;39(5 suppl 1): I215–21.
26. Van Praagh R, Van Praagh S, Vlad P, Keith JD. Anatomic types of congenital dextrocardia. Diagnosis and embryologic implications. Am J Cardiol. 1964;13:510–31.
27. Van Praagh R. Terminology of congenital heart disease. Glossary and commentary. Circulation. 1997;56:139–41.

Congenital venous anomalies are subdivided into systemic and pulmonary venous anomalies. Classical radiological assessment comprises chest radiograph, angiography, and echocardiography. These anomalies are difficult to diagnose on echocardiography, and angiography is not devoid of risks; moreover, it is no longer justified in view of the *excellent* performances of MRI, which allows precise morphological description of the anomalies [1–9].

MRI and CT have greatly improved the depiction of extracardiac congenital vascular anomalies, in large part because of their multiplanar and cross sectional ability to depict the anatomy. Moreover, they do not have the limitations of echocardiography (poor depiction of vascular structures and poor acoustic window) [10] or angiography (catheter-related complications, overlap of adjacent structures, and difficulties in depicting the systemic and pulmonary vascular systems simultaneously) [11, 12].

The development of multiple row detectors CTs allows for faster acquisition, higher spatial resolution, and simultaneous assessment of cardiovascular structures and lung parenchyma [11–13]. Some researchers have described encouraging results for the use of CT angiography in anomalous pulmonary venous connections (APVC) [14–17]. However, helical CT angiography has limitations in the pediatric patients. These are mainly related to the small size of patients, nonbreath-hold imaging, and slow infusion rates of contrast media [13, 18]. CT is also limited in depicting associated congenital cardiac anomalies in comparison to MRI. Moreover, the repeated exposure to high doses of ionizing radiation (the effective radiation dose from ECG-gated CT of the heart is estimated to be approximately 15 mSv (19)) over time is of great concern in the pediatric population and in young women. Thus, because of all these drawbacks, CT is not, at our institution, the imaging modality of choice for the depiction of the congenital anomalous venous connections.

In this chapter, we describe the MR features of the main anomalies of systemic and pulmonary venous connections:

- Left superior vena cava, double superior vena cava and azygos continuation of the inferior vena cava (IVC).
- Total anomalous pulmonary venous connection and partial anomalous pulmonary venous connection.

Each anomaly is described separately, but it must be kept in mind that several anomalies can coexist in the same patient, as they often constitute elements of various congenital heart diseases.

4.1 Examination Techniques

The examination always starts with a series of mediastinal axial ECG-gated *black blood sequences* (fast spin-echo or *double IR sequences)* that must always be completed in this type of disease by coronal and when pertinent sagittal and oblique imaging planes (see Chap. 1) to ensure optimal visualization of certain anomalies (course of vessels, connections, etc.).

The slice thickness is adapted to the size of the patient: 3–5 mm in the very young and 5–8 mm in older children and adults. Optimal visualization of small vascular structures and the tracheobronchial tree can be obtained by performing stacks of intertwined and overlapping images, 3–5 mm thick (i.e., slice interval of 2–3 mm, see Chap. 2).

For bright blood imaging, gradient-echo cine-MRI sequence, recently replaced by balanced-SSFP sequences (higher SNR, shorter imaging time, optimal flow enhancement not relying on inflow effects) are performed in complement to black blood sequences to confirm vascular nature or patency. Gadolinium enhanced magnetic resonance angiography sequences displaying the anomalies on a large 3D Fov are also essential in this context.

4.2 Anomalous Systemic Venous Connections

Two paired, symmetrical venous systems give rise to the superior vena cava system (SVC): the common cardinal veins and the anterior cardinal veins. The left cardinal veins regress, while the SVC is derived from the right common cardinal vein (right Cuvier duct) and the terminal portion of the right anterior cardinal vein. Anastomosis of anterior cardinal veins forms the left brachiocephalic vein. The coronary sinus (CS) is a remnant of the left common cardinal vein.

Four paired, symmetrical venous systems give rise to the IVC and azygos system. Normal development is a complex process, marked by the appearance of transverse anastomoses between the various systems and disappearance of left venous channels in favor of right venous channels.

The retrohepatic segment of the IVC is formed by the hepato-subcardinal anastomosis (between the right subcardinal vein and the network of vitelline veins). The left subcardinal vein disappears and the prerenal segment of the IVC is formed by the right subcardinal vein. With caudal development of the embryo, a third system of sacrocardinal veins appears. The right sacrocardinal vein forms the distal portion of the IVC and the anastomosis between the two sacrocardinal veins forms the left common iliac vein.

During involution of the posterior cardinal veins, a fourth system appears – the supracardinal system. The trunk of the azygos vein is formed by the suprarenal segment of the right supracardinal vein and the arch of the azygos vein is formed by the superior segment of the right posterior cardinal vein. The left supracardinal vein forms the inferior and superior hemiazygos veins and the left intercostal vein (and its anastomosis with the left brachiocephalic vein is also formed by the superior segment of the left posterior cardinal vein as well as the left common cardinal vein).

4.3 Left Superior Vena Cava

Persistent left SVC is observed with a frequency of 0.3% in the general population and in 4.4% of subjects with congenital heart disease [19–21]. It is the most frequent variant of systemic venous connections.

Embryologically, persistence of the left SVC is due to absence of involution of the left anterior cardinal vein. This anomaly can be subdivided (Figs. 4.1–4.4) into isolated left SVC when the right anterior cardinal vein involutes (inducing atresia, or even absence of the right SVC) or double SVC (about 90% of cases) [19]. Absence of the left brachiocephalic vein is observed in about 40% of cases [21–24]. The left SVC travels anteriorly to the left pulmonary artery and enters the right atrium via a dilated CS [23, 24]. Persistence of the left SVC can be associated with an atrial septal defect and azygos continuation of the IVC [19, 25], anomalies of cardiac and visceral symmetry[1] and various forms of congenital heart disease. In 10% of cases, the left SVC is connected to the roof of the left atrium [26] (Fig. 4.5).

Persistent left SVC (Figs. 4.1–4.3) must be distinguished from *left* partial APVC [27, 28] via an anomalous vertical vein (with the same mediastinal course *lateral the aortic arch*) connecting the left superior pulmonary vein to the homolateral brachiocephalic vein (see below and Fig. 4.21). However, in left SVC, two vessels are present anterior to the left main bronchus (the left SVC and the left superior pulmonary vein), whereas in left partial APVC to the brachiocephalic vein, no vessel is present anterior to the bronchus (as the left superior pulmonary vein drains upward via the vertical vein). Unlike persistent left SVC, the anomalous vertical vein can pass behind the left pulmonary artery and, most importantly, does not drain into the CS.[2] Also see paragraph on cor triatriatum and Fig. 4.23 for a rare case of venous drainage via a vertical vein.

---

[1]Especially in the case of right isomerism, in which persistence of right-sided structures explains the presence of two SVC (53%) or even double IVC each connecting with an atrium (see Chap. 3). The presence of two SVC is less frequent (33%) in left isomerism.

[2]This criterion is more reliable, hence the value of oblique images to confirm or exclude connection with the coronary sinus – see below.

Fig. 4.1 Diagram of the various forms of persistent left superior vena cava draining into the coronary sinus and right atrium (RA) (above) or more rarely into the left atrium (LA) (below). (**a**) Double SVC. (**b**) Double SVC and absence of left brachiocephalic vein. (**c**) Single left SVC. Right superior vena cava (RSVC), left superior vena cava (LSVC) left brachiocephalic vein (LBCV), coronary sinus (CS)

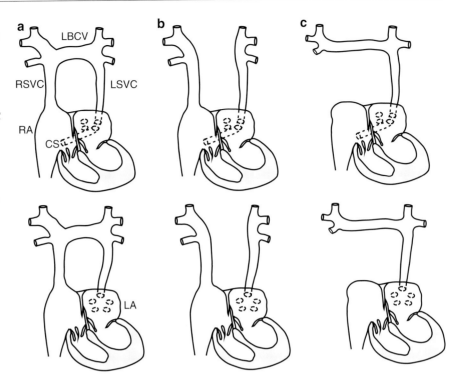

4.3.1 Clinical Features

In the absence of other associated anomalies, persistent left SVC has no clinical repercussions [19]. It is generally an incidental finding at adolescence or during adulthood (chest radiograph, chest CT, or MRI). However, it is important to recognize this anomaly when planning cardiac surgery or pacemaker implantation.

4.3.2 Imaging

• Chest radiograph

The left SVC usually presents with widening of the left superior mediastinum. In some cases, the chest radiograph can be normal [29].

• Echocardiography

B-mode echocardiography shows dilatation of the CS [24]. Color-coded Doppler echocardiography facilitates detection of the left SVC [30], which nevertheless remains difficult because of the extracardiac mediastinal site of the anomaly.

• Computed tomography

The anomaly is sometimes discovered on chest CT, which provides the same information as MRI (axial images) [25, 30–32], visualizing the left SVC in the form of a left mediastinal tubular opacity situated in front of the aortic arch, draining into the CS and presenting vascular contrast enhancement kinetics.

• Angiography

Angiography is *at present* useless for the diagnosis of isolated forms of persistent left SVC. During right transfemoral cardiac catheterization [29], the catheter ascends in the left SVC via the dilated CS. Left brachial catheterization with injection of contrast agent into the origin of the left brachiocephalic vein opacifies the left SVC, its connection to the CS, and the communication with the contralateral SVC.

4.3.3 MRI

MR imaging of the left SVC (Figs. 4.2–4.5 and 4.15, also see Chap. 3, Fig. 3.6 and Chap. 5, Fig. 5.23) does

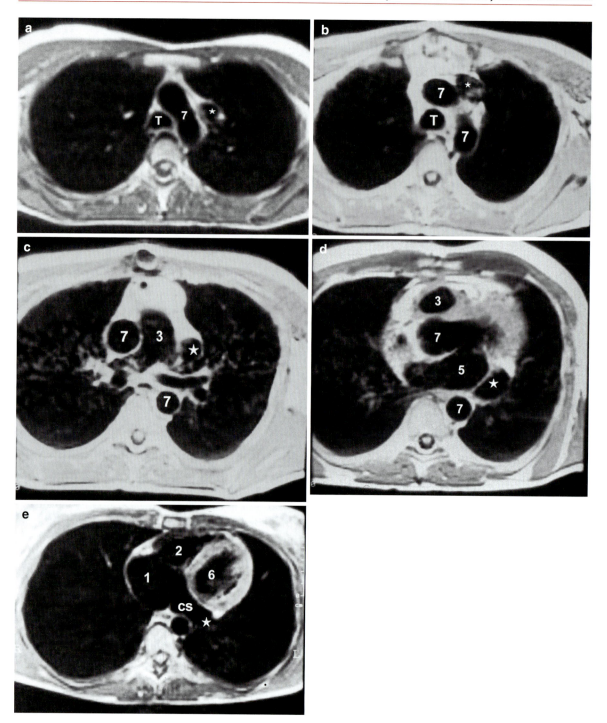

Fig. 4.2 Isolated left superior vena cava. Follow-up MRI after incidental intraoperative discovery of a left superior vena cava during mitral valve replacement in a 37-year-old patient. (**a–e**) Axial images, craniocaudad series, showing the mediastinal course of the left SVC (*asterisks*) anteriorly to the aortic arch (aorta-7) and left hilum (pulmonary artery-3), as far as its anastomosis in the dilated coronary sinus (cs). (**f, g**) LAO (short-axis) images confirming abnormal drainage of the left superior vena cava (*asterisks*) into the right atrium (*1*) via the dilated coronary sinus (situated in the left inferior atrioventricular groove); trachea (T), right ventricle (*2*), left atrium (*5*), left ventricle (*6*)

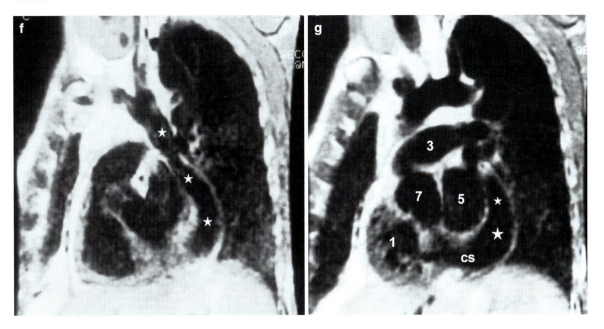

Fig. 4.2 (continued)

not require injection of contrast agent. In the superior mediastinum, the left SVC is situated laterally to the common carotid artery and anteriorly to the left subclavian artery. It has a vertical descending course, anteriorly and to the left of the aortic arch and left hilum. MRI axial especially LAO images clearly visualize the terminal intrapericardial part of the left SVC, which travels in the posterior atrioventricular groove before draining into the dilated CS. Coronal images demonstrate the two SVC on the same slice in the case of double SVC (Fig. 4.4). This view is also useful when the left SVC drains into the left atrium (Fig. 4.5). *Contrast enhanced MRA displays the anomaly on a large Fov* (Fig. 4.4).

4.4 Azygos Continuation of the Inferior Vena Cava

Azygos continuation of the IVC is the second most frequent anomaly of systemic venous connections after persistent left SVC (Figs. 4.6, 4.7 and 4.19). It is also the commonest congenital anomaly of the IVC [33–35], observed in 0.6% of cases of congenital heart disease. Due to the absence of formation of the hepato-subcardinal anastomosis, blood from the caudal part of the embryo is drained by the right supracardinal vein, which subsequently becomes the azygos vein [21]. Azygos continuation of the IVC occurs above the level of the renal veins. Right azygos continuation via the azygos vein is the more usual form. In this case, the hepatic veins drain directly into the right atrium due to the absence of the retro hepatic IVC [32].

Hemiazygos continuation of a left side IVC is a much less common anomaly. Routes for the blood to reach the right atrium are as follows: Drainage of the hemiazygos vein to azygos vein, the accessory hemiazygos vein, a persistent left SVC, or via left superior intercostal vein into the brachiocephalic trunc and SVC.

Azygos continuation of the IVC is usually (84% of cases) associated with left isomerism (or polysplenia syndrome),[3] much less frequently with right isomerism (Ivemark syndrome or asplenia) [36, 37], and in cardiac malpositions and abdominal situs inversus [35]. It can also be associated with APVC (see Chap. 3, Figs. 3.6 and 3.7). A rare variant of anomalous connection of the IVC consists of direct drainage into the left atrium [38].

---

[3]In left isomerism, often associated with polysplenia, azygos continuation of the IVC is present in 84% of cases (see Chap. 3).

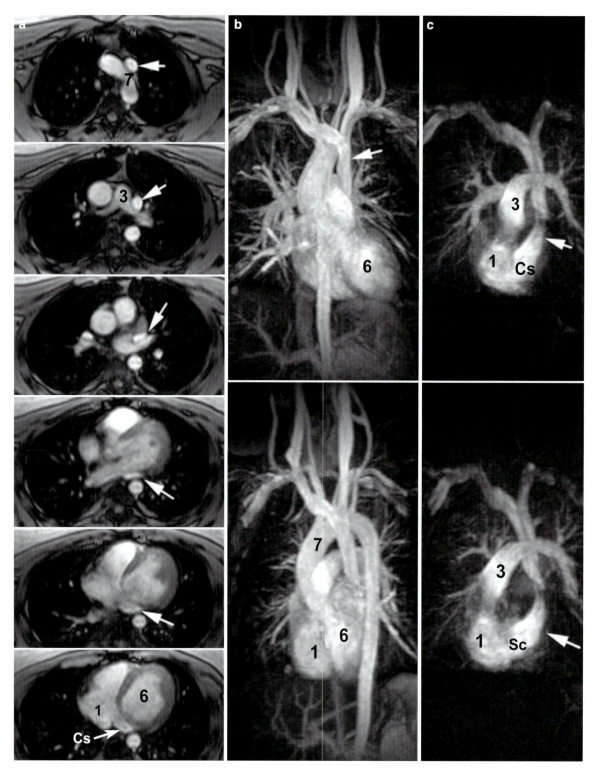

Fig. 4.3 Persistent left superior vena cava (*arrowhead*). Gradient-echo (**a**) column. MR contrast-enhanced angiography (Dota-Gd, Guerbet, France). (**b**) middle and (**c**) right columns. These latter multiplanar and MIP reconstructions allow 180° cine-loop viewing on a large Fov.

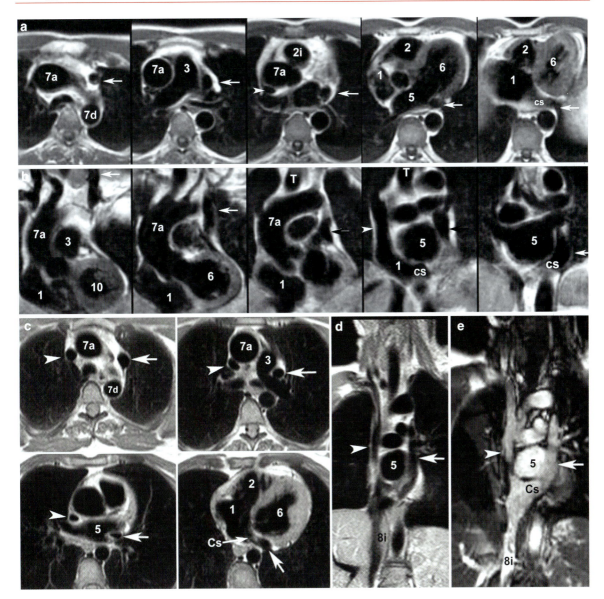

Fig. 4.4 (**a**, **b**) Persistent left superior vena cava. Follow-up MRI, after intraoperative fortuitous discovery of a left superior vena cava in a 37-year-old male patient. (**a**) *upper row*: axial spin-echo images, craniocaudal series, showing the mediastinal course of the left SVC (*arrows*) anteriorly to the aortic arch (ascending aorta-*7a*, descending aorta *7d*) and left hilum (pulmonary artery-*3*), as far as its anastomosis in the dilated coronary sinus (cs). (**b**) *lower row*: coronal spin-echo images confirming abnormal drainage of the left superior vena cava (*arrows*) into the right atrium (*1*) via the dilated coronary sinus (cs-situated in the left inferior atrioventricular groove); the normal course of the right superior vena cava is also displayed (*arrowhead*); trachea (T), right ventricle (*2*), pulmonary infundibulum (*2i*), left atrium (*5*), left ventricle (*6*). Persistent left SVC may be confused with partial anomalous pulmonary venous connection of the left superior pulmonary vein into the left brachiocephalic vein which has the same mediastinal course. This latter, however, has a cranial course and does not drain into the coronary sinus (see Fig. 4.21). (**c–e**) Double superior vena cava: unexpected finding at echography in a young female patient. (**c**) Four axial spin-echo images, craniocaudal series, showing the mediastinal course of the left SVC (*arrows*) anteriorly to the aortic arch (ascending aorta-*7a*, descending aorta *7d*) and left hilum (pulmonary artery-*3*), as far as its anastomosis in coronary sinus (sc). Coronal spin-echo (**d**) and gradient-echo (**e**) images confirming abnormal drainage of the left superior vena cava (*arrows*) into the right atrium (*1*) via the dilated coronary sinus (cs-situated in the left inferior atrioventricular groove); right superior vena cava (*arrowhead*) right atrium (*1*), aorta (*7*), pulmonary artery (*3*), right ventricle (*2*), pulmonary infundibulum (*2i*), left atrium (*5*), left ventricle (*6*), inferior vena cava (*8i*). (**f**, **g**) Double superior vena cava in a child with coarctation of the aorta. The right superior vena cava (*arrowhead*) and left superior vena cava (*arrows*) are visible on the axial (**f**) and LAO (short) (**g**) images; right atrium (*1*), pulmonary artery (*3*), left atrium (*5*), aorta (*7*) (see Fig. 4.22, Chap. 6, Fig. 6.2 and Chap. 5, Fig. 5.23

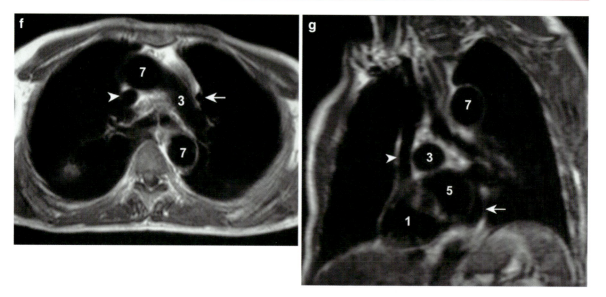

Fig. 4.4 (continued)

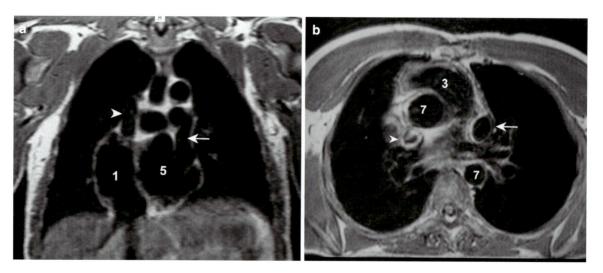

Fig. 4.5 Double superior vena cava with left SVC draining into the roof of the left atrium. The right superior vena cava (*arrowhead*) and left superior vena cava (*arrows*) are visible on the axial (**a**) and coronal (**b**) images. The LSVC drains into the left atrium (*5*); right atrium (*1*), pulmonary artery (*3*), aorta (*7*) (also see Chap. 7, Fig. 7.22)

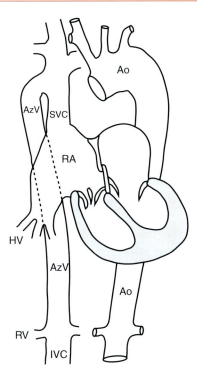

Fig. 4.6 Diagram of right azygos continuation of the inferior vena cava. The inferior vena cava (IVC) continues in the dilated azygos vein (AzV), which drains into the superior vena cava (SVC) above the right hilum. Right atrium (RA), renal veins (RV), hepatic veins (HV), aorta (Ao)

4.4.1 Clinical Features

Isolated azygos continuation of the IVC has no clinical repercussions and may be an incidental finding on thoracic or abdominal radiological examinations.

4.4.2 Imaging

- Chest radiograph

The AP chest radiograph shows dilatation of the azygos vein, causing lateral shift of the right paravertebral line and prominence of the azygos arch in the angle between the trachea and right main bronchus [39].

- Echocardiography

Echocardiography demonstrates absence of the retrohepatic IVC and drainage of hepatic veins into a short IVC segment or directly into the right atrium.

- Computed tomography

Contrast-enhanced CT findings are similar to those of MRI.

- Cavography

Cavography, when it is performed in the context of another disease, visualizes infrahepatic interruption of the IVC. Insertion of a catheter via a femoral vein advances with difficultly and follows an unusual posterior course via the azygos vein as far as the SVC and right atrium; the lateral view shows dilatation of the azygos vein and its arch, giving a "candy cane" appearance [40].

4.4.3 MRI

MRI (Fig. 4.7, also see Fig. 4.19c) shows a dilated azygos vein formed from a venous anastomotic network between the IVC and the azygos vein at the level of the renal veins [34]. Coronal images [41] demonstrate interruption of the superior part of the IVC at the renal pedicle, an azygos vein almost as large as the aorta, and drainage of hepatic veins directly into the atrium due to the absence of the retrohepatic IVC. The dilated azygos arch is symmetrical to the aortic arch.

Thoraco-abdominal coronal and sagittal images visualize all or most of the course of the azygos vein on either side of the diaphragm. Associated anomalies of situs and the spleen are easily recognized [36]. The prognosis of azygos continuation of the IVC depends on the associated congenital heart disease.

4.5 Anomalous Pulmonary Venous Connection or Return

APVC is defined by drainage of one or several pulmonary veins into structures other than the left atrium. Depending on the site of drainage (supracardiac, cardiac, or infracardiac), the number of veins involved (defining the magnitude of the pulmonary drainage territory), and the presence or absence of obstruction of the abnormal venous connection, many anatomical variants and clinical syndromes are encountered, ranging from partial APVC discovered incidentally to obstructed total APVC, which represents a dramatic neonatal emergency.

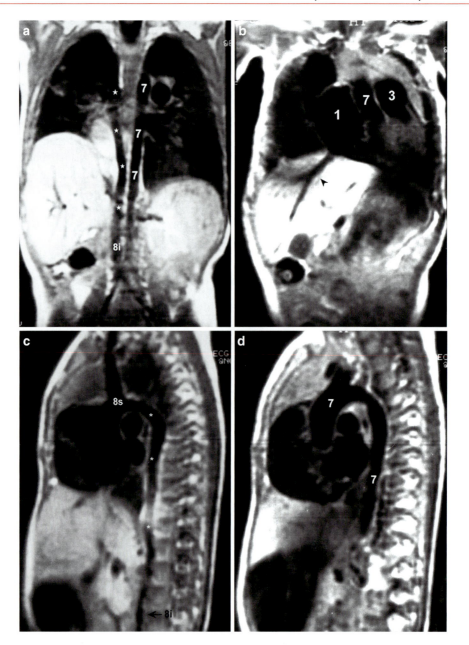

Fig. 4.7 (**a–d**) Azygos continuation of the inferior vena cava (right-sided via the azygos vein – *asterisks*). Female neonate: cesarean section for acute fetal distress. Complementary assessment after postnatal echocardiography showed absence of the retrohepatic IVC and a right diaphragmatic defect. (**a, b**) Coronal images. (**a**) The inferior vena cava (*8i*) continues in the dilated azygos vein (*asterisks*). The arches of the azygos and aorta (*7*) are side by side at the top of the image. (**b**) Hepatic veins (on the right, *arrowhead*) drain directly into the right atrium (*1*) due to the absence of the retrohepatic IVC. (**c, d**) Sagittal images showing azygos continuation of the inferior vena cava (8i *black arrows*) with a dilated azygos vein (*asterisk*). The arch of the azygos passes above the right pulmonary hilum and drains into the superior vena cava (*8s*); aorta (*7*). (**e–h**) Other case of azygos continuation of the inferior vena cava. Rows (**e**) and (**f**) axial gradient-echo images, craniocaudal series. The IVC continues in the dilated azygos vein (*asterisks*) which courses first behind the right atrium (*1*), then describes its arch, which is dilated (*12*), over the right hilum and merges at last into the superior vena cava. A left SVC (*arrow head*) is also present coursing down toward the coronary sinus. MR contrast-enhanced angiography (Dota-Gd, Guerbet, France): (**g**) Left column sagittal and (**h**) right column coronal MIP projections display adequately the dilated continuation of azygos vein (*asterisks*) and aorta (*7*)

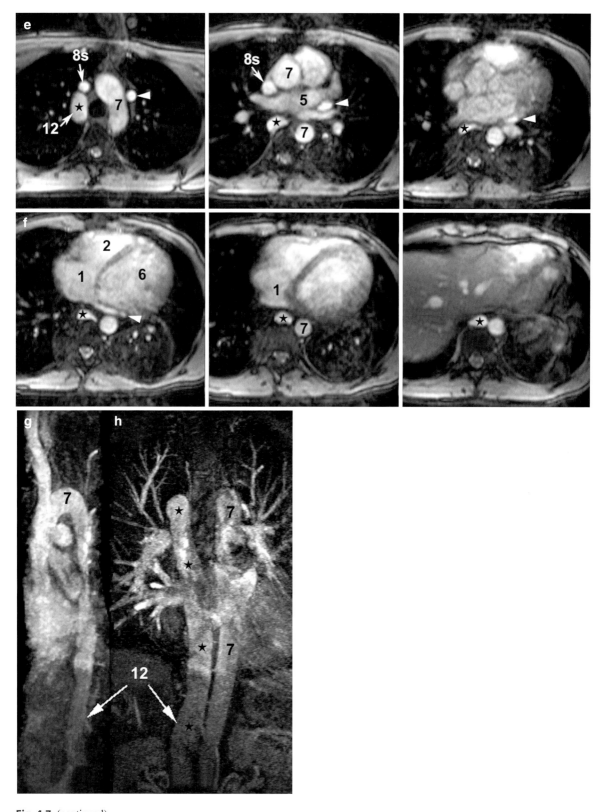

Fig. 4.7 (continued)

Embryologically, development of normal pulmonary venous connection requires anastomosis between the primitive pulmonary veins, the pulmonary venous plexus, the common pulmonary vein and the left atrium [42–44]. In APVC, the pulmonary venous plexus preserves part or all of its primitive connections with cardinal or umbilicovitelline veins.

4.5.1 Total Anomalous Pulmonary Venous Connection or Return (TAPVC)

TAPVC represents 2% of all cases of congenital heart disease [45]. The defect occurs as a consequence of the common pulmonary vein not incorporating into the left atrium. There is no connection between the pulmonary venous system and the left atrium, that is, all pulmonary veins drain directly into the right atrium or via a systemic vein. A patent foramen ovale or ostium secundum atrial septal defect is constantly observed to allow blood to reach the left cardiac chambers. Apart from asplenia or polysplenia[4] syndromes, in which TAPVC is only one element of a series of severe multiple malformations, it is generally an isolated anomaly. TAPVC with obstructed venous return[5] is a neonatal diagnostic and therapeutic emergency.

4.5.2 Anatomical Classification of TAPVC

According to the various levels of connection of the venous confluence TAPVC can be divided grossly in three categories: supracardiac, cardiac, and infracardiac (Fig. 4.8).

- Supracardiac TAPVC into the superior vena cava system

This form represents 50% of all cases of TAPVC. In 80% of cases, the venous confluence, situated posteriorly to the left atrium, is connected to the left brachiocephalic vein via a vertical vein, which can be compressed during its passage between the pulmonary artery (anteriorly) and the left main bronchus (posteriorly) or, more proximally, between the right pulmonary artery (anteriorly) and the trachea (posteriorly). Extrinsic compression is generally not observed when the venous confluence passes anteriorly to the pulmonary artery (the most frequent case) (Fig. 4.9). In the remaining 20% of cases, the venous confluence drains into the right SVC or, more rarely, the azygos vein.

- Cardiac TAPVC

This form represents 25% of all cases of TAPVC. The pulmonary veins usually drain into the right atrium via the CS, or, less frequently, directly into the right atrial chamber (separately or via a venous confluence).

- Infracardiac TAPVC

This form represents 20% of all cases of TAPVC. A transdiaphragmatic draining vein passes through the esophageal hiatus of the diaphragm and connects the left retroatrial confluence of the pulmonary veins to the portal vein or to one of its tributaries (ductus venosus, left gastric vein). There is a marked male predominance with about 3–6 boys for 1 girl [46]. The venous confluence can be narrowed as it passes through the diaphragm and its wall can become hypertrophied [47]; these two mechanisms can lead to obstruction of venous return.

- Mixed TAPVC

The pulmonary venous return cannot be classified in 5% of cases.

4.5.3 Clinical Features

The age of onset and the severity of the cardiorespiratory symptoms and signs vary according to the type of TAPVC and the presence or absence of obstruction to venous return.

Obstructed TAPVC in a neonate requires cardiorespiratory resuscitation and urgent surgical correction [48] under hypothermia and cardiopul6monary bypass. Surgical correction consists of anastomosis of the venous confluence to the left atrium. The prognosis is related to the presence of pulmonary artery hypertension, which increases the early postoperative mortality [49]. The major complication is restenosis of the venous confluence

---

[4]In left isomerism, the right and left pulmonary veins frequently depend on each of their respective atria (morphologically left), which is logical anatomically, but which creates hemodynamic abnormalities. In right isomerism, there is "always" an anomalous venous connection, as, even if all of the pulmonary veins converge onto the atrium situated to the left, this atrium (like the atrium on the right) has a right-sided morphology.

[5]It may have an extrinsic origin (compression) but also an intrinsic origin (stenosis of the venous confluence or drainage into a high-resistance channel i.e., the portal system).

Fig. 4.8 Diagram of the various *anatomical* levels of anastomosis of the venous confluence in total anomalous pulmonary venous connection (TAPVC). (**a**) Normal, (**b**) Supracardiac, (**c**) Infracardiac and (**d**) Cardiac (see text). Superior vena cava (SVC), vertical vein (VV), left brachiocephalic vein (LBCV), inferior vena cava (IVC), portal vein (PV), right atrium (RA), coronary sinus (CS)

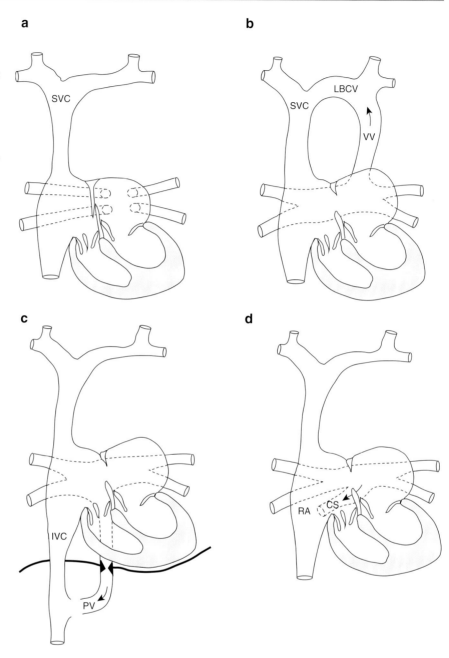

or the anastomosis, associated with a poor prognosis due to the need for a difficult operation.

4.5.4 Imaging

• Chest radiograph

The appearance on the standard chest radiograph depends on the anatomical type of anomaly: "fog lung" or "cathedral glass" appearance with a normal-sized

heart shadow corresponds to neonatal obstructed TAPVC (e.g., infradiaphragmatic TAPVC). A "snowman" [50] or "figure of eight" appearance with dilatation of the right heart and pulmonary hypervascularization is observed in the case of TAPVC with a vertical vein in a neonate or child.

• Echocardiography

B-mode echocardiography visualizes dilatation of the right chambers and pulmonary arteries, the absence

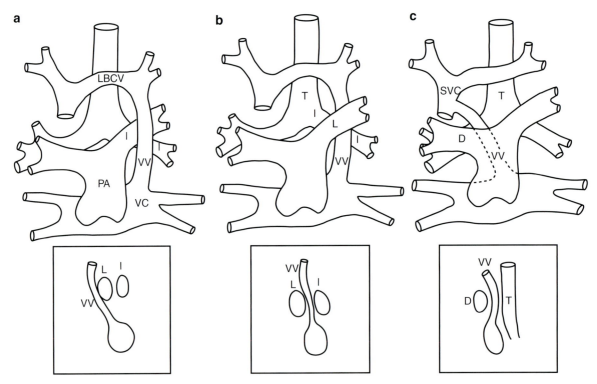

Fig. 4.9 Diagram of the sites of compression in supracardiac TAPVC into a vertical vein. The mediastinal course of the vertical vein (VV) connecting the venous confluence (VC) to the left brachiocephalic vein (LBCV) (**a, b**) or superior vena cava (SVC) (**c**) determines the possibilities of compression. (**a**) Vertical vein anterior to the left (L) pulmonary artery (PA) (no compression).

(**b**) Vertical vein between the left pulmonary artery anteriorly and the left main bronchus posteriorly (g) (possible site of compression). (**c**) Vertical vein between the right (R) pulmonary artery anteriorly and the trachea (T) posteriorly (possible site of compression). Figures lower row Figures: sagittal views

of connection of pulmonary veins to the small left atrium, and possibly the venous confluence in the form of a left retroatrial echo-free space [51, 52]. The site of drainage of the TAPVC may be visualized [53, 54]. Color-coded Doppler echocardiography can sometimes demonstrate the infradiaphragmatic vein, in the form of a midline vascular structure with continuous venous flow in the same direction as aortic blood flow [55].

- Computed tomography

CT-scan requires injection of contrast agent and is ionizing. Therefore, we prefer to perform MRI [45] in neonates and infants as part of the assessment of TAPVC. However, the long imaging time and/or restricted access to an MR imager may preclude MRI in favor of multidetector CT scanning.

- Angiography

Pulmonary angiography visualizes the venous confluence and its systemic connection. Angiography is associated with certain risks in the neonatal period and is, therefore, not *usually* performed *for diagnostic evaluation.*

4.5.5 MRI

- Supracardiac TAPVC into a vertical vein

The diagnosis is confirmed by MRI (Fig. 4.10), which shows the left retroatrial venous confluence; the vertical vein arises from the left part of the venous confluence and ascends anteriorly to the left hilum and aortic arch according to the course of the persistent left SVC as far as the origin of the left brachiocephalic vein [3, 4, 56, 57]. More rarely, the vertical vein travels between the left pulmonary artery and the left main bronchus, which can be a source of obstruction. Coronal images show all the vascular structures involved in their long-axis as well as their connections.

• Infracardiac TAPVC into ductus venosus

Axial, coronal and left anterior oblique images (Fig. 4.11) demonstrate the left retroatrial venous confluence, which gives rise to a vein that crosses the diaphragm to connect with hepatic veins [45].

4.6 Partial Anomalous Pulmonary Venous Connection or Return (PAPVC)

In partial anomalous pulmonary venous connection or return (PAPVC) some of the pulmonary veins normally drain into the left atrium, while the others drain into the right atrium or one of its tributaries (vena cavae, azygos vein, CS, left vertical vein). An atrial septal defect is associated in 15% of cases. PAPVC accounts for 70% of all cases of APVC [58] and is found in 0.6% of cases in autopsy series [59]. There is a higher prevalence of PAPVC in subjects with congenital heart disease (0.5–7% of patients) [59, 60].

4.6.1 Classification of Partial Anomalous Pulmonary Venous Connection (PAPVC)

In almost all cases (Fig. 4.12), the anomalous pulmonary vein drains into the closest systemic vein (drainage into a structure homolateral to the corresponding lobes or lung).

• Right PAPVC

Right PAPVC represents 66% of all cases of PAPVC [27]. One or several right pulmonary veins drain into the SVC, IVC, portal vein or, more rarely, the azygos vein or right atrium.

• PAPVC into the right SVC

In this second most common PAPVC, the right superior pulmonary vein drains into the SVC-right atrium junction, directly above a sinus venosus atrial septal defect. A variant of this form consists of PAPVC into the azygos vein [61]. A sinus venosus atrial septa defect is present in up to 90% of cases (Figs. 4.13–4.15).

• PAPVC into the IVC

The abnormal drainage concerns all of the right lung (60% of cases) or only the lower and/or middle lobes. An atrial septal defect is present in 20% of subjects. The scimitar or Halasz syndrome [62–64] usually also comprises dextrocardia, pulmonary hypoplasia with right diaphragmatic defect and partial or complete systemic vascularization of the right lung from the abdominal aorta (pulmonary sequestration). In PAPVC, the pulmonary vein is connected to the infradiaphragmatic IVC or to the IVC-right atrium junction.

• Left PAPVC

Left PAPVC is half as frequent as right PAPVC. It drains into the left brachiocephalic vein or, more rarely, the CS.

• PAPVC into the left brachiocephalic vein

An anomalous vertical vein connects the left superior pulmonary vein (and sometimes also the left inferior vein) to the left brachiocephalic vein [27, 28] (Fig. 4.21). This should be distinguished from persistent left SVC with a similar mediastinal[6] left to the aortic arch – Figs. 4.2–4.3 (see below).

4.6.2 Clinical Features

The age of diagnosis and the severity of the clinical signs depend on the number of pulmonary veins that drain into right cardiac chambers and the presence or absence of an atrial septal defect. If isolated it is often an incidental finding or is discovered at a later age. Surgery is indicated in the case of a major shunt: the

---

[6]The left SVC crosses the left pulmonary artery anteriorly, while the anomalous vertical vein can pass behind the pulmonary artery, between the pulmonary artery and the left main bronchus with a risk of compression (see Figs. 4.4–4.9).

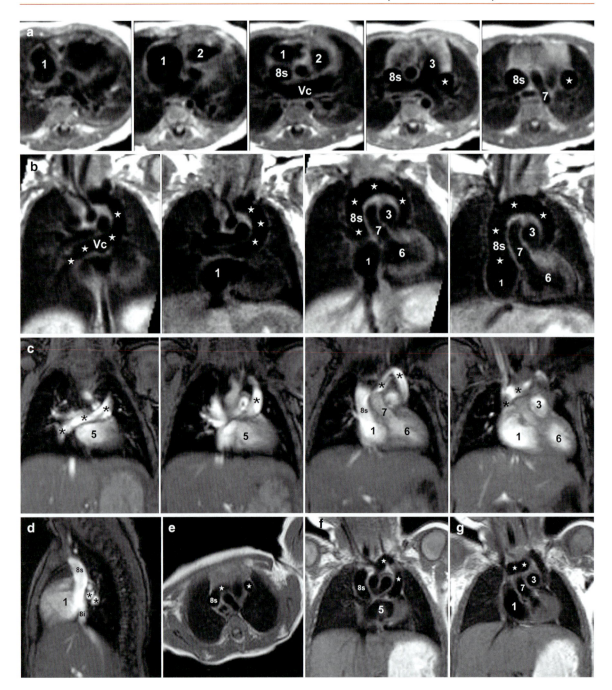

Fig. 4.10 (**a**, **b**) Supracardiac total anomalous pulmonary venous connection in a 30-month-old hospitalized for dyspnea and progressive cyanosis [35].Rows (**a**) axial, and (**b**) coronal fast spin-echo images, clearly showing the venous confluence (Vc), the draining vein (*asterisks*) merges into the left brachiocephalic vein and then into the dilated right atrium (*1*) via the SVC (*8s*); ascending aorta (*7*). The draining vein runs anterior to the left pulmonary artery (*3g*) (no compression); right atrium (*1*), right ventricle (*2*), pulmonary artery (*3*). (**c**–**g**) Other example of supracardiac total anomalous pulmonary venous connection (*asterisks*) depicted on coronal (**c**), sagittal (**d**) gradient-echo images and axial (**e**) and coronal (**f**, **g**) fast spin-echo images

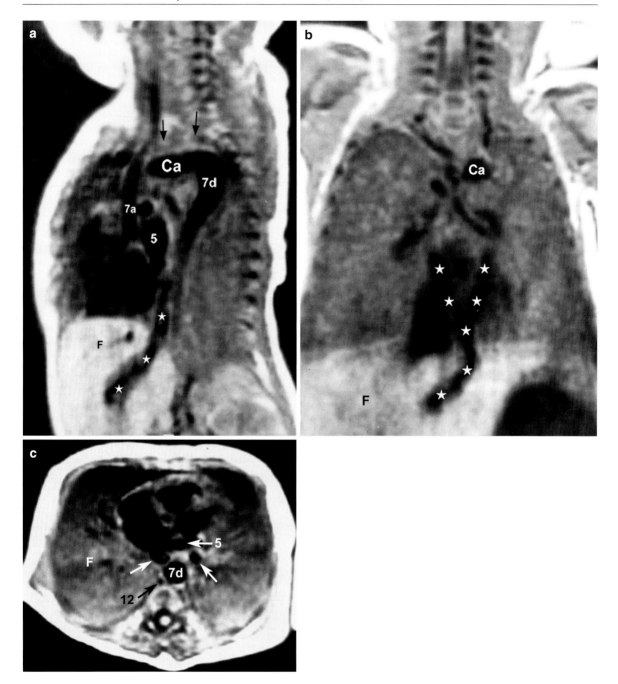

Fig. 4.11 Infradiaphragmatic total anomalous pulmonary venous connection. Emergency MRI performed in a neonate in cardiorespiratory failure [25]. (**a**) Left anterior oblique image showing the infradiaphragmatic venous return (*asterisks*). Also note the interrupted aortic arch (*arrows*) above the ascending aorta (*7a*). The "pseudo-arch" is formed by a very large patent ductus arteriosus (Ca) joining the descending aorta (*7d*); left atrium (*5*) (also see Chap. 6, Fig. 6.21). (**b**) Coronal image visualizing the Y-shaped confluence (*asterisks*) of the right and left pulmonary venous collectors through the diaphragm towards the portal vein (see Fig. 4.7c); liver (F). (**c**) Axial image: the two right and left pulmonary collectors (*arrows*) are also visualized behind the heart; descending aorta (*7d*); azygos vein (*12*). Note the small size of the left atrium (*5*)

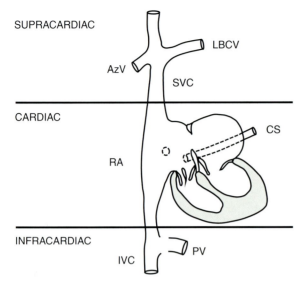

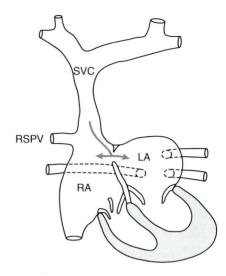

Fig. 4.12 Diagram of the various levels of connection of right and left partial anomalous pulmonary venous connection (PAPVC). Supracardiac: superior vena cava (SVC), left brachiocephalic vein (LBCV), azygos vein (AzV); cardiac: right atrium (RA); coronary sinus (CS) and infracardiac: inferior vena cava (IVC) and portal vein (PV)

Fig. 4.13 Diagram of partial anomalous pulmonary venous connection of the right superior pulmonary vein (RSPV) into the superior vena cava (SVC) with sinus venosus (high ASD – *double-headed arrow*). Right atrium (RA) and left atrium (LA)

general principle consists of directing the venous return toward the left atrium via a Dacron® conduit, if necessary, and closure of the atrial septal defect, when present. The major surgical complication is shunt thrombosis.

4.6.3 Imaging

- Chest radiograph

Chest radiograph is normal in minor forms. In other cases, dilatation of the right heart, pulmonary artery hypertrophy and pulmonary hypervascularization may be observed. The standard **AP** chest radiograph can sometimes suggest the type of PAPVC. For example, in Halasz syndrome or scimitar syndrome, chest radiograph demonstrates the characteristic scimitar appearance of the right pulmonary veins draining into the IVC associated with dextrocardia [42, 64].

- Echocardiography

B-mode echocardiography only rarely shows the PAPVC, but raises a suspicion of PAPVC in the case of high-flow left-right shunt by demonstrating signs of

diastolic overload with right ventricular dilatation on M-mode.

- Computed tomography

The diagnosis may be made incidentally or during CT performed for a suspicious mediastinal or hilar image on chest radiograph, corresponding to PAPVC [61, 65].

- Angiography

Angiography is an invasive examination that is not devoid of risks and provides less information than MRI for the diagnosis of PAPVC; it is no longer used in our department [1, 2]. Opacification of the abnormal vein is obtained by contrast agent injection into the pulmonary artery trunk.

4.6.4 MRI

Chest MRI with ECG-gated black blood sequences (fast spin-echo or double IR) visualizes the PAPVC and associated cardiac malformations [1, 66, 67].

- Anomalous connection of the right pulmonary vein into the superior vena cava

The right superior pulmonary vein drains into the SVC and the fusion of the two vessels (signal void) induces loss of the lateral wall of the SVC (intermediate signal) and adjacent mediastinal fat (high signal intensity). This corresponds to Julsrud's "broken ring" sign [1, 66, 67] (Figs. 4.14 and 4.15). The APVC is also visible in the coronal plane. However, the small right superior vein converging abnormally to the SVC may be difficult to differentiate from a right superior vein reaching, as is supposed, the right atrium because of partial volume effect: numerous incidences and thin contiguous overlapped slices may be necessary (Fig. 4.15).

• Anomalous connection of the right superior pulmonary vein into the azygos vein

Coronal spin-echo images reveal a hypointense tubular structure communicating with the azygos vein. Gradient-echo flow compensation sequences may be useful confirm the vascular to nature of this rather small structure (presence of high signal intensity, indicating blood flow) (Figs. 4.16 and 4.17).

• Anomalous connection of the right inferior pulmonary vein into the IVC [68, 69]

Figures 4.18–4.20 present a diagram and MR images of this anomaly. Coronal fast spin-echo and gradient-echo images (Fig. 4.19) show the venous confluence (arrows), which drains into the IVC stump, at the junction with the right atrium.

In another 8-year-old patient (Fig. 4.20), axial gradient-echo images show the presence of an anomalous venous confluence on the right (associated with absence of normal connection of the right pulmonary veins into the left atrium). Axial images show an inflow enhancement effect (paradoxical enhancement phenomenon). Coronal gradient-echo flow compensation sequences confirm the vascular nature of this structure (presence of high signal intensity, indicating after blood flow) which drains into the IVC at its junction with the right atrium. The appearance of the anomalous pulmonary vein (resembling a Turkish curved saber) is responsible for the characteristic scimitar sign on the X-ray chest image.

• Anomalous connection of the right inferior pulmonary vein into the left brachiocephalic vein [27, 28]

Axial MR images at the level of the aortic arch with velocity mapping (Fig. 4.21) can identify the anomalous vertical vein connecting to the left superior pulmonary vein coursing upward to the left brachiocephalic vein.

This formerly allows distinguishing this entity from persistent left SVC with the same mediastinal[7] course (similarly placed left to the aortic arch – Figs. 4.2 and 4.3). However, this latter anomaly communicates with the CS,[2] which is usually dilated. Also, in this type of anomaly, no vessel is present anterior to the left main bronchus (as the left superior pulmonary vein drains upward in the vertical vein). On the contrary, in persistent left SVC, two vessels are present anterior to the bronchus (the left SVC and the left superior pulmonary vein).

4.7 Other Pulmonary Venous Anomalies

Three entities other than APVCs also need to be described here: supernumerary or absent pulmonary veins, pulmonary vein stenoses and cor triatriatum.

4.7.1 Supernumerary or Absent Pulmonary Veins

There are normally two right pulmonary veins and two left pulmonary veins. The most frequent anomaly is absence of a pulmonary vein on the right or on the left [70]. Rarely, the four pulmonary veins form a venous confluence that drains normally into the left atrium. One (more rarely two) supernumerary pulmonary vein is encountered in 2% of cases [70]. These isolated anomalies have no clinical expression and are generally discovered incidentally. Like persistent left SVC, they must be identified prior to surgery in the region or before radio-ablation of atrial fibrillation.

4.7.2 Pulmonary Vein Stenosis

As we have seen, stenosis can be observed on a vein or venous confluence with an abnormal course (possibly responsible for obstruction of venous return). Stenosis of one or even several pulmonary veins with a normal course may also be observed. Short stenoses

---

[7]The left SVC crosses the left pulmonary artery anteriorly, while the anomalous vertical vein can pass behind the pulmonary artery, between the pulmonary artery and the left main bronchus with a risk of compression (see Figs. 4.4–4.9).

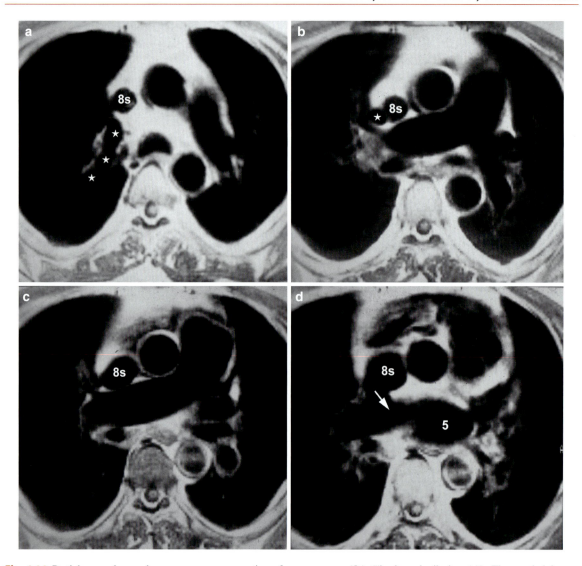

Fig. 4.14 Partial anomalous pulmonary venous connection of the right superior pulmonary vein into the superior vena cava with sinus venosus. Examination performed in a former miner with longstanding dyspnoea. MRI and cardiac angiography led to surgical correction. (**a–e**) Axial images, craniocaudad series: the right superior pulmonary vein (*asterisks*) has an abnormally anterior course in contact with and draining into the superior vena cava (*8s*) ("broken ring" sign (**c**)). The caudad image (**d**) demonstrates the high sinus venosus ASD (at the arrival of the SVC, *arrow*) confirmed on short-axis images (**f**) and (**g**). On a more caudad axial image (**e**), the interatrial septum is intact. (**f**, **g**) Short-axis images: the superior vena cava (*8s*) communicates (*arrows*) with both the right atrium (*1*) and the left atrium (*5*) (via the sinus venosus)

usually involve the connection with the left atrium, while longer stenoses with a pulmonary or extrapulmonary course are described as segmental aplasia. Finally, stenosis of a venous confluence connecting with an accessory chamber corresponds to cor triatriatum.

4.7.3 Cor Triatriatum

Cor triatriatum or stenosis of the common pulmonary venous chamber was first described in 1868 by Church [82]. A common pulmonary venous chamber enters an accessory chamber and then the left atrium via a

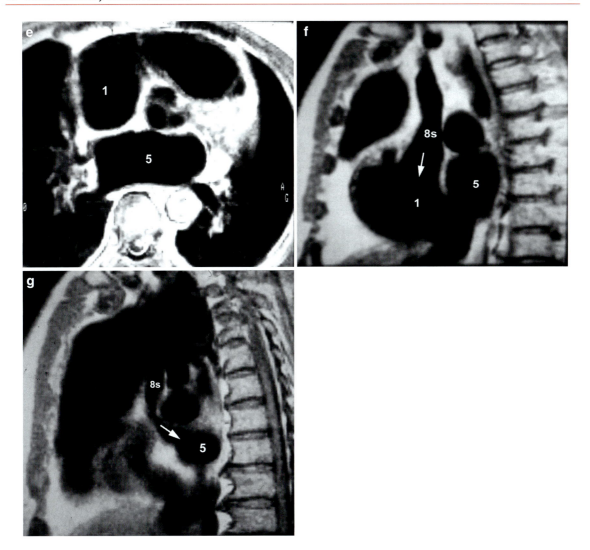

Fig. 4.14 (continued)

septum with one or several ostia (Fig. 4.22). Autopsy series on patients with congenital heart disease reveal an estimated frequency of 0.4% Niwayama, Jegier [71, 72]. The most widely accepted embryological origin (defect of incorporation of the common pulmonary vein into the left atrium) was proposed by Edwards [73]. Many variants have been reported [71–75], especially concerning the anastomosis, which can be direct into the left atrium or indirect via the anomalous pathways already considered in the context of TAPVC (vertical vein, CS, IVC, etc.). There may be a partition

of this accessory chamber. Each of its compartments then receives part of the pulmonary veins and is connected separately to an atrium or anomalous venous confluence – vertical vein – Fig. 4.23). Finally, these variants can also be associated with atrial septal defect (Fig. 4.23). The diagnosis is suggested by echocardiography which shows the accessory chamber with its diaphragm over the left atrium. The anomaly can also be clearly identified by MRI, which is useful to determine the variant of cor triatriatum as part of the preoperative workup [76–80].

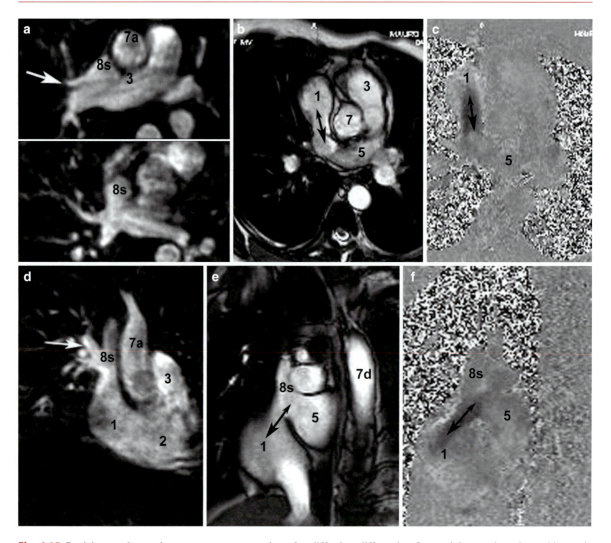

Fig. 4.15 Partial anomalous pulmonary venous connection of the right superior pulmonary vein into the superior vena cava. (**a–c**) Axial, (**d**) coronal and (**e, f**) sagittal slices. The abnormal anastomosis of the right superior pulmonary vein (*arrows*) directly into the right superior vena cava (*8s*) is clearly visualized on these images; right atrium (*1*), left atrium (*5*). This small right superior vein converging abnormally to the SVC may be difficult to differentiate from a right superior vein reaching, as is supposed, the right atrium because of partial volume effect: numerous incidences and thin contiguous overlapped slices may be necessary. The sinus venosus (*double-headed arrow*) is confirmed here by velocity mapping technique: image (**c**) (matches with **b**) and image (**f**) (matches with **e**); pulmonary artery (*3*), ascending aorta (*7a*), descending aorta (*7d*)

4.8 Conclusion

MRI allows precise anatomical analysis of congenital venous anomalies by allowing multiplanar vascular imaging 1–7]. MRI also provides precise 3 D mapping of the mediastinum in multiple imaging planes. It has been established for decades as a fundamental imaging modality for the diagnosis and assessment of congenital heart disease [79–81]. CE-MRA sequences displaying the anomalies on a large Fov are also essential in this context [8, 9]. It is more reliable than echocardiography to visualize (extra cardiac) congenital anomalous systemic and pulmonary venous connections, which is particularly useful for the surgeon by avoiding intraoperative discovery of anomalies not detected on the conventional preoperative workup.

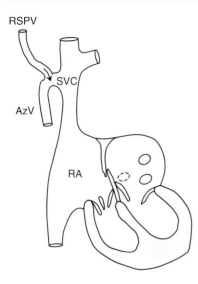

Fig. 4.16 Diagram of partial anomalous pulmonary venous connection of the right superior pulmonary vein (RSPV) into the azygos vein (AzV). Superior vena cava (SVC); right atrium (RA)

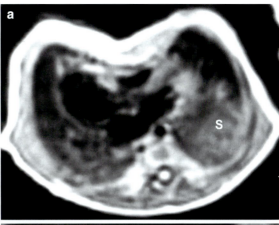

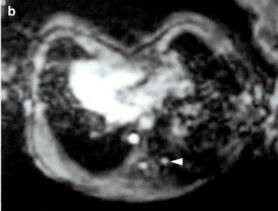

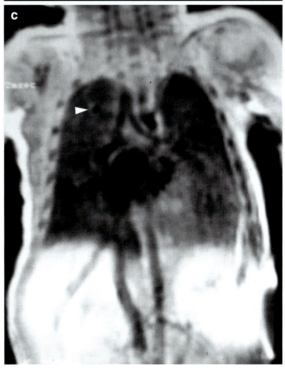

Fig. 4.17 Partial anomalous pulmonary venous connection of the right upper lobe vein into the azygos vein. Referred for MRI to confirm pulmonary sequestration. (**a**, **b**) Axial spin-echo and gradient-echo flow compensation images, showing an iso-intense mass of the lower part of the left lung. Left posterobasal extralobar sequestration (S) is confirmed by the presence of a draining vessel with a white circulating flow signal on the flow sequence (**b**: *white arrowhead*). Note the associated pectus excavatum. (**c**) Coronal spin-echo image: an abnormal right upper lobe annular structure is revealed (*arrowhead*). (**d**) Coronal gradient-echo flow compensation image, confirming the vascular structure (*arrowhead*: white circulating flow). (**e**) Coronal spin-echo image: the right upper lobe vein presents an abnormal course (*arrowhead*) and drains into the azygos vein (AzV)

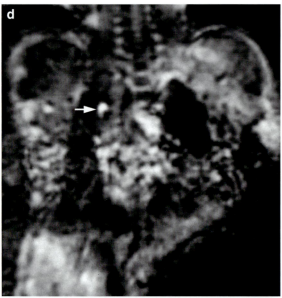

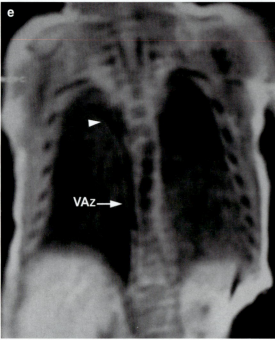

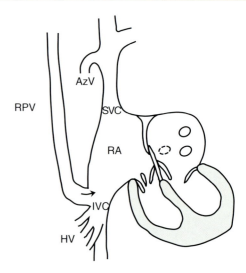

Fig. 4.18 Diagram of partial anomalous pulmonary venous connection of the right inferior pulmonary vein (RIPV) into the inferior vena cava (IVC) responsible for the "scimitar" sign on AP chest radiograph (and MRI!). Right atrium (RA), hepatic veins (HV), azygos vein (AzV), superior vena cava (SVC)

Fig. 4.17 (continued)

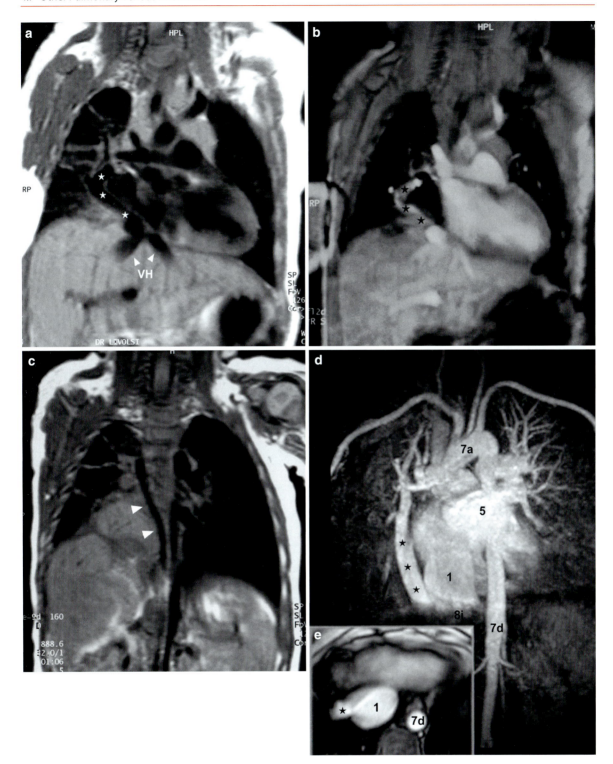

Fig. 4.19 (**a–c**) Right partial anomalous pulmonary venous connection with drainage of all of the right lung into the inferior vena cava. The venous confluence drains into the IVC stump at the junction with the right atrium (*asterisks*). (**a**) Coronal fast spin-echo image. (**b**) Gradient-echo image. This patient also presents azygos continuation of the IVC (*arrowhead* in **c**). Hepatic veins (HV) drain directly into the IVC stump (absence of retrohepatic IVC) (**a**). (**d, e**). Other examples using MR contrast-contrast enhanced angiography (Dota-Gd, Guerbet, France) in a 45-year-old female with scimitar syndrome: (**d**) 3D coronal projection and (**e**) axial native reconstruction display adequately the anomalous right pulmonary veins (*asterisks*) into the inferior vena cava (*8i*) ("scimitar" sign), ascending and descending aorta (*7a* and *7d*); right atrium (*1*), left atrium (*5*)

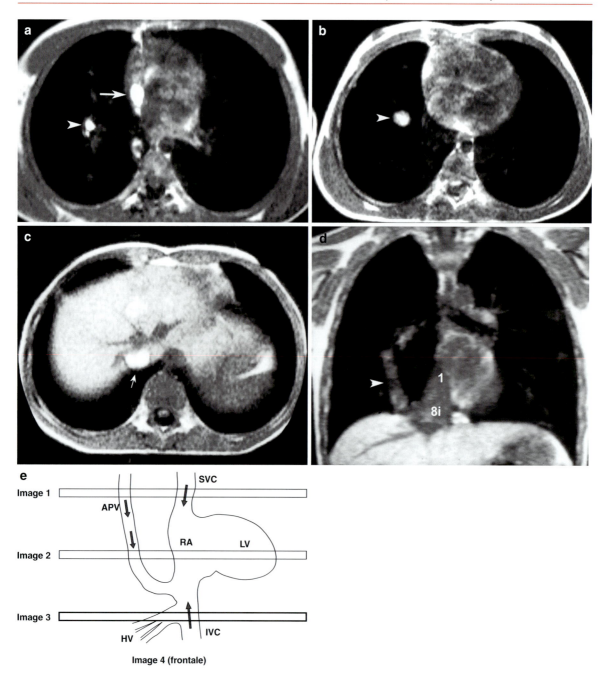

Fig. 4.20 Right partial anomalous pulmonary venous connection with drainage of all of the right lung into the inferior vena cava. Demonstration of the inflow effect (formerly named "paradoxical enhancement phenomenon"). Multislice gradient-echo sequence with flow compensation. On the first "entry of flow" axial image (craniad image, **a**), the vena cava (*arrow*) and aberrant pulmonary vein (*arrowhead*) have an enhanced signal ("entry" of fresh spins on craniocaudad flow by inflow effect "paradoxical enhancement"); a similar appearance is observed on the more caudad axial image (**c**), where the inferior vena cava (*arrow*) has a high signal intensity ("entry" of fresh spins on caudocraniad flow with paradoxical enhancement). Note the absence of signal enhancement of the three hepatic veins (as they are parallel to the imaging plane with partially saturated spins). On intermediate images (**b**), the aberrant vein (*arrowhead*) no longer has such a high signal intensity (protons have been previously stimulated by successive pulses to proximal slices and are therefore partially saturated). On the coronal image (**d**), the venous confluence (*arrowhead*) drains into the inferior vena cava (*8i*) at the junction with the right atrium (*1*) ("scimitar" sign). (**e**) Diagram illustrating the inflow effect ("paradoxical enhancement") on aberrant pulmonary vein (APV) and inferior vena cava (IVC); superior vena cava (SVC); right atrium (RA); hepatic veins (HV)

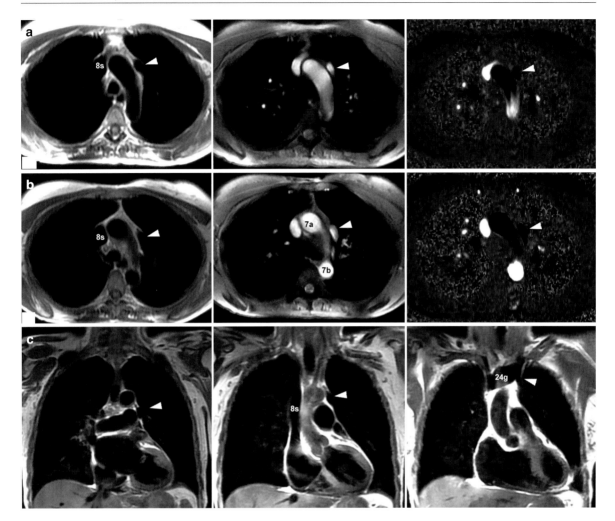

Fig. 4.21 Partial anomalous pulmonary venous connection (*arrowheads*) of the left superior pulmonary vein via a vertical vein into the left brachiocephalic vein. Axial MR images at the level of the aortic arch (**a** upper row) and slightly below (**b** lower row). From left to right black blood IR, cine-MR and velocity mapping images. This abnormal mediastinal vertical vein is coursing cranially as is confirmed by the velocity mapping images (through plane black signal similar to the ascending aorta = blood flow cranial direction). This criteria allows the formal differentiation of an anomalous pulmonary venous connection of the left superior pulmonary vein (converging abnormally via a cranial course to the left brachiocephalic vein) from a persisting left superior vein (coursing caudally – blood flow caudal direction-to the coronary sinus which is usually dilated and the right atrium because – see Figs. 4.2 and 4.3. The abnormal course of the left superior pulmonary vein (*arrowheads*) via a vertical vein directly into the left brachiocephalic vein (*24 g*) and the right superior vena cava (*8s*) is clearly visualized on these coronal black blood IR images (**c**); right atrium (*1*), left atrium (*5*), superior vena cava (*8i*), ascending and descending aorta (*7a* and *7d*)

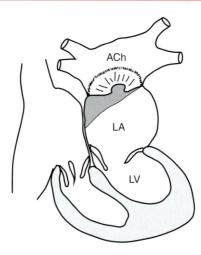

Fig. 4.22 Diagram of cor triatriatum (classical form, *see text*). Accessory chamber (ACh), left atrium (LA), left ventricle (LV)

Fig. 4.23 Axial (**a**, **b**) and sagittal oblique (**c**) spin-echo images. Particular form of cor triatriatum with partition of the accessory chamber: one compartment receiving a pulmonary venous collector (VC) drains into the left atrium (*5*) via a perforated septum (**a**) and the other compartment receiving the pulmonary venous collector (VC) via a vertical vein (*arrowhead* image **b**) into the left brachiocephalic vein and left superior vena cava. The vertical vein (*arrowheads* images **a–c**) has same mediastinal course as a left superior vena cave see Fig. 4.2, 4.3, and 4.21). Note also the atrial septal defect. This patient also presents complex heart disease with a left dominant ventricle (*6*) and rudimentary right ventricle (*2*) (also see Fig. 7.23, Chap. 7), malposition of the great vessels and tubular hypoplasia of the aorta (see Chap. 6, Fig. 6.9); right atrium (*1*)

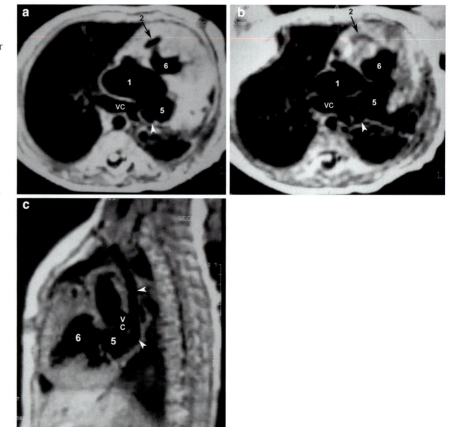

Table 4.1 Anomalous systemic and pulmonary venous connections

Anomalous systemic venous and pulmonary connection (caval)	Morphology	Imaging planes centered on the anomaly (always axial)
Anomalous systemic venous connections		
Persistent left superior vena cava	LSVC → RA via coronary sinus (10% to roof of LA) Double superior vena cava: separate or joined by brachiocephalic vein	Axial Coronal LAO (short-axis) in the axis of the coronary sinus
Azygos continuation of IVC	Absence of retrohepatic IVC: IVC → azygos vein → arch → SVC → RA	Axial Coronal Sagittal
Total anomalous pulmonary venous connection (TAPVC)	*All PVs drain into systemic veins*	
Supracardiac (50%)	Venous confluence posterior to LA → Vertical vein → brachiocephalic vein 80% → Directly into SVC or azygos 20%	Axial Coronal
Cardiac (25%)	PV drains directly → RA or via coronary sinus → Portal vein or tributary	Axial Coronal LAO
Infracardiac (20%)	Venous confluence posterior to LA	Axial Coronal
Partial anomalous pulmonary venous connection (PAPVC)	*One or several PVs drain into homolateral systemic vein*	
Right PAPVC (66%) Supracardiac Cardiac Infracardiac (20%)	→ SVC (sinus venosus ASD) → Azygos vein → RA (rare) → Portal vein or IVC (all right PVs (60%) or right superior PV (40%))	Axial (sinus venosus) Coronal
Left PAPVC (34%)	Right superior PV → vertical vein → left brachio-cephalic vein → SVC Rarely → coronary sinus	Axial Coronal and LAO (short-axis) in axis of coronary sinus

RA right atrium; *LA* left atrium; *SVC* superior vena cava; *IVC* inferior vena cava; *PV* pulmonary vein; *ASD* atrial septal defect

References

1. Julsrud PR. Magnetic resonance imaging of the pulmonary arteries and veins. Sem US, CT/MR. 1990;11:184–205.
2. Masui T, Seelos KC, Masui T, Kersting-Sommerhoff BA, Higgins CB. abnormalities of the pulmonary veins: evluation with MR imaging and comparison with cardiac angiography and echocardiography. Radiology. 1991;181:645–9.
3. Kastler B, Gangi A, Klinkert A, Livolsi A, Germain P, Dietemann JL. Contribution of MRI in systemic and pulmonary venous anomalies. RSNA,Chicago, Novr 29–Dec 4. Radiology 1992;suppl:353.
4. Klinkert A, Kastler B, Gangi A, AHRAN JM, Livolsi A, et al. Diagnoctic IRM des anomalies congénitales des veines caves et des veines pulmonaires. Feuillets de Radiologie. 1994;34:319–29.
5. White CS, Baffa JM, Haney PJ, Pace ME, Campbell AB. MR imaging of congenital anomalies of the thoracic veins. Radiographics. 1997;17(3):595–608.
6. White CS. MR imaging of thoracic veins. Magn Reson Imaging Clin N Am. 2000;8(1):17–32.
7. Kastler B, Clair C, Delabrousse E, Klinkert A, Livolsi A, Sarlieve P, Allal R, Vetter D, Germain P, Bernard Y. Retours veineux systémiques et pulmonaires anormaux: aspects IRM et classification Encycl Méd Chir, Radiodiagnostic- Cœur-Poumon, 32-016-A-20, 2002, 15 p.
8. Fitoz S, Unsal N, Tekin M, Tutar E. Contrast-enhanced MR angiography of thoracic vascular malformations in children. Int J Cardiol. 2007;123(1):3–11.

9. Rahmani N, White CS. MR Imaging of thoracic veins. Magn Reson Imag Clin N Am. 2008;16:249–62.

10. Glickstein JS, Haramati LB, Issenberg HJ, et al. MR imaging and CT of vascular anomalies and connections in patients with congenital heart disease: significance in surgical planning. RadioGraphics. 2002;22:337–47. discussion, 348–349.

11. Goo HW, Park IS, Ko JK, et al. CT of congenital heart disease: normal anatomy and typical pathologic conditions. RadioGraphics. 2003;23(Spec Issue):S147–65.

12. Leschka S, Oechslin E, Husmann L, et al. Pre- and postoperative evaluation of congenital heart disease in children and adults with 64-section CT. Radiographics. 2007;27(3):829–46. Review.

13. Oh KH, Choo KS, Lim SJ, et al. Multidetector CT evaluation of total anomalous pulmonary venous connections: comparison with echocardiography. Pediatr Radiol. 2009;39:950–4.

14. Kawano T, Ishii M, Takagi J, et al. Three-dimensional helical computed tomographic angiography in neonates and infants with complex congenital heart disease. Am Heart J. 2000;139:654–60.

15. Kim TH, Kim YM, Suh CH, et al. Helical CT angiography and three-dimensional reconstruction of total anomalous pulmonary venous connections in neonates and infants. AJR Am J Roentgenol. 2000;175(5):1381–6.

16. Goo HW, Park IS, Ko JK, et al. CT of congenital heart disease: normal anatomy and typical pathologic conditions. Radiographics. 2003;23 Spec No:S147–65. Review.

17. Hopkins KL, Patrick LE, Simoneaux SF, Bank ER, Parks WJ, Smith SS. Pediatric great vessel anomalies: initial clinical experience with spiral CT angiography. Radiology. 1996;200:811–5.

18. Hausleiter J, Meyer T, Hadamitzky M, et al. Radiation dose estimates from cardiac multislice computed tomography in daily practice: impact of different scanning protocols on effective dose estimates. Circulation. 2006;113: 1305–10.

19. Cha EM, Khouri GH. Persistent left superior vena cava. Radiologic and clinical significance. Radiology. 1972; 103:375–81.

20. Campbell M, Deuchar DC. The left-sided superior vena cava. Br Heart J. 1994;18:423–39.

21. Webb WR, Gamsu G, Speckman JM, Kaiser JA, Federle MP, Lipton MJ. Computed tomographic demonstration of mediastinal venous anomalies. AJR Am J Roentgenol. 1982; 139(1):157–61.

22. Winter FS. Persistent left superior cava. Survey of world literature and report of thirty additional cases. Angiology. 1954;5:90–132.

23. Dillon EH, Camputaro C. Partial anomalous pulmonary venous drainage of the left upper lobe vs duplication of the superior vena cava: distinction based on CT findings. AJR Am J Roentgenol. 1993;160(2):375–9.

24. Gonzalez-Juanatey C, Testa A, Vidan J, Izquierdo R, Garcia-Castelo A, Daniel C, et al. Persistent left superior vena cava draining into the coronary sinus: report of 10 cases and literature review. Clin Cardiol. 2004;27(9):515–8.

25. Cormier MG, Yedlicka JW, Gray RJ, Moncada R. Congenital anomalies of the superior vena cava: a CT study. Semin Roentgenol. 1989;24:77–83.

26. Park HY, Summoror MH, Preues K, et al. Anomalous drainage of the right superior vena cava into the left atrium. J Am Coll Cardiol. 1983;2:358–62.

27. Peene P, Verschakelen J, Wilms G, Baert AL. Abnormal pulmonary venous return associated with partially persistent left superior vena cava. Röfo. 1991;154:337–9.

28. Edwards JE, Dushane JW. Thoracic venous anomalies: vascular connnection on the left atrium and the innominatc vein (levoatriocardinal vein) associated with mitral atresia and premature closure of the foramen oval (case 1). Arch Pathol. 1950;49:517–28.

29. Pastor BH, Blumberg BI. Persistent left superior vena cava demonstrated by angiocardiography. Am Heart J. 1958; 55:120–5.

30. Ellis JH, Denham JS, Bies JR, Olson EW, Cory DA. Magnetic Resonance Imaging of systemic venous anomalies. Computerized Radiol. 1986;10:15–22.

31. Huggins TJ, Lesar ML, Friedman AC, Pyatt RS, Thane TT. CT appearance of persistent left superior vena cava. J Comput Assist Tomogr. 1982;6:294–7.

32. Kellman GM, Alpern MB, Sandler MA, Craig BM. Computed tomography of vena cava anomalies with embryologic correlation. Radiographics. 1988;8:533–56.

33. Schultz CL, Morrison S, Brian PG. Azygos continuation in the inferior vena cava: demonstration by NMR. J Comput Assist Tomogr. 1984;8:774–6.

34. Coulomb M, Rose-Pittet L, Dalsoglio S, Lebas JF, Paillasson F, Gros CH, et al. Continuation azygos droite de la veine cave inférieure. A propos de 3 observations avec étude IRM. J Radiol. 1987;68:45–50.

35. Pernot C, Hoeffel JC, Worms AM, Auguste JP. La continuation azygos de la veine cave inférieure. Ann Radiol. 1978;21:525–30.

36. Jelinek JS, Stuan PL, Done SL, Ghaed N, Rudd SA. MRI of polysplenia syndrome. Magn Res Imag. 1989;7:681–6.

37. Anderson C, Devine WA, Anderson RH, Debich DE, Zuberbuhler JR. Abnormalities of the spleen in relation to congenital malformations of the heart: a survey of necropsy findings in children. Br Heart J. 1990;63:122–8.

38. Venables AW. Isolated drainage of the inferior vena to the left atrium. Br Heart J. 1963;25:545–8.

39. Berdon WE, Baker DH. Plain film findings in azygos continuation of the inferior vena cava. AJR Am J Roentgenol. 1968;104:452–7.

40. Rey C. Anomalie du retour systémique. Encycl Méd Chir 1990, Radiodiagnostic, 3:32-016-A-15.

41. Bank ER, Hernandez RJ. CT and MR of congenital heart disease. Radiol Clin North Am. 1988;26:241–62.

42. Bennet J, Remy J. Le syndrome de Halasz. Ann Radiol. 1975;18:271–6.

43. Oropeza G, Hernandez FA, Callard GM, Jude JR. Anomalous pulmonary venous drainage of the left upper lobe. Ann Thorac Surg. 1970;9(2):180–5.

44. Pennes DR, Ellis JH. Anomalous pulmonary venous drainage of the left upper lobe shown by CT scans. Radiology. 1986;159(1):23–4.

45. Livolsi A, Kastler B, Marcellin L, Casanova R, Bintner M, Haddad J. MR diagnosis of subdiaphragmatic anomalous pulmonary venous drainage in a newborn. J Comput Assist Tomogr. 1991;15:1051–3.

46. Dupuis C, Kachaner J, Freedom RM, Payot M, Davignon A. Cardiologie pédiatrique. Flammarion 2e édition. 1991.

47. Haworth SG. Total anomalous plumonary venous return. Prenatal damage to pulmonary vascular bed and extrapulmonary veins. Br Heart J. 1982;48:513–24.

48. Sano S, Brawn WJ, Mee RBB. Total anomalous pulmonary venous drainage. J Thorac Cardiovasc Surg. 1989;97:886–92.

49. Ninet J, Gordillo M, Vigneron M, et al. Retour veineux pulmonaire anormal total. Résultats de la correction chez 50 nourrissons. Arch Mal Coeur. 1990;83:217–21.

50. Gathman GE, Nadas AS. Total anomalous pulmonary venous connection: clinical and physiologic observations of 75 pediatric patients. Circulation. 1970;42:143–54.

51. Paquet M, Gutgesell H. Echocardiographic features of total anomalous pulmonary venous connection. Circulation. 1975;51:599–605.

52. Rey C, Lablanche IM, Deloche A. Apport de l'échocardiographie au diagnostic du retour veineux pulmonaire anormal total infradiaphragmatique. Arch Mal Coeur. 1977;70: 997–1001.

53. Chin AJ, Sanders SP, Sherman F, Lang P, Norwood WI, Castaneda AR. Accuracy of subcostal two-dimensional echocardiography in prospective diagnosis of total anomalous pulmonary venous connection. Am Heart J. 1987;113:1153–9.

54. Sahn DJ, Allen HD, Lange LW, Goldberg SJ. Cross-sectional echocardiographic diagnosis of the sites of total anomalous pulmonary venous drainage. Circulation. 1979;60:1317–25.

55. Cooper MJ, Teitel DF, Silverman NH, Enderlein MA. Study of the infradiaphragmatic total anomalous pulmonary venous connection with cross-sectional and pulsed Doppler echocardiography. Circulation. 1984;70:412–6.

56. Boxer RA, Singh S, Lacorte MA, Goldman M, Stein HL. Cardiac magnetic resonance imaging in congenital heart disease. J Pediatr. 1986;109:460–4.

57. Kastler B, Livolsi A, Germain P, et al. Contribution of MRI in supracardiac total anomalous pulmonary venous drainage. Pediat Radiol. 1992;22:262–3.

58. Snellen HA, Van Ingen HC, Hoefsmit ECM. Patterns of anomalous pulmonary venous drainage. Circulation. 1968; 38:45–63.

59. Healy JE. Anatomic survey of anomalous pulmonary veins: thier clinical significance. Thorac Surg. 1952;23:443–4.

60. Kalke BR, Carlson RG, Ferlic RM, Sellers RD, Lillehei CW. Partial anomalous pulmonary venous connections. Am J Cardiol. 1967;20:91–101.

61. Schatz SL, Ryvicker MJ, Deutsch AM, Cohen HR. Partial anomalous pulmonary venous drainage of the right lower lobe shown by CT scans. Radiology. 1986;159:21–2.

62. Neill CA, Perenez C, Sabiston DC, Sheldon H. The familial occurence of hypoplastic right long with systemic arterial supply and venous drainage: Scimitar syndrome. Bull John Hopkins. 1960;107:1–21.

63. Kuiper-Oosterwal CH, Moulaert A. The scimitar syndrome in infancy and childhood. Eur J Cardiol. 1973;1:55–61.

64. CIRILLO RL. The scimitar sign. Radiology. 1998;206:623–4.

65. Pennes DR, Ellis JH. Anomalous pulmonary venous drainage of the left upper lobe shown by CT scan. Radiology. 1986;159:23–4.

66. Julsrud PR, Ehman RL. The " broken ring " sign in magnetic resonance imaging of partial anomalous pulmonary venous connection at the superior vena cava. Mayo Clin Proc. 1985;60:874–9.

67. Vesely TM, Julsrud PR, Brown JJ, Hagler DJ. MR imaging of partial anomalous pulmonary venous connections. J Comput Assist Tomogr. 1991;15:752–6.

68. Baxter R, McFadden PM, Gradman M, Wright A. Scimitar syndrome: cine magnetic resonance imaging demonstration of anomalous pulmonary venous drainage. Ann Thorac Surg. 1990;50(1):121–3.

69. Kivelitz DE, Scheer I, Taupitz M. Scimitar syndrome: diagnosis with MR angiography. AJR Am J Roentgenol. 1999; 172(6):1700.

70. Healey JE. Anatomic survey of anomalous pulmonary veins: their clinical significance. J Thorac Cardiovas Surg. 1952; 23:433.

71. Niwayama G. Cor triatriatum. Am Heart. 1960;J 59:291.

72. Jegier W, Gibbons JE, Wiglesworth FW. Cor triatriatum: clinical, hemodynamic, and pathologic studies: surgical correction in early life. Pediatrics. 1963;31:255.

73. Edwards JE. Malformations of the coronary vessels: anomalies of the coronary sinus. In: Gould SE, editor. Pathology of the heart. 2nd ed. Springfield: Charles C Thomas; 1960. p. 431.

74. Loeffler E. Unusual malformation of the left atrium: pulmonary sinus. Arch Pathol. 1949;48:371.

75. Grondin C, Leonard AS, Anderson RC, Amplatz KA, Edwards JE, Varco RL. Cor triatriatum: a diagnostic surgical enigma. J Thorac Cardiovasc Surg. 1964;48:527.

76. Ono Y, Fukuki K, Munakata M, Narita J, Takahata T, Sudo Y, et al. Usefulness of the preoperative MRI for diagnostic and operative method in a case of cor triatriatum. Kyobu Geka. 1996;49(11):921–3.

77. Horike K, Matsumura C, Egawa Y, Kirino A, Ohshio T, Kawahito T, et al. A case report of cor triatriatum benefit of MRI for preoperative diagnostic and surgical method. Kyobu Geka. 1993;46(12):1063–5.

78. Sakamoto I, Matsunaga N, Hayashi K, Ogawa Y, Fukui J. Cine-magnetic resonance imaging of cor triatriatum. Chest. 1994;406(5):1586–9.

79. Kastler BA, Livolsi A, Germain P, et al. MRI in the management of congenital heart disease in newborns and s. Hospimedica. 1991;9:31–41.

80. Sieverding L, Klose U, Apitz J. Morphological diagnosis of congenital and acquired heart disease by magnetic resonance imaging. Pediat Radiol. 1990;20:311–9.

81. Didier D, Higgins CB, Fisher MR, Osaki L, Silverman NH, Cheitlin MD. Congenital heart disease: gated MR imaging in 72 patients. Radiology. 1986;158:227–35.

82. Church WS. congenital malformation of the heart: abnormal septum in left auricle. Trans Pathol Soc (Lond). 1868; 19:188.

5.1 Introduction

Aortic arch anomalies represent a group of various congenital malformations that share a common embryological origin [1] as they involve the vessels derived from the primitive branchial arches.

It is difficult to establish the overall frequency of these anomalies, as many cases are asymptomatic and not diagnosed. They represent about 30% of all cases of congenital heart disease, observed in 7 per 1,000 births [2].

Tracheal compression and stenosis, due to non-vascular causes, are also described in this chapter because the clinical features, diagnostic approach, and management of these patients present a number of similarities.

5.2 Clinical Features

The circumstances of discovery of the anomalies are variable and can be classified into three groups:

- The vascular malformation is responsible for a vascular ring encircling the trachea and oesophagus, inducing respiratory and/or gastrointestinal symptoms and signs. This form often corresponds to neonates or toddlers presenting with unresolved pulmonary symptoms and stridor, dyspnoea that may be mistaken for early-onset asthma, respiratory distress, recurrent bronchopneumonia with chronic cough and episodes of cyanosis with dying spells or even sudden death. Endoscopic examination is frequently requested in this context and indicates a diagnosis of vascular compression of the lower airways. In other cases, gastrointestinal symptoms are predominant with dysphagia, reflux and poor weight gain.

- The anomaly is part of a broader context of congenital heart disease and is discovered during assessment of this disease [3].
- Finally, the diagnosis is established on routine radiological examination in an asymptomatic child or adult [4].

5.3 Anatomical Diagnosis by Imaging

5.3.1 Chest Radiograph

The first examination to be performed in the case of suspicion of aortic arch anomaly is AP and lateral chest radiograph. In children and adults, analysis of the AP view of the mediastinum, following the site of the aortic knob, may raise a suspicion of left or right aortic arch. In infants and young children, the position of the trachea constitutes a very useful indirect sign: it is normally deviated to the right in the case of left aortic arch (and vice versa). The right or left position of the descending aorta is deduced from the position of the para-aortic line, most easily visible in its superior part. On the lateral radiograph, the tracheal edges are normally straight and parallel, except in infants, in whom a slight anterior compression of the superior intrathoracic trachea may be observed where it is crossed by the brachiocephalic trunk (BCT) (innominate artery).

5.3.2 Barium Swallow

In the past, this used to be an important examination. It must be performed according to a rigorous technique

B. Kastler, *MRI of Cardiovascular Malformations*,
DOI: 10.1007/978-3-540-30702-0_5, © Springer-Verlag Berlin Heidelberg 2011

with a half-filled oesophagus (abnormal indentations may be masked when the oesophagus is over-full or inadequately filled), with AP, lateral, RAO and LAO views. The site, size and pulsatile nature of any abnormal indentations are analyzed. A retro-oesophageal subclavian artery or ligamentum arteriosum causes a small indentation, while an aortic arch causes a large indentation. Barium swallow can, therefore, indirectly confirm the presence of a vascular ring. However, it is unable to specify the exact anatomical type of sometimes very complex anomalies. Since the arrival of MRI, it is admitted that barium swallow is of lesser importance.

5.3.3 Echocardiography

Echocardiography is a minimally invasive, but disappointing and unreliable method for the study of aortic arch anomalies. The diagnosis is rarely established on echocardiography [5, 6], which is mainly useful for the assessment of associated cardiac malformations.

5.3.4 Bronchoscopy

Bronchoscopy can be carried out in children, whatever the age or the underlying condition, provided it is performed in a specialized unit by an experienced and fully equipped operator. However, it is highly desirable to perform bronchoscopy close to a radiology department, paediatric intensive care unit, and an operating room specialized in paediatric surgery.

5.3.5 Techniques

Two complementary techniques are available depending on the type of equipment:

- Fiberoptic bronchoscopy

Fiberoptic bronchoscopes, composed of flexible and orientable optical fibres connected to a cold light source, are now available in various diameters and allow complete exploration of the respiratory tract among every age group [7]. The most widely used outer diameters are:

- 2.2 mm: premature babies
- 2.8 and 3.6 mm: full-term newborn babies and toddlers
- 5 mm: schoolchildren

Apart from life-threatening situations, the procedure can be conducted in outpatients under conscious sedation and lidocaine topical anaesthesia. For an experienced operator the whole central airway can be checked in less than 1 min.

If required, fiberoptic bronchoscopes can also be passed through most paediatric endotracheal and tracheotomy tubes without interrupting mechanical ventilation.

- Rigid tube bronchoscopy

Rigid bronchoscopes are hollow metal tubes through which various operating instruments can be passed: suction probes and catheters, optical telescopes, forceps, fiberoptic laser beams, cryodes, stents, etc. The rigid tube is introduced into the airways by placing the child in the supine position with the neck hyperextended ("sword-swallowing position"). As the side port of the bronchoscope allows gas intake (oxygen, anaesthetic gases), the examination is usually performed under general anaesthesia (oxygen, anaesthetic gases), with close monitoring of vital parameters (pulsed oxymetry, end tidal CO_2) [8–11]. Rigid bronchoscopes are available in various lengths and diameters to be used in all age groups, even in premature infants (smaller tubes outer diameters: 3 mm).

Videos can be recorded with both types of bronchoscopes by means of a CCD camera connected to the instrument eyepiece. The camera is connected to a unit including a video monitor providing a magnified image, a video cassette recorder allowing dynamic recording of the procedure, and a colour printer to obtain real-time images. Saving images and/or video clips is essential when longitudinal follow-up of a lesion is required, and in order to compare endoscopic findings with radiological findings in the same cross-sectional area (short-axis MR images).

- Choosing the technique

Choosing between the rigid or the flexible bronchoscope depends on the purpose of the procedure and the underlying condition. Schematically, fiberoptic bronchoscopy is performed first because it is easier. It is essentially used for diagnostic purpose or for assistance in tracheal intubation (mandibulofacial malformations). The indications for rigid tube bronchoscopy are limited by the relative complexity of the procedure, which is usually restricted to interventional purposes: for removal of foreign bodies, airway disobstruction, laser photoresection, stenting and dilatation of rigid strictures, and management of tracheo-oesophageal fistula.

Both endoscopy techniques can be used intraoperatively in order to assess the effects of mediastinal surgical repair on the central airway.

Bronchoscopy can reveal central airway compression in children with unresolved respiratory symptoms, raising the problem of the underlying aetiology. The observed level and type of compression (pulsatile or non-pulsatile) usually guide the diagnosis, but rarely provide sufficient information. In our experience, analyzing the endoscopic and MRI findings together is enough to define the compression mechanism in the great majority of cases. Apart from its diagnostic role, bronchoscopy remains essential to evaluate the degree of endoluminal narrowing ("stenotic ratio") and the stenosis dynamic behaviour during the respiratory phase (airway dyskinesia), as in case of absence of dynamic data, MRI frequently underestimates the stenosis due to the absence of signal of the respiratory mucosa; However, evaluation of this stenotic ratio together with the clinical data and tolerance are essential to guide therapeutic options (surgery, interventional bronchoscopy, conservative management).

5.4 Magnetic Resonance Imaging

MRI provides a complete and precise anatomical assessment of cardiovascular anomalies and their consequences on the tracheobronchial tree and oesophagus. It provides a global view of the mediastinum [12] (see below) and identifies the mechanisms of respiratory tract compression responsible for the patient's symptoms [6, 13–20].

MRI comprises a series of mediastinal axial and coronal ECG-gated black blood images, completed in this type of disease by sagittal images and possibly coronal oblique images allowing optimal visualization of the trachea (see Chap. 2, atlas S2).

The slice thickness is adapted to the size of the child, 3–5 mm in young infants and 5–8 mm in older children. The small vascular structures and tracheobronchial tree are optimally visualized by acquiring stacks of intertwined and overlapping images, 3–5 mm thick (i.e. slice increment of 2–3 mm – see Chap. 1, Examination Technique).

We also sometimes perform dynamic bright-blood cine-MRI sequences to confirm patency of a vessel or the pulsatile nature of tracheal compression, or a gadolinium-enhanced MR angiography sequence to obtain a global view of the vascular system. Real-time imaging, available on more recent machines, is also very useful in this context to assess the dynamic appearance of a lesion (pulsatility, respiratory collapse, etc.). The total examination time ranges from 20 to 40 min.

Schematically, four types of anomalies can be encountered:

- A congenital anomaly of vessels (double aortic arch, anomalous left pulmonary artery, etc.) directly responsible for compression of the tracheobronchial tree and the clinical features, with or without an intrinsic lesion of the tracheobronchial tree.
- A malformation of cardiac chambers, such as ventricular septum defect, patent ductus arteriosus, pulmonary atresia, congenital aortic stenosis, responsible for dilatation of the pulmonary arteries or the aorta and its branches, inducing tracheal or bronchial compression.
- Intrinsic tracheal anomalies such as tracheomalacia or subglottic stenosis, resulting in tracheal compression by a vessel in a normal position on an abnormal trachea; typical example, BCT (innominate artery).
- A frequent form comprises a vessel in an abnormal position with abnormal trachea and bronchi. It is always difficult in these cases to determine the predominant factor responsible for the patient's symptoms.

It should also be mentioned that non-vascular mediastinal mass responsible for tracheal compression must also be excluded.

5.4.1 Computed Tomography-Scan

Computed tomography (CT) as well as MRI, plays a valuable role in bridging the gaps created by echocardiography and angiography, specifically with regard to extracardiac arterial and venous anatomy and connections in patients with congenital heart disease [21–24]. CT has the advantages of easy availability and very short scanning times. Contrast material-enhanced helical CT allows the precise timing necessary for accurate extracardiac arterial and venous vascular imaging. Dynamic CT imaging techniques and postprocessing techniques such as multiplanar reformatting, volume rendering and virtual bronchoscopy assist in surgical planning by providing a better representation of three-dimensional (3D) anatomy and decrease the inherent disadvantage of CT image acquisition exclusively in the transaxial plane [25–27]. In comparison to MRI, CT is faster, less often requires sedation, has better spatial resolution, and is less compromised in the presence of metallic devices. However, the major drawbacks of CT include patient exposure to ionizing radiation and the risks of iodinated contrast material, which are of particular concern in the paediatric population [25–27].

The decision to image with CT versus MRI should be based on institutional equipment, scheduling, and availability as well as the patient's ability to cooperate. The need to tailor the examination to answer the specific questions being asked may also guide the choice of CT versus MRI [25].

5.4.2 Angiography

Angiography used to be performed for diagnosis and preoperative assessment, but is an invasive method in children, often requiring general anaesthesia [29–32]. It is no longer useful for the diagnosis of aortic arch anomalies and the preoperative assessment is now based on MR slice imaging and angiography.

5.4.3 Aortic Arch Anomalies

The embryology of aortic arch anomalies is essentially based on the studies conducted by Edwards [2]. The six primitive aortic arches (numbered from the cephalic extremity of the embryo) form junctions between ventral and dorsal pairs of aortas.

Normally:

- The first two primitive aortic arches involute completely.

- The third arches develop to form the carotid arteries.
- The fifth arches involute completely.
- The sixth arches form the pulmonary artery and its branches and the ductus arteriosus.
- The fourth primitive aortic arches have a different outcome on the right and on the left. The left fourth arch contributes to form the left portion of the aortic arch between the common carotid artery and left subclavian artery. The right fourth arch involutes between the right subclavian artery and descending aorta and the remaining segment gives rise to the proximal portion of the right subclavian artery (the distal portion and left subclavian artery are derived from the seventh intersegmental arteries).

The normal anatomy of the aortic system, but also most of the known malformations of the aorta and its branches are therefore due to various combinations of atresia or patency of various segments of the aortic arches of the embryo.

5.5 Classification

Classification of aortic arch anomalies is illustrated by the diagram proposed by Corone [1], based on the various possible sites of involution of the right or left fourth aortic arches. This diagram has been entirely modified, completed and adapted to modern tomographic imaging[1] (Fig. 5.1).

The right or left fourth primitive aortic arches can be seen on this diagram between the ascending aorta (AAo) anteriorly and the descending aorta (DAo) posteriorly.

Sites of involution are numbered in an Counterclockwise direction from the normal site of involution on the right arch (indicated by N) by increasing number for sites of involution on the right arch (→ left arch). Sites of involution on the left arch (→ right arch) are identified by negative numbers (symmetrical or mirror image variants of the sites of involution on the right arch).

---

[1]On which the left is on the right of the image (right-left inversion compared to usual anatomical sections and transoesophagal US).

There are many possible sites of involution on the right arch and, apart from the typical examples of left or right arch, they must also include the possibility of ligamentum arteriosum situated on the right (RLA) and/or on the left (LLA):

- When the ligamentum arteriosum is situated on the same side as the aortic arch, it generally does not cause a vascular ring (Fig. 5.1a).
- When the ligamentum arteriosum is situated on the opposite side to the aortic arch, there is a risk of vascular ring. These anomalies, some of which are more difficult to understand at first reading (Fig. 5.1b), are shown in italics in the following

discussion. Vascular rings on a right arch are described in detail below (also see Fig. 5.9).

5.5.1 Involution of the Right Arch Resulting in Left Aortic Arch

The normal aortic arch results from involution at point N between the right subclavian artery (anteriorly) and the descending aorta (posteriorly). Involution on the right at −3, between the common carotid artery (anteriorly) and the right subclavian artery (posteriorly) results in an aberrant right subclavian artery arising

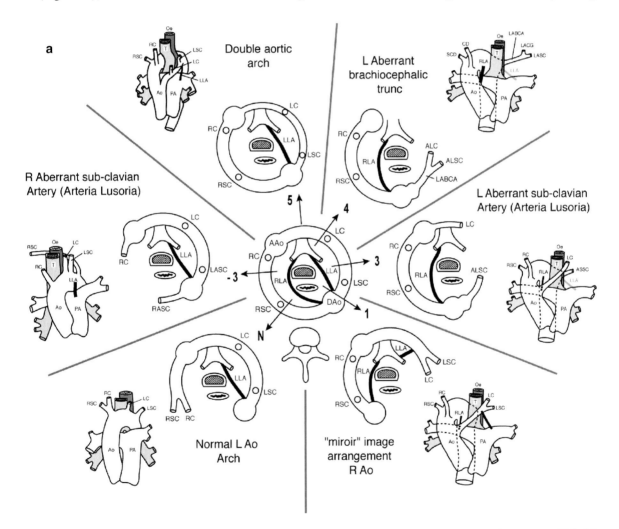

Fig. 5.1 Aortic arch anomalies: (**a** and **b**) diagrams of the various possible sites of involution of the left and right fourth primitive aortic arches (see text and Fig. 5.9). R (right), L (left), AAo (ascending aorta), DAo (descending aorta), PA (pulmonary artery), C (common carotid artery), SC (subclavian artery), APBS (AP barium swallow), LBS (lateral barium swallow); right ligamentum arteriosum (RLA), left ligamentum arteriosum (LLA), if RLA or LLA remain patent: residual persistant ductus arteriosum

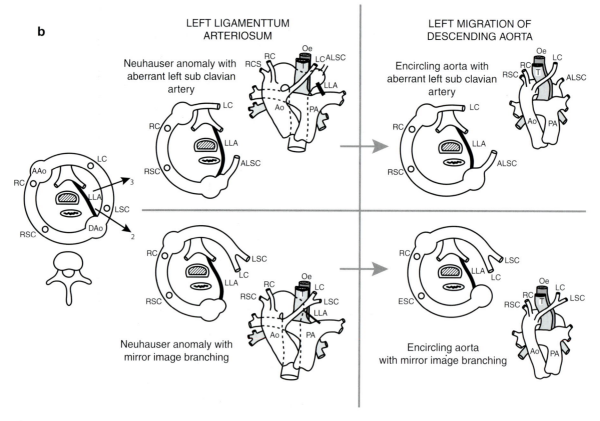

Fig. 5.1 (continued)

from the distal part of the aortic arch and reaching the right upper limb via a retro-oesophageal course.

5.5.2 Total or Partial Absence of Involution of the Two Arches (no Involution at 5)

This results in double aortic arch, generally with a dominant right arch (exceptionally the two aortae do not merge, and travel side by side and, subsequently, bifurcate to form their respective iliac arteries).

5.5.3 Involution of the Left Aortic Arch Resulting in Right Aortic Arch

Involution at 1 between the left subclavian artery (anteriorly) and the descending aorta (posteriorly) with

right ligamentum arteriosum (RLA) results in a mirror image (also see Fig. 5.9).

Less frequently, the ligamentum arteriosum is on the left (LLA); there is no vascular ring when involution occurs posterior to the LLA, as the LLA is then inserted anteriorly onto the subclavian artery.

There is also a rarer variant with involution at 2, between the left subclavian artery (anteriorly) and the descending aorta (posteriorly), but anterior to the LLA, which, by insertion into the LLA, becomes compressive: There is a mirror image arrangement of supra-aortic vessels and a potential vascular ring. This variant belongs to the group of Neuhauser anomalies (Neuhauser anomaly with mirror image branching).

Involution at 3 between the left common carotid artery (anteriorly) and the left subclavian artery (posteriorly) with RLA leads to a right arch with aberrant (retro-oesophageal) left subclavian artery.

The presence of a right arch and a compressive left ligamentum arteriosum attached to a vascular enlargement at the origin of the retro-oesophageal left subclavian artery (Kommerell diverticulum) forms a compressive vascular ring, which also belongs to the group of Neuhauser anomalies (Neuhauser anomaly with arteria lusoria, which is much more frequent than Neuhauser anomaly with mirror image branching).

The encircling aorta is a consequence of a right arch with migration of the dorsal arch to the left with a retro-oesophageal aortic segment and left descending aorta (hence the term "encircling"). It is generally due to involution at 3 (with retro-oesophageal left subclavian artery) or more rarely involution at 2 with mirror image branching.

Involution at 4 between the ascending aorta and the left common carotid results in a right arch with aberrant left BCT (innominate artery).

The same sites of involution, symmetrical or mirror image variants of the sites of involution on the right arch can also be observed on the left:

Involution at 3 on the right arch is the mirror image of involution at −3 on the left arch, described above.

Involution at −4 (left arch with aberrant right BCT) is the mirror image of involution at 4.

As discussed below, mirror image of the encircling left aorta is also possible: encircling aorta with right arch, retro-oesophageal aortic segment and left descending aorta.

5.5.4 Other Anomalies

Other anomalies must be added to this classification:

- Anomalous (retrotracheal) left pulmonary artery, due to involution of the proximal part of the sixth left arch.
- Congenital atresia of one of the pulmonary arteries.
- Cervical aorta, due to absence of involution of the third aortic arch (Fig. 5.19).
- Isolation of a subclavian artery with congenital subclavian steal syndrome (double involution at 1 and 3 (Fig. 5.21).
- Persistent fifth left arch, resulting in a normal aortic arch, duplicated in its concavity by a second aortic arch (Fig. 5.22). These last two anomalies are exceptional.

5.6 Double Aortic Arch

Double aortic arch is due to persistence of both the left and right aortic arches (patency of the segment of the right dorsal aorta between the origin of the seventh right segmental artery and its junction with the left dorsal aorta). It represents the most frequent type of symptomatic vascular ring (40–50% of cases) as the arches encircle the trachea and oesophagus. This anomaly is characterized (Fig. 5.2) by the persistence of two aortic arches arising from the ascending aorta. After crossing the trachea laterally and the two main bronchi superiorly, the two arches join to form the descending aorta behind the oesophagus. The common carotid and subclavian arteries each arise independently from their respective arch (there are always 4 supra-aortic vessels, i.e. "four artery sign").

The double arch usually is usually complete and comprises a larger and more cephalad right arch, a left descending aorta and left ligamentum arteriosum between the distal part of the left arch and the left pulmonary artery (Fig. 5.2) [33].

The other anatomical variants depend on the diameter of the arches, and partial or complete involution (atresia) of one of the two arches, usually the smaller one on the left [34]. This form (with involution of the left arch) is difficult to distinguish from Neuhauser anomaly with arteria lusoria, but it is more symptomatic as it comprises two compressive elements on the left (left aortic arch and LLA, see Figs. 5.2c and 5.12b and Neuhauser anomalies). It is seldom associated with congenital heart disease such as ventricular septal defect or tetralogy of Fallot.

5.6.1 Clinical Features

Infants are often seen before the age of 3 months, as symptoms usually start from birth, ranging from mild respiratory obstruction to severe respiratory distress. Stridor, feeding troubles (dysphagia, dyspnoea during feeding), chest overdistension, anoxic spells or recurrent respiratory tract infections are suggestive [33]. Asthma-like symptoms are frequently reported but patients are unresponsive to bronchodilators. Gastrointestinal signs such as reflux or hypersialorrhoea are rarely observed.

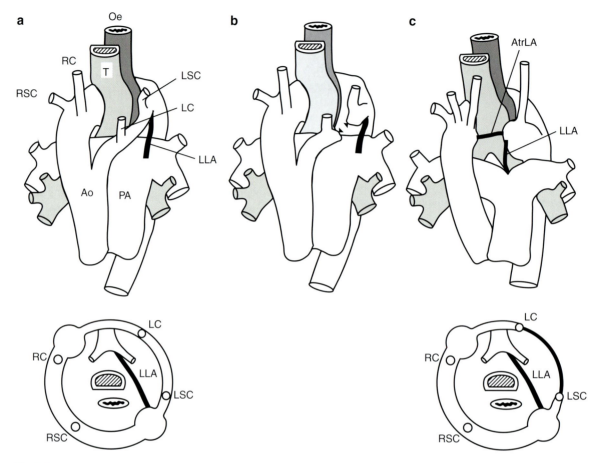

Fig. 5.2 (**a**) Diagram of double aortic arch: The ascending aorta (*Ao*) gives rise to left and right aortic arches that encircle the trachea (*T*) and oesophagus (*Oe*). (**b**) Diagram of surgical correction of double aortic arch. Section of the thinner arch (in this case the left arch) between the carotid and subclavian arteries with end-to-end suture, combined with section of the ligamen-tum arteriosum. (**c**) Diagram of double aortic arch with atresia of the left arch (*AtrLA*). Left ligamentum arteriosum (*LLA*). This form is difficult to distinguish from Neuhauser anomaly with arteria lusoria, but potentially comprises two compressive elements on the left (AtrLA and LLA) (also see Fig. 5.12)

Treatment is usually surgical and consists of sectioning the thinner arch with end-to-end suture (after verification of the absence of hypoplasia on the dominant arch) (Fig. 5.2c). Ligamenta arteriosa often need to be sectioned. The post-operative course is generally uneventful, but transient inspiratory dyspnoea can persist for several weeks.

5.6.2 Imaging

• Radiography

The AP chest radiograph often shows bilateral pulmonary distension due to obstructive emphysema, or disorders of ventilation such as atelectasis. Absence of the aortic knob (left superior arch) and the para-aortic line (midline or right-sided aorta) are very useful signs, which must be systematically investigated. In young children, on good quality radiographs, the trachea and main bronchi are often clearly visible in contrast with the surrounding mediastinal structures. Consequently, loss of the tracheal radiolucency can be observed in the supracarinal region in the case of double aortic arch. Severe tracheal obstruction is associated with bilateral lung overdistension.

• Barium swallow

If performed, the AP barium swallow shows a double indentation: a deep indentation on the right border of the oesophagus over T3 corresponding to the right arch, and another less marked and lower indentation on the left corresponding to the left arch. The lateral view shows a clearly visible, large posterior oesophageal notch, corresponding to the right posterior arch, which is usually dominant [35]. Note that if one of the segments is atresic, particularly on the right (requiring right lateral thoracotomy), oesophageal indentations are also generally observed. Atresia of the left arch raises the problem of Neuhauser anomaly with arteria lusoria, as indicated above.

- Echocardiography

Echocardiography is especially useful to confirm or exclude associated congenital heart disease, but usually does not contribute to the diagnosis of double aortic arch [5].

- Bronchoscopy

Bronchoscopy performed in this context generally raises the suspicion of the diagnosis, by demonstrating extrinsic anteroposterior or circumferential compression of the supracarinal trachea (Fig. 5.3). The cross-sectional area is pulsatile and the tracheal lumen is usually severely narrowed. The tracheal cartilages in contact with the vascular ring are regularly malacic so that the extrinsic compression is associated with segmental dyskinesia responsible for expiratory collapse and mucociliary clearance impairment. This dyskinesia is best visualized by post-operative bronchoscopy, explaining persistence of respiratory symptoms after

surgical correction of double aortic arch. The endoscopic appearance of the double arch is not specific and can be confused with Neuhauser anomaly or anomalous left pulmonary artery.

- Angiography

X-ray angiography is no longer performed [29–32], and has been replaced, when necessary, by gadolinium-enhanced MR angiography (Fig. 5.5c). The two arches, each of which gives rise to a carotid artery and a subclavian artery, are visualized; luminal images may reveal an atresic segment.

- MRI

MRI provides a precise 3D anatomical assessment of the anomaly and its relations with the tracheobronchial tree (Figs. 5.4 and 5.5) [13, 36–39].

Anterior coronal images visualize the origin of the aorta from the left ventricle and the two arches encircling the trachea laterally. They are be used to assess the respective diameter of the two arches and determine the surgical approach by depicting the dominant and smaller arch and possible hypoplasia or atresia of one arch, particularly the posterior segment of the right arch (which will thus require right lateral thoracotomy instead of left thoracotomy) [40, 41].

Posterior coronal images show fusion of the two arches posteriorly to form the descending aorta and indicate the side of the descending aorta. They demonstrate the complete or incomplete nature of the double arch and the presence or absence of a Kommerell diverticulum. These images are important for assessment of extent and degree tracheal compression and the integrity of the rest of the trachea.

Axial images visualize the two arches and their relations with the trachea and oesophagus.

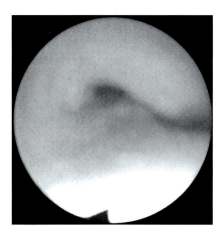

Fig. 5.3 Bronchoscopy in a 4-month-old child with severe dyspnoea related to double aortic arch. View of the intrathoracic trachea showing a circumferential constriction ring (pulsatile and dyskinetic), which totally masks the main carina (left and right are reversed compared to MRI axial images)

5.7 Left Aortic Arch with Aberrant Right Subclavian Artery (or Right Aortic Arch with Aberrant Left Subclavian Artery)

This anomaly, also called retro-oesophageal right subclavian artery or arteria lusoria (with dysphagia lusoria) is the most frequent anomaly of involution of the right arch (site of involution 3, see summary diagram, Fig. 5.9), affecting 0.5% of subjects [42].

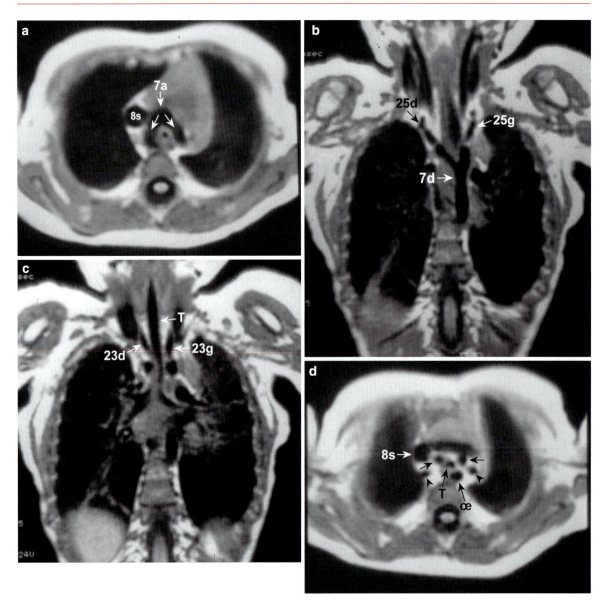

Fig. 5.4 (a–d). Double aortic arch in a 6-week-old child presenting with stridor and dyspnoea. (**a**) Axial fast spin-echo images of the aortic arches: The ascending aorta (*7a*) gives rise to left and right arches (*arrows*), which encircle the trachea and oesophagus; superior vena cava (*8s*). The two arches appear to have essentially the same calibre. Coronal images allow more accurate assessment of the respective diameters of the two arches. (**b**) Axial fast spin-echo image situated just above the two arches, demonstrating the symmetrical origin of the common carotid arteries (*arrows*) and right and left subclavian arteries (*arrowheads*), separately from each of the arches (there is no brachiocephalic trunk). The left brachiocephalic vein can be seen anteriorly; it merges with the right brachiocephalic vein to form the superior vena cava (*8s*); dilated oesophagus (Oe), trachea (T), left atrium (*5*). (**c**) Coronal spin-echo images: the trachea (*T*) is compressed by the two arches which give rise, superiorly, to left and right common carotid arteries (the left arch is dominant). The right (*23d*) and left (*23g*) subclavian arteries also arise from the two arches. (**d**) The two arches join to form the descending thoracic aorta (*7d*); right subclavian artery (*25d*), left subclavian artery (*25g*), right pulmonary artery (*3d*) and left pulmonary artery (*3g*). In this patient (unlike the usual case, Figs. 5.4e–g and 5.5), the left arch is larger, consequently requiring section of the thinner right arch.

Fig. 5.4 (**e–g**) Double aortic arch in an infant presenting with stridor and dyspnoea. Upper row (**e**) and middle row (**f**): coronal fast spin-echo anteroposterior series and lower row axial and sagittal fast spin-echo images (**e**), demonstrate the compression of the trachea (*T*) and oesophagus (*black arrows*) by the two arches (*white arrows* and *arrowheads*). The right arch as usual is dominant (*arrowheads*); right atrium (*1*), right ventricle (*2*), left atrium (*5*), left ventricle (*6*), ascending aorta (*7a*), descending aorta (*7d*), azygos vein (*12*).

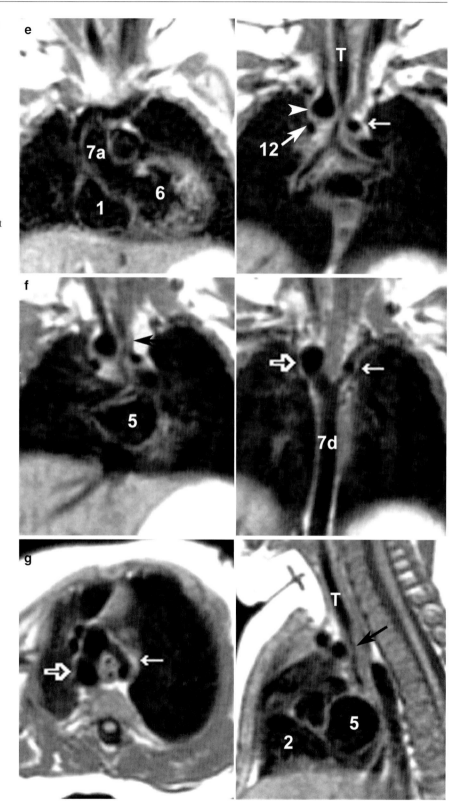

Fig. 5.4 (**h**, **i**). Double aortic arch in an adult patient discovered fortuitously on an MRI requested because of mediastinal enlargement on Chest radiograph. The two arches have here the same calibre (*arrows* on fast spin-echo and contrast-enhanced images; ascending aorta (*7a*), descending aorta (*7d*), right atrium (*1*), left ventricle (*6*))

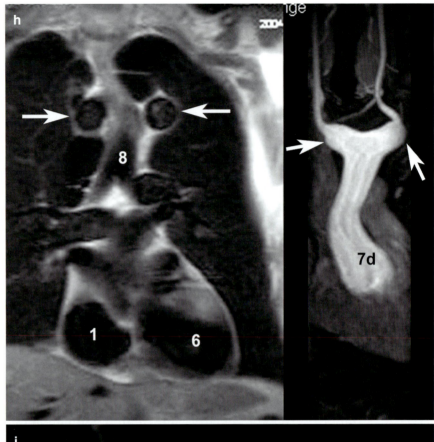

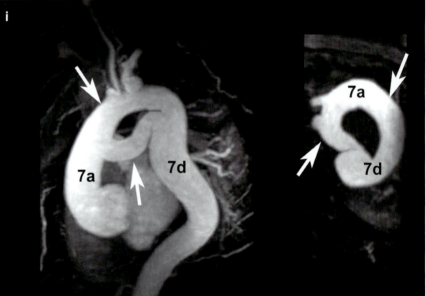

The right subclavian artery (or more rarely the left subclavian artery in the case of right arch), arises as the last branch of the aortic arch, at the junction between the aortic arch and the descending aorta (Fig. 5.6 and also see Chap. 7, Fig. 7.12 and Chap. 8, Fig. 8.25).

This artery, with a right superior oblique course, supplies the right upper limb and passes behind the oesophagus in 80% of cases, between the trachea and the oesophagus in 15% of cases and in front of the trachea in 5% of cases.

A large diverticulum may be present at the origin of the aberrant right subclavian artery, corresponding to a remnant of the right arch (Kommerell diverticulum). There is no vascular ring, as the ligamentum arteriosum is generally situated on the side of the aortic arch. When the ligamentum arteriosum is situated on the opposite side to the arch, The vascular ring is however loose.

In the forms with right arch and LLA, a vascular ring can be formed depending on the site of posterior insertion and tightness of the ligamentum arteriosum, which can encircle the supra-aortic vessels or descending aorta; these forms, which may be symptomatic, belong to the group of Neuhauser anomalies, discussed below (Fig. 5.11a, also see summary diagram, Fig. 5.9 for configurations of the right aortic arches with arteria lusoria, which can be observed on the left arch).

Aberran right or left subclavian artery are generally isolated, but can be associated with congenital heart disease in 12% of cases [42, 43]. The most frequent associated anomalies are tetralogy of Fallot, coarctation of the aorta and interrupted aortic arch (see Chap. 6, Fig. 6.12), while rarer anomalies are aortic stenosis, VSD and tricuspid atresia.

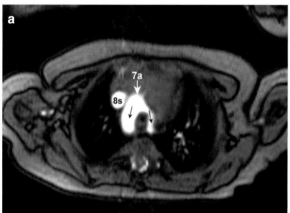
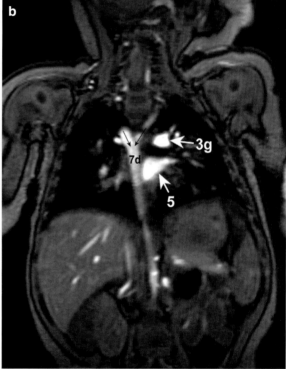

Fig. 5.5 Double aortic arch in a 2-month-old infant presenting with severe dyspnoea and abnormal respiratory noises. Contrast enhanced images (Dota-Gd, Guerbet, France). (**a**) Axial image: The ascending aorta (*7a*) gives rise to left and right arches (*arrows*) which encircle the trachea and oesophagus that are barely visible; superior vena cava (*8s*). As usual, the right arch is dominant, as confirmed on coronal images. (**b**) Posterior coronal image through the descending aorta: The right arch is dominant and travels to the left to join the left arch (*arrows*) to form the descending thoracic aorta (*7d*), which is initially right-sided, then rapidly regains a "left-sided" position in mid-thorax; left atrium (*5*), left pulmonary artery (*3g*). (**c**) Gadolinium-enhanced MR angiography: MIP reconstruction and detail of the two arches (*arrows*). This patient was treated by section of the thinner left arch (via left thoracotomy)

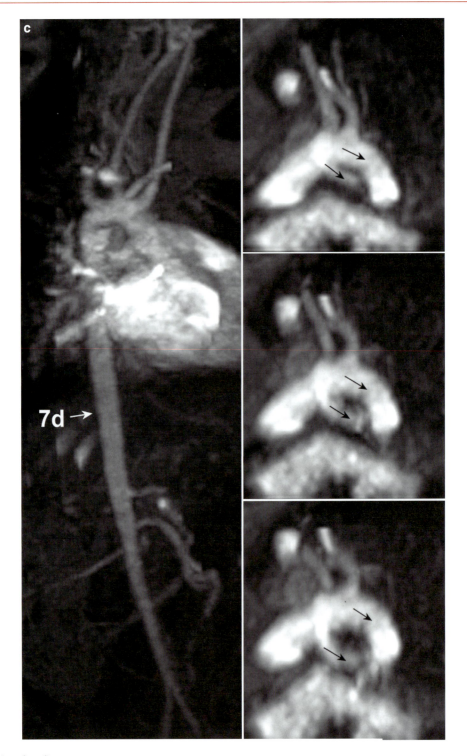

Fig. 5.5 (continued)

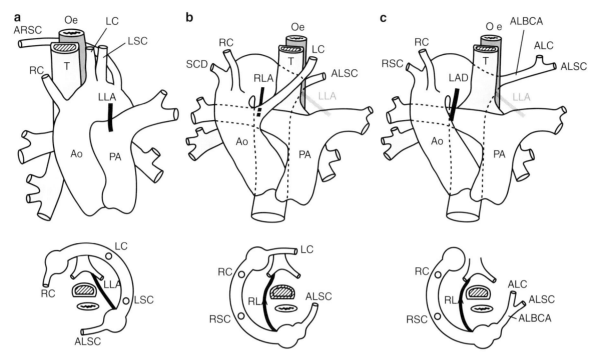

Fig. 5.6 Diagram of the variants of aberrant subclavian arteries (see Figs. 5.1 and 5.9). (**a**) Right subclavian artery on left arch (involution at −3). The aberrant right subclavian artery (ARSC), the fourth supra-aortic vessel, arises abnormally from the aortic isthmus and usually passes behind the oesophagus to reach the right upper limb. (**b**) Left subclavian artery on right arch (involution at 3). The aberrant left subclavian artery (ALSC), at its origin on the aorta, can present an enlargement or Kommerell diverticulum. N.B.: The ligamentum arteriosum can be compressive when it is situated on the left (LLA, *pale gray*) on a right arch (see Neuhauser anomaly, Fig. 5.12a, b). (**c**) Left subclavian artery with aberrant left brachiocephalic trunk (innominate artery) (LABCT ALBCA) (involution at 4). This rarer form is due to more anterior involution of the left arch in front of the origin of the left common carotid artery (LC). Ascending aorta (Ao), pulmonary artery (PA), right common carotid artery (RC), left common carotid artery (LC), right subclavian artery (RSC), left subclavian artery (LSC), trachea (T), oesophagus (Oe), right ligamentum arteriosum (RLA), left ligamentum arteriosum (LLA)

When the right common carotid artery is isolated posteriorly with the aberrant right subclavian artery, this variant constitutes an aberrant right (or left in the case of right arch) BCT (site of involution 4, type 4 right arch – see Figs. 5.1 and 5.9).

Conservative management is generally sufficient. Surgical treatment may be proposed in the presence of disabling and life-threatening (repeated vomiting, weight loss) symptoms (Fig. 5.8) and consists of section and reimplantation of the right subclavian artery.

5.7.1 Clinical Features

This malformation is rarely symptomatic. However, dysphagia can be observed and is thus frequently associated with patent gastro-oesophageal reflux symptoms. Respiratory symptoms related to tracheal compression are exceptionally reported. These forms are almost never life-threatening and usually resolve in the growing child.

5.7.2 Imaging

• Chest radiograph

Chest radiograph is generally normal.

• Barium swallow

Barium swallow confirms the diagnosis: AP views show a right superior oblique linear depression, slightly displacing the oesophagus, giving a bayonet appearance above the normal notch at the level of T3, to the left of the aortic arch. Lateral views are more specific, by showing a posterior triangular, deep and narrow notch with the left main bronchus indenting the oesophagus anteriorly over T3 and T4 [44].

- Echocardiography

Echocardiography is not contributive in this disease.

- Bronchoscopy

Bronchoscopy is usually not indicated unless respiratory symptoms are reported. A minor degree of posterior pulsatile compression can be observed at the middle part of the trachea in this case.

- CT

As already mentioned above, with the advent of modern multi-slice CT scan and the use of post-processing techniques, CT imaging is now able to accurately depict the extracardiac arterial and venous anomalous connections [21–24]. However, its major drawbacks compared to MRI include patient exposure to ionizing radiation and the risks of iodinated contrast material, which are of particular concern in the paediatric population [25–27]. It may be discovered incidentally in older children or adults.

- MRI

MRI usually confirms the absence of significant tracheal compression (Figs. 5.7 and 5.8) [45]. The diagnosis is easy on a posterior coronal image showing the origin of an abnormal vessel from the isthmus of the aorta and its right superior oblique course towards the right upper limb (in the case of the right variant on a left arch). Sagittal images visualize the aberrant vessel, generally situated behind the trachea, and assess the state of the trachea and the presence of any compression. The retro-oesophageal subclavian artery, its posterior origin and its aberrant course can also be identified on several successive axial images (as with computed tomography).

5.8 Right Aortic Arch

In this type of anomaly [46], the left arch involutes, resulting in three main forms: right aortic arch with right descending aorta (and mirror image of supra-aortic vessels), Neuhauser anomalies (comprising a compressive tight left ligamentum arteriosum), and right aortic arch with encircling retro-oesophageal left descending aorta.

However, in order to understand the numerous possible variants, we need to describe the embryology of the various sites of involution of the left arch in relation to the left supra-aortic vessels and the site of implantation of the left ligamentum arteriosum when it persists (see summary diagram, Fig. 5.9, modified and adapted from the classification by Shuford and Sybers [35]). As already mentioned, a number of the anomalies described above on a right arch can also present mirror image forms on a left arch.

Fig. 5.7 Aberrant (or retro-oesophageal) subclavian artery; right variant on left aortic arch in a 7-week-old presenting with reflux and recurrent episodes of bronchopulmonary infection. (**a**) Coronal spin echo image: The aberrant right subclavian artery (*25′dA*) arises abnormally on the left in the aortic isthmus and travels to the right (with a retro-oesophageal course, see **d**) to reach the right upper limb. The aortic arch and descending aorta (*7d*) are in a normal position on the left. Note the azygos vein, which runs parallel on the right (*12d*) and which describes an arch slightly lower than the aortic arch (see Fig. 5.1 and type 3, summary diagram Fig. 5.9). (**b**) Aberrant (or retro-oesophageal) subclavian artery; left variant on right aortic arch in a 9 month-old. Right variant on left aortic arch; coronal spin echo image: The aberrant subclavian artery (*25′gA*) arises from an aortic Kommerell diverticulum (*K*) and travels to the left (with a retro-oesophageal course) to reach the left upper limb. The descending thoracic aorta (*7′d*) is almost continuous with the right arch and lies on the right. The right subclavian artery and the origin of the vertebral arteries (arrowheads) are also clearly visualized (dominant right); brachiocephalic trunk (*22′*). (**c, d**) Aberrant subclavian artery, right variant on left aortic arch in a 9-month-old presenting with dyspnoea who underwent surgical correction of ventricular septum defect. Left aortic arch and course of right aberrant subclavian artery (arrows) are depicted on both fast spin-echo and gradient-echo images (rows d and e). No tracheal compression is present. Aortic arch (*7*), ascending aorta (*7a*), descending aorta (*7d*), right atrium (*1*), right ventricle (*2*), pulmonary artery (*3*), left atrium (*5*), left ventricle (*6*). (**e**) Aberrant subclavian artery, unusual form of right variant on left aortic arch in a 15-month infant with right lung agenesia and both heart and left aortic arch heart shifted to the right. Left aortic arch and course of right aberrant subclavian artery (arrows) are depicted on coronal and axial gradient-echo images; ascending aorta (*7a*), descending aorta (*7d*)

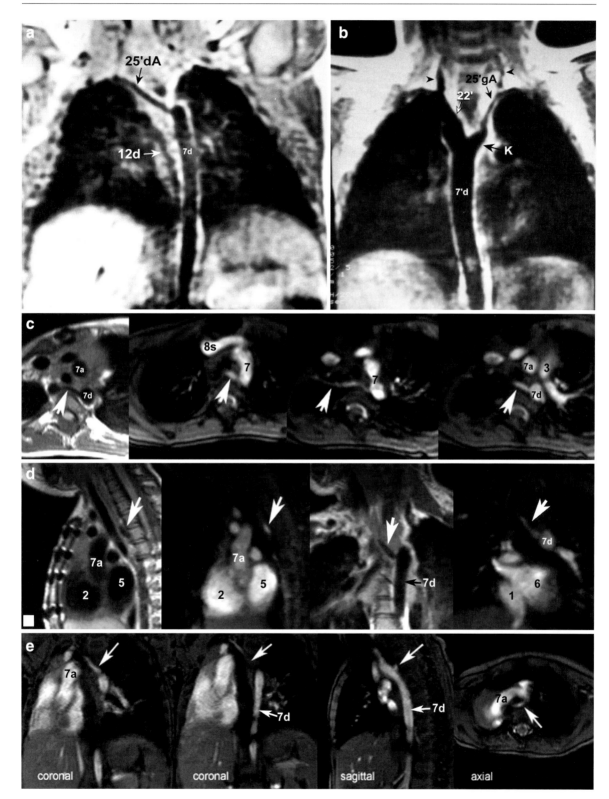

The ligamentum arteriosum can be situated on the right, on both sides, or on the left. A right ligamentum arteriosum is not associated with a vascular ring, but when it is situated (or persists) on the left, the site of interruption determines the type of arch and the possibility of a vascular ring.

- Interruption between the descending aorta and the ligamentum arteriosum

The ligamentum arteriosum is implanted on the subclavian artery (site of involution 1): type 1 right arch or right aortic arch with mirror image branching and no vascular ring (Fig. 5.10b). The same applies when the ligamentum arteriosum is situated on the right.

- Interruption between ligamentum arteriosum and the subclavian artery (site of involution 2)

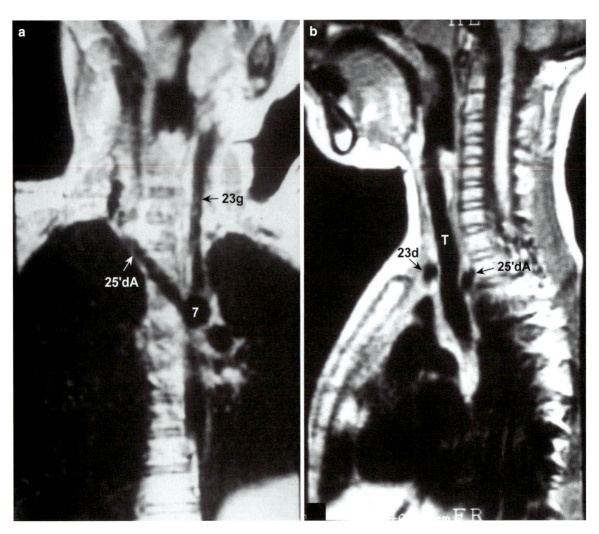

Fig. 5.8 (**a–c**) MRI in a 4-year-old child presenting with dysphagia, vomiting and weight loss: aberrant or retro-oesophageal right subclavian artery. (**a**) Posterior coronal image shows the right subclavian artery (25'dA) arising abnormally from the aortic isthmus (aorta-7) and travelling towards the right upper limb. Note the absence of diverticulum at its origin. (**b**) The sagittal image shows that this artery crosses the oesophagus posteriorly and induces a slight posterior indentation on the trachea (*T*). (**c**) On an anterior coronal image, the right common carotid artery (*23d*) crosses the trachea anteriorly. (**d, e**) Aberrant subclavian artery (*arrows*), right variant on left aortic arch. Two cases are presented: Residual narrowing in a patient with coarctation corrected by a Crawford procedure (**d**) and typical coarctation in a female teenager presenting with arterial hypertension (**e**): Bright-blood gradient-echo images on the right and MR contrast-enhanced angiography (Dota-Gd, Guerbet, France) images on the left. The latter are of better diagnostic quality displaying the vessels on a larger Fov. Descending aorta (*7d*) (also see Chap. 6, Fig. 6.18d, e and Chap. 8, Figs. 8.23b and 8.24 for the Crawford procedure)

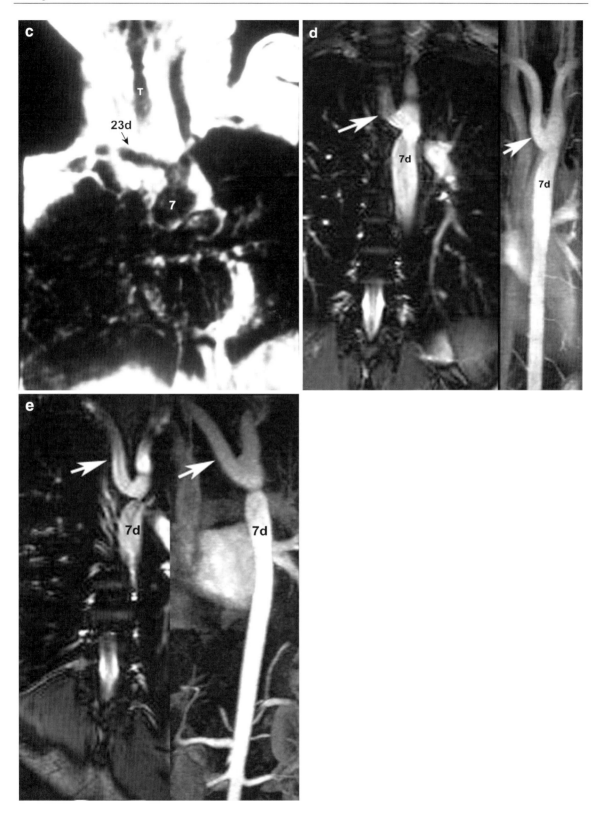

Fig. 5.8 (continued)

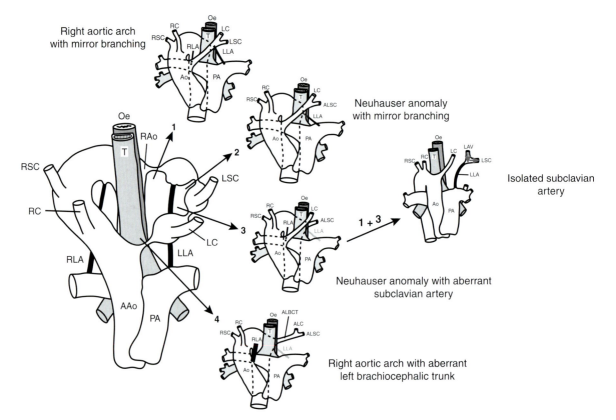

Fig. 5.9 Summary diagram of the various sites of interruption of the left aortic arch with right aortic arch (modified version of the classification of Shuford and Sybers [28]). Involution at 1 with right ligamentum arteriosum (RLA) (Fig. 5.10a), or less frequently, posteriorly to a left ligamentum arteriosum (LLA), which is then inserted onto the left subclavian artery (LSC): type 1 right aortic arch with mirror image branching (Fig. 5.10b), no vascular ring. Involution at 2 between the descending aorta (DAo) with LLA inserted on the DAo and the LSC: type 2 right aortic arch or Neuhauser anomaly with mirror image branching (Fig. 5.12c) and vascular ring. Involution at 3 between the LSC and left common carotid artery (LC) and right ligamentum arteriosum (RLA): right aortic arch with aberrant LSC artery (Fig. 5.6b) and no vascular ring. Involution at 3 and compressive LLA inserted on the aorta: type 3 right aortic arch (with aberrant LSC) or Neuhauser anomaly with arteria lusoria and vascular ring (Fig. 5.12a, b). Involution at 3 and left retro-oesophageal course of the aorta after having described a right arch: encircling aorta generally associated with a loose vascular ring (Fig. 5.14). Involution at 4 between the LC and the ascending aorta and RLA: type 4 right aortic arch with aberrant left brachiocephalic (innominate artery) trunk and no vascular ring (Fig. 5.6c); possibility of vascular ring with LLA (Fig. 5.6c). Involution at 1 and 3 and LLA: type 5 right aortic arch, isolated left subclavian artery with congenital subclavian steal syndrome and no vascular ring (Fig. 5.21). Ascending aorta (AAo), pulmonary artery (PA), descending aorta (DAo), right common carotid artery (RC)

The ligamentum arteriosum is implanted more distally on the aorta (usually but not always via a Kommerell diverticulum): Type 2 right arch or right aortic arch with unusual mirror image branching and possible vascular ring. This form belongs to the group of Neuhauser anomalies (Neuhauser anomaly with mirror image branching, Fig. 5.12c).

- Interruption between the subclavian artery and the left common carotid artery (site of involution 3)

This corresponds to type 3 right arch or right aortic arch with aberrant left subclavian artery and loose or absent vascular ring, as the ligamentum arteriosum is generally situated on the right (type 3 with arteria lusoria and right ligamentum arteriosum, Fig. 5.6b).

If the ligamentum arteriosum is on the left, it is implanted more posteriorly on the descending aorta, generally via a Kommerell diverticulum. This anomaly is similar to type 2, but also comprises an aberrant left subclavian artery (type 3 with arteria lusoria and left ligamentum arteriosum). It belongs to the group of Neuhauser anomalies (Neuhauser anomaly with arteria lusoria and more or less prominent Kommerell diverticulum).

- Interruption anteriorly to the right common carotid artery (site of involution 4).

This corresponds to type 4 right arch or right aortic arch with aberrant left BCT (innominate artery): There is a possibility of vascular ring if the ligamentum arteriosum is situated on the left (LLA). This ring is loose or absent if the ligamentum arteriosum is situated on the right.

- Double interruption

In the case of double interruption between the descending aorta and the left subclavian artery posterior to the left ligamentum arteriosum (site of involution 1), and between the subclavian artery and the left common carotid artery (site of involution 3): Type 5 right arch or right aortic arch with isolated left subclavian artery and possible congenital subclavian steal syndrome, and no vascular ring (Fig. 5.21). Similarly, a double interruption at 1 and 4 and 3 and 4 can lead to isolation of a BCT (innominate artery) or left common carotid artery.

- Other Variants

After describing a right arch, the aorta migrates to the left, obliquely crossing the posterior surface of the oesophagus to become a left-sided structure, therefore forming a tracheo-oesophageal ring. This variant, with a generally loose vascular ring (the ligamentum arteriosum and descending aorta are on the left), is called encircling aorta. Depending on the level of interruption, involution at 3 (usual) or at 2, this variant may or may not be associated with aberrant left subclavian artery.[2]

5.8.1 Right Aortic Arch with Mirror Image Branching and Right Descending Aorta

Right aortic arch with mirror image branching results from complete involution of the left arch between the left subclavian artery and the descending aorta [47]. The first artery arising from the aorta is therefore a left BCT, (innominate artery) followed successively by the right common carotid artery and the right subclavian artery[3] (Fig. 5.10). The descending aorta is on the right and only crosses over to the left side in the inferior part of the thorax. As the ligamentum arteriosum is generally on the right, there is no vascular ring. More rarely, the ligamentum arteriosum is situated on the left, but there is no vascular ring if it is implanted on the left subclavian artery (site of involution 1, type 1 right aortic arch with mirror image branching, see Fig. 5.9).

However, when the ligamentum arteriosum is implanted more posteriorly on the aorta, generally via a Kommerell diverticulum, it can contribute to form a vascular ring (site of involution 2, type 2 right aortic arch with mirror image branching, see Fig. 5.9). This variant is very rare [48] and is part of the group of Neuhauser anomalies (Neuhauser anomaly with mirror image branching, Fig. 5.12a, b) that will be discussed below.

- Clinical features

In its usual form (with right or even left ligamentum arteriosum implanted on the subclavian artery), this malformation is asymptomatic. However, it is almost constantly associated with congenital heart disease (98% of cases), particularly tetralogy of Fallot (48% of cases) (also see Chap. 7, Fig. 7.7b), pulmonary atresia with VSD (Fig. 5.11a–c, and see Chap. 8, Fig. 8.4), tricuspid atresia (Fig. 5.11d, e) and atresia of the left pulmonary artery. This disease is usually discovered during assessment of associated congenital heart disease. In combination with tetralogy of Fallot, a large right aortic arch can compress the right main bronchus that it crosses superiorly (in the absence of a real vascular ring) [49] (see Sect. 5.11.4). Also in combination with tetralogy of Fallot, when Blalock-Taussig shunt is indicated, it must be performed on the left (and not on the right, as is usually the case, see Chap. 8), to avoid kinking of the subclavian artery.

- Imaging

Chest radiograph may show a right aortic knob.

---

[2]See Fig. 5.1.

[3]As indicated above, this type of right aortic arch can be accompanied by aberrant left subclavian artery (*see* Fig. 5.1).

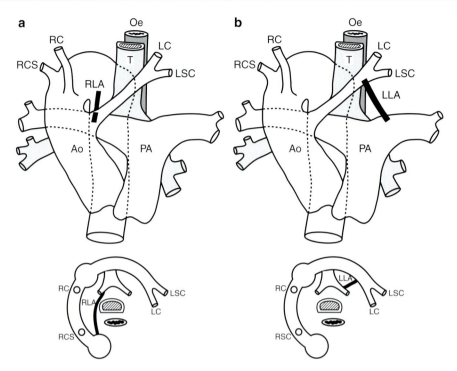

Fig. 5.10 Diagram of the variants of type 1 right aortic arch with mirror image branching (see Figs. 5.1 and 5.9). The ligamentum arteriosum can be situated on the right (RLA) (no vascular ring, (**a**), on both sides, or on the left (LLA). When it is situated on the left, the site of interruption of the left aortic arch determines the site of implantation of the ligamentum arteriosum and the presence or absence of a vascular ring (also see Fig. 5.9). Involution at 1 and implantation of the LLA on the left subclavian artery (LSC): No vascular ring (**b**); involution at 2 and implantation of the LLA on the aorta (vascular ring), very rare form which corresponds to Neuhauser anomaly with mirror image branching (see Fig. 5.12c). Ascending aorta (Ao), pulmonary artery (PA), trachea (T), oesophagus (Oe), right common carotid artery (RC), left common carotid artery (LC), left subclavian artery (LSC) (also see Chap. 7, Fig. 7b)

Barium swallow shows a right lateral oesophageal indentation by the aortic arch with no abnormal posterior indentation.

Echocardiography establishes the diagnosis, especially infants; the suprasternal window shows the ascending aorta and the right aortic arch.

Bronchoscopy is normal in most cases.

MRI provides the same information as angiography. Axial and oblique images visualize the origin of the supra-aortic vessels with a left BCT, a right common carotid artery and then a right subclavian artery. MRI is particularly useful for assessment of associated congenital heart disease, which is often complex (Fig. 5.11) and for analysis of the trachea, which can be compressed by a residual left ligamentum arteriosum inserted onto the aorta (type 2 right arch and vascular ring), which corresponds to a Neuhauser anomaly with mirror image branching (Fig. 5.12c). A left lateral notch on the coronal view of the trachea is suggestive of a compressive left ligamentum arteriosum.

MR angiography, as well as CT-angiography, demonstrates the malformation; the left anterior oblique view shows the mirror image of the vessels arising from the arch and the coronal view shows the arch and the descending aorta on the right. In neonates, umbilical artery catheterization reveals the right-sided descending aorta.

5.8.2 Neuhauser Anomaly

Neuhauser anomaly, a variant of right aortic arch [44], represents 15–20% of all cases of symptomatic aortic arch due to encircling of the trachea and oesophagus. This anomaly is less frequent than simple type 1 right aortic arch (or right aortic arch with mirror image

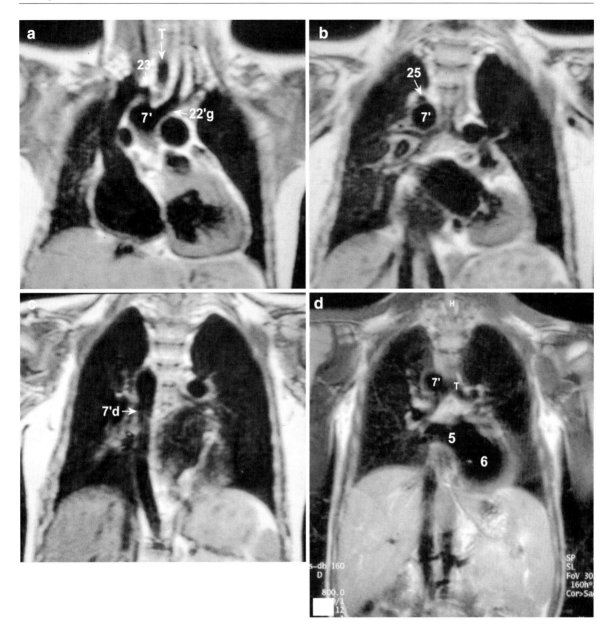

Fig. 5.11 (**a**–**e**) Right aortic arch in two children with cyanotic heart disease. (**a**–**c**) Pulmonary atresia with VSD. Anteroposterior series of coronal spin-echo images. The aorta (7′) forms an arch on the right of the trachea (T), giving rise to a left brachiocephalic trunk (22g′); a right common carotid artery (23d′) and a right subclavian artery (25d′) (see Chap. 8, Fig. 8.19). (**d**, **e**) Type 1b tricuspid atresia. The aorta (7′) forms an arch on the right of the trachea (T) (**d**: coronal spin-echo image); left atrium (5), left ventricle (6) (see Chap. 8, Figs. 8.10 and 8.26 and Chap. 8, Fig. 8.10 for correction by bidirectional cavopulmonary shunt; also see Chap. 6, Fig. 6.4 and Chap. 8, Figs. 8.4 and 8.17). (**e**) Gadolinium-enhanced MR angiography and MIP reconstruction (Dota-Gd, Guerbet, France). (**f**) Right aortic arch (7′) with aberrant LSC artery (*arrows*) arising from a Kommerel diverticulum (Kd) in a young female patient. MR contrast-enhanced angiography (Dota-Gd, Guerbet, France) displays the region of interest on a large on multiplanar and MIP reconstructions on a 180° cine-loop. Although MRI does not explicitly visualize ligamentum arteriosus and its implantation, as this anomaly was discovered incidentally in an adult patient who presented no symptoms, there is no vascular ring and the ligamentum arteriosum is certainly located on the right; descending aorta (7d). For further explanation compare the diagram of two forms of right aortic arches: The right arch with aberrant left subclavian artery and RLA, Fig. 5.11b (similar to the case here Fig. 5.11f, with no vascular ring, nor symptoms) and the Neuhauser anomaly with with LLA, Fig. 5.12b (potential vascular ring and usually symptomatic in the young age – also refer to Fig. 5.13)

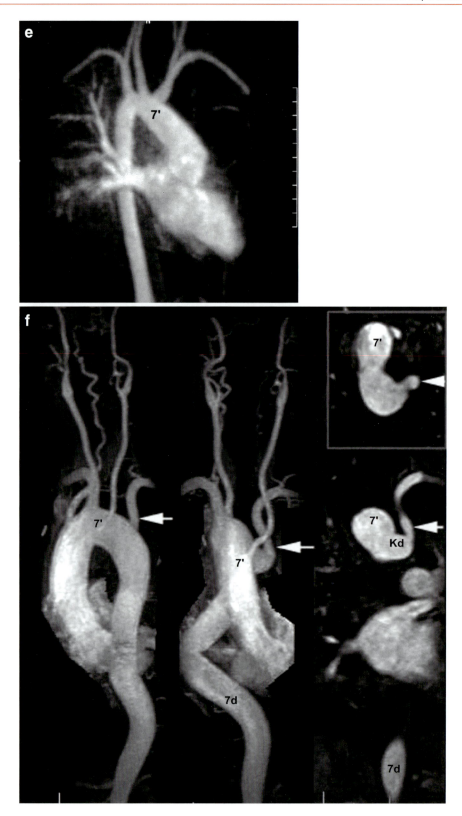

Fig. 5.11 (continued)

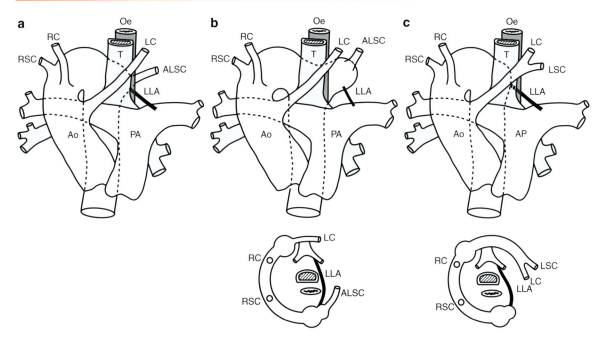

Fig. 5.12 Diagram of Neuhauser anomaly. The ligamentum arteriosum is inserted posteriorly on the aorta forming a vascular ring. There are two forms. (**a**) Usual form with arteria lusoria; involution at 3 and implantation of the left ligamentum arteriosum (LLA) on the aorta generally via a Kommerell diverticulum (KD) (also see involution at 3, Figs. 5.1 and 5.9). This form, particularly when the diverticulum is prominent (**b**), is difficult to distinguish from double aortic arch with partial atresia of the left arch. The vascular ring is generally looser than in double arch, which comprises two potentially compressive structures (see Figs. 5.2c, 5.6b). (**c**) Very rare form with mirror image branching; involution at 2 and implantation of the LLA on the aorta (also see Fig. 5.10b and also involution at 2, Fig. 5.9). The Kommerell diverticulum can also be prominent as in (**b**). Ascending aorta (Ao), pulmonary artery (PA), right common carotid artery (RC), left common carotid artery (LC), left subclavian artery (LSC), aberrant left subclavian artery (ALSC), trachea (T), oesophagus (Oe)

branching and no vascular ring). It actually corresponds to forms of right arch with compressive left ligamentum arteriosum. There are two variants: the usual form with presence of arteria lusoria and the rarer form with mirror image branching.

In the usual form, there is an aberrant left subclavian artery (interruption between the subclavian artery and the right common carotid artery: site of involution 3, type 3 right arch with left ligamentum arteriosum). The vascular ring is formed by the right aortic arch, the Kommerell diverticulum (of variable size), which gives rise to the retro-oesophageal left subclavian artery, and the residual left ligamentum arteriosum (Fig. 5.12a). In most cases, involution is incomplete and the distal portion of the left arch, giving rise to the left subclavian artery, therefore persists in the form of a prominent Kommerell diverticulum forming a large posterior notch that may be suggestive of double arch (Fig. 5.12b). This anomaly is frequently associated with congenital heart disease, such as VSD (rarely in the context of tetralogy of Fallot), transposition of the great vessels, atrioventricular septal defect and cor triatriatum [46].

The other, much rarer variant consists of interruption of the left arch between the ligamentum arteriosum and the subclavian artery resulting in mirror image branching with the left ligamentum arteriosum inserted onto the aorta, generally also via a Kommerell diverticulum (site of involution 2 with type 2 right arch or right aortic arch with mirror image branching and vascular ring or Neuhauser anomaly with mirror image branching, see Fig. 5.12c).

Finally, if the interruption occurs between the left subclavian artery and the left common carotid artery (site of involution 3), as in Neuhauser anomaly with arteria lusoria, but when the ligamentum arteriosum is on the right, there is no vascular ring: This corresponds to right arch with aberrant left subclavian artery (already considered in the paragraph on aberrant left subclavian artery see Figs. 5.6b and 5.13g).

• Clinical features

The vascular ring is generally looser than in double aortic arch and causes minimal or non-specific symptoms: Chronic cough, dyspnoea at exertion, recurrent respiratory tract infections and wheezing. However, the tolerance can be poor when the ligamentum arteriosum is short. In this case, the symptoms are the same as those observed in the double aortic arch (*see this paragraph*).

• Imaging

The AP chest radiograph may show obstructive ventilatory disorders. Absence of the aortic knob (left superior arch) and para-aortic line (midline or right-sided aorta) must be investigated. In young children, on good quality radiographs, the trachea and main bronchi are often clearly visible in contrast with the surrounding mediastinal structures. Consequently, loss of the tracheal radiolucency can be observed in the supracarinal region in the case of Neuhauser anomaly.

Barium swallow if performed, on the AP film, depicts a large right indentation at T3 corresponding to the aortic arch and a lower acute-angled triangular notch situated on the left border, corresponding to compression by a residual ligamentum arteriosum. A left superior oblique draped appearance is suggestive of aberrant left subclavian artery. The lateral film shows the triangular indentation of the compressive ligamentum on the posterior surface of the oesophagus and/or a very large indentation related to Kommerell diverticulum.

Bronchoscopy reveals supra- or juxtacarinal pulsatile anteroposterior flattening of the trachea. The endoscopic appearance is difficult to distinguish from that of double aortic arch. Post-operative bronchoscopy must be performed to verify the condition of the tracheal wall, which generally presents less tracheomalacia than in double arch.

MRI (Fig. 5.13) shows a right arch with right descending aorta and a bulb-shaped Kommerell diverticulum at the origin of the aberrant left subclavian artery. Tracheal compression with left lateral indentation is suggestive of Neuhauser anomaly, but MRI does not explicitly visualize the ligamentum arteriosum and its implantation. Consequently, Kommerell

diverticulum with Neuhauser anomaly of the ligamentum arteriosum can be confused with atresia of the left aortic arch, although this second entity potentially comprises two compressive elements on the left (atresic arch and left ligamentum arteriosum, also see Fig. 5.2c). Neuhauser anomaly (usual form) is, therefore, difficult to distinguish preoperatively from double aortic arch with atresia of the left arch. Signs suggestive of Neuhauser anomaly are associated cardiac anomalies and, to a lesser degree, the descending aorta, which generally remains strictly on the right. MR angiography visualizes an arch on the right with Kommerell diverticulum. It is also difficult to confirm the Neuhauser anomaly due to the difficulty to demonstrate the compressive ligamentum arteriosum.

Finally, it should be remembered that double arch is more frequent, and Neuhauser anomaly with mirror image branching is very rare.

In any event, surgery is formally indicated in both of these anomalies. In the presence of lower airway compression, preoperative MRI assessment of the lesions is generally necessary to determine the surgical incision: Right lateral thoracotomy in the case of diverticulum and/or aberrant left subclavian artery [40, 41, 50] and left lateral thoracotomy in the case of simple anomaly (such as double arch with atresia of the left arch).

5.8.3 Right Aortic Arch with Encircling (or Circumflex) Left Descending Aorta

This malformation is due to a right aortic arch with migration of the posterior segment of the aortic arch to the left. The aortic arch passes to the right of the trachea and the descending aorta obliquely crosses the posterior surface of the oesophagus to lie on the left side (hence the term encircling) [35]. Involution of the right arch generally occurs between the left common carotid and left subclavian arteries (site of involution 3) and the left subclavian artery is then retro-oesophageal,

Fig. 5.13 (**a–f**) Neuhauser anomaly in an infant with reflux. Axial fast spin-echo (**a**, **c**) and gradient-echo (**b**, **d**) images. The right aortic arch (7′) is clearly visualized, together with the Kommerell diverticulum (K), which gives rise to the aberrant left subclavian artery (25′gA). The left common carotid artery is situated anteriorly (23′g). Between the two, there is no real left aortic arch. Anteroposterior series of coronal images (**e**, **f**). The

aortic arch is situated to the right of the trachea (T); left atrium (5), right pulmonary artery (3d) and left pulmonary artery (3g). The aberrant left subclavian artery (25′gA) arises from the Kommerell diverticulum (K). The descending thoracic aorta (7′d) is almost continuous with the right aortic arch and is situated on the right (in the thorax)

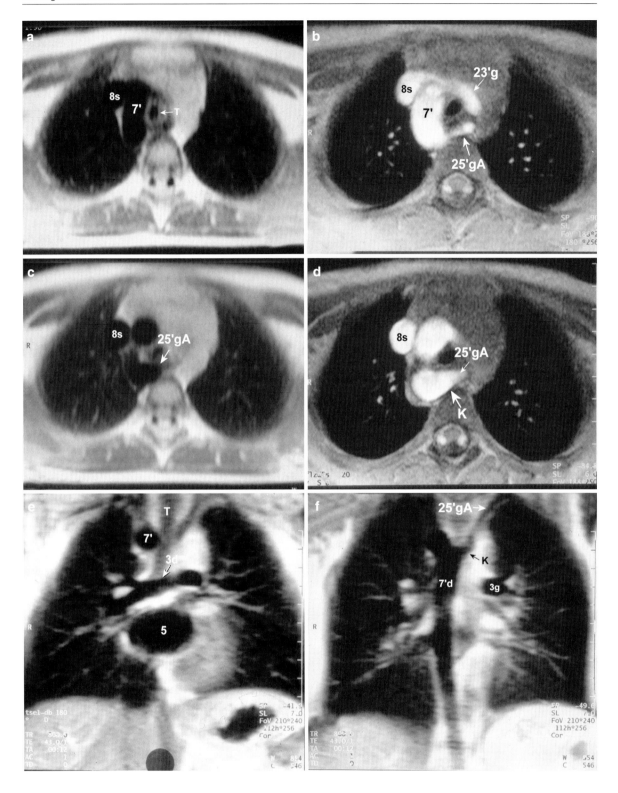

or more rarely between the descending aorta at the site of implantation of the left ligamentum arteriosum and the left subclavian (site of involution 2 with mirror image) (also see Figs. 5.1 and 5.9). Encircling aorta is a rare anomaly, frequently associated with congenital heart disease such as tetralogy of Fallot. There is a risk of tracheo-oesophageal compression due to the retro-oesophageal course of the aorta, sometimes completed by a left ligamentum arteriosum (Fig. 5.14). The vascular ring is generally loose. Migration can also be incomplete with midline retro-oesophageal aorta. A mirror image anomaly also exists with right descending aorta and right ligamentum arteriosum, but it is

very rare. One case was recently reported emphasizing the value of MRI [51].

• Clinical features

In most cases, this anomaly is asymptomatic. When present, symptoms are often gastrointestinal, such as dysphagia or reflux. Patients are usually treated conservatively and section of a vascular ring is rarely necessary.

• Imaging

AP barium swallow shows a very large left inferior oblique indentation corresponding to the retro-

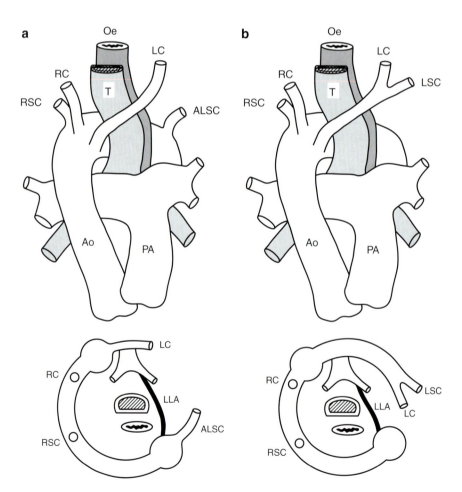

Fig. 5.14 Diagram of right aortic arches with encircling left descending aorta. (**a**) Involution at 3: Aberrant retro-oesophageal left subclavian artery. (**b**) Involution at 2 with mirror image branching. Ascending aorta (Ao), pulmonary artery (PA), right common carotid artery (RC), left common carotid artery (LC), right subclavian artery (RSC), left subclavian artery (LSC), aberrant left subclavian artery (ALSC), trachea (T), oesophagus (Oe). Ligamentum arteriosum can be situated on the right (RLA) or on the left (LLA) (also see Figs. 5.1 and 5.9)

oesophageal segment of the aorta and the lateral film shows a posterior indentation over T5.

Echocardiography does not provide any information.

MRI (Fig. 5.15) with axial and coronal images visualizes the course of the aorta, which describes a right arch before passing behind the oesophagus to form left descending aorta. Narrowing of the tracheal may suggest a complete vascular ring. Sagittal images show the relations of the retro-oesophageal segment of the aorta with the oesophagus.

5.9 Anomalies of the Sixth Aortic Arch

5.9.1 Anomalous Left Pulmonary Artery

Anomalous (retrotracheal) left pulmonary artery is a rare anomaly, which forms a pulmonary artery sling often severely compressing the trachea. In this malformation, the right pulmonary artery is continuous with the pulmonary artery trunk, while the left pulmonary artery arises from either the right pulmonary artery, or

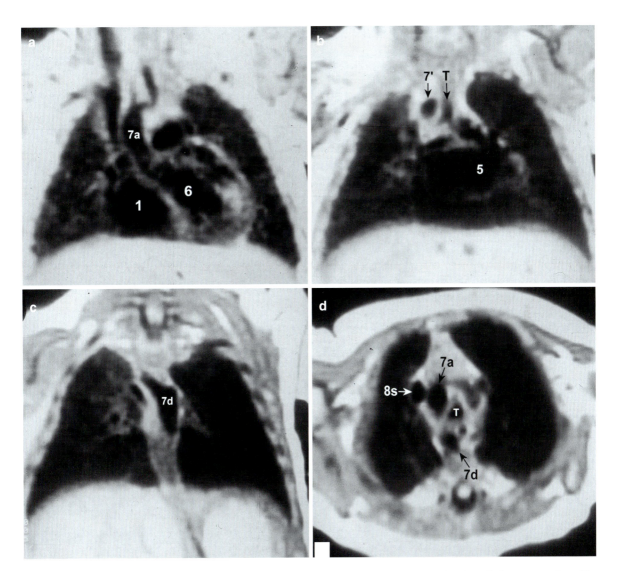

Fig. 5.15 Right aortic arch with encircling left descending aorta in a 3-month-old with reflux. (**a–c**) Anteroposterior series of coronal spin-echo images. The ascending thoracic aorta (*7a*) describes its arch (*7′*) on the right of the trachea (*T*), then passes behind the trachea to gain its normal position on the left (descending thoracic aorta *7d*). These findings are confirmed by axial images (**d**) and (**e**); superior vena cava (*8s*), right atrium (*1*), left atrium (*5*), left ventricle (*6*), pulmonary artery (*3*), trachea (*T*), left main bronchus (*11g*), and right main bronchus (*11d*)

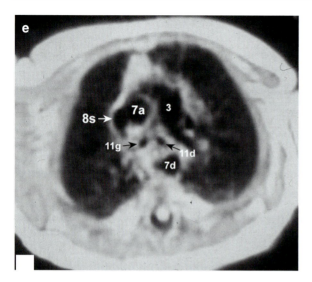

Fig. 5.15 (continued)

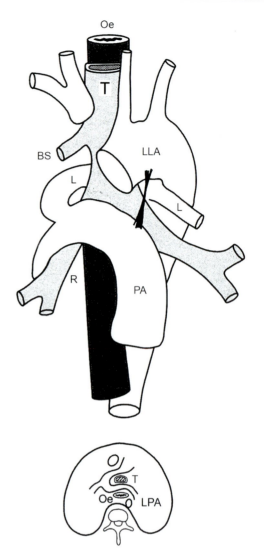

Fig. 5.16 Diagram of anomalous (retrotracheal) left pulmonary artery. Origin of the left pulmonary artery (L and LPA) from the right pulmonary artery (R), sometimes associated with stenosis at this level. The left pulmonary artery then encircles the trachea (T) posteriorly by crossing the oesophagus (Oe) anteriorly and rejoining the left hilum. Aorta (Ao), pulmonary artery (PA), bronchus suis (BS) originating directly from the trachea on the right

the middle of the pulmonary artery trunk. It then travels posteriorly, forming an arch over the right main bronchus and to the right of the trachea (or bronchus intermedius in the case of *bronchus suis*[4]). The artery then crosses the oesophagus anteriorly and the trachea posteriorly to reach the left lung (Fig. 5.16). It compresses the right main bronchus superiorly at its origin and the right and posterior margin of the trachea and induces anterior indentation of the oesophagus. This extrinsic tracheobronchial compression is often accentuated by intrinsic malformations (complete tracheal rings, "chicken" trachea, *bronchus suis*, etc.), which determine the prognosis [52–55].

This malformation can be isolated, but, in more than one half of cases, it is associated with cardiac anomalies [54–56] such as dextrocardia, VSD, tetralogy of Fallot, double outlet right ventricle, interrupted aortic arch and pulmonary artery stenosis.

- Clinical Features

Symptoms in relation with airway central obstruction are usually present very early, at birth or during the first 6 months of life [53, 55]. They are severe: Abnormal respiratory noises, dyspnoea, choking episodes, intermittent cyanosis and recurrent respiratory tract infections. These symptoms are often associated with low birth weight and growth retardation [57].

The surgical reimplantation of the left pulmonary artery is carried out under cardiopulmonary bypass. Various types of surgical tracheoplasty can be proposed at the same operative time in the case of an associated intrinsic tracheal anomaly. The prognosis depends on the extent of the cartilage stenosis and the quality of the tracheal reconstruction. The forms

---

[4]Right upper lobe bronchus – also called "tracheal bronchus - arises directly from the trachea.

without cartilage complete rings or with short-segment stenosis have the better one.

• Imaging

The chest radiograph must be of very good quality. It can show bilateral lung distension (obstructive emphysema), hyperlucency on the right or atelectasis, stenosis of the right and posterior margins of the trachea with deviation to the left and compression at the origin of the right main bronchus [55, 58].

Lateral (or preferably LAO) barium swallow shows a marked anterior concave notch over the tracheal bifurcation [56, 57], but is unable to formally exclude bronchogenic cyst, oesophageal duplication, tumour or lymphadenopathy [53]. It can also be normal in 20% cases.

Echocardiography provides no clear information about the anomaly. It is especially useful for assessment of the associated cardiac anomalies.

Bronchoscopy, often performed under difficult conditions, can show two different types of lesions:

• Anteroposterior flattening of the main carina and the ostia of both mainstem bronchi, with variable evidence of pulsatility (as the pulmonary artery is a low-pressure vessel). This endoscopic appearance of extrinsic compression is always present in the case of anomalous left pulmonary artery.

• Intrinsic stenosis of the tracheal wall due to complete cartilage rings over a variable length. It can affect the whole lower airways ("chicken" trachea), but usually only involves the lower tracheal rings and both mainstem bronchi ostial rings ("funnel" stenosis). The endoscopic appearance is that of rigid circumferential stenosis, stopping the metal rigid tube's course. This particular feature is inconstantly associated with the anomalous left pulmonary artery and worsens the prognosis. The combination of these two types of stenosis has been called "ring-sling complex".

Before MRI and CT, angiography was the only examination able to provide a precise diagnosis of the lesions (Fig. 5.18b).

MRI (Fig. 5.17) in neonates [59, 60] generally visualizes the right and left pulmonary arteries on the same axial image. The origin of the left pulmonary artery to the right of the trachea and its retrotracheal course are easily identified (Figs. 5.17 and 5.18a) [61]. Coronal

and sagittal images confirm the presence of the aberrant vessel and assess its effects on the trachea and bronchi and the presence of an intrinsic anomaly and can also demonstrate associated congenital heart disease.

5.9.2 Congenital Atresia of One of the Two Pulmonary Arteries

This entity is described in Chap. 7.

5.10 Other Clinical Forms

Other clinical forms do not have any major functional repercussions on the trachea and oesophagus (except for right arch with mirror image branching).

5.10.1 Cervical Aortic Arch

Cervical aortic arch is a rare malformation [62, 63] corresponding to persistence of the third arch. The aortic arch ascends to the base of the neck, usually on the right, and crosses the mediastinum generally behind the oesophagus to form the descending aorta which is situated on the left. By definition, an aortic arch is said to be cervical when it exceeds the manubrium sternae (Figs. 5.19 and 5.20) [64, 65]. It is frequently associated with anomalies of the origins of the supra-aortic vessels, particularly aberrant subclavian artery[5] (Fig. 5.19) or coarctation.[6]

• Clinical Features

Cervical aorta is responsible for a pulsatile, expansive mass in the supraclavicular fossa and sometimes in the cervical region. It is exceptionally associated with symptoms such as stridor, expiratory dyspnoea or recurrent tracheitis. We have observed one case with

---

[5]Comprising direct origin of the external and internal carotid and/or vertebral arteries from the aortic convexity.
[6]Reciprocally, the aortic arch is often abnormally high in the case of coarctation of the aorta or pseudo-coarctation (see Chap. 6).

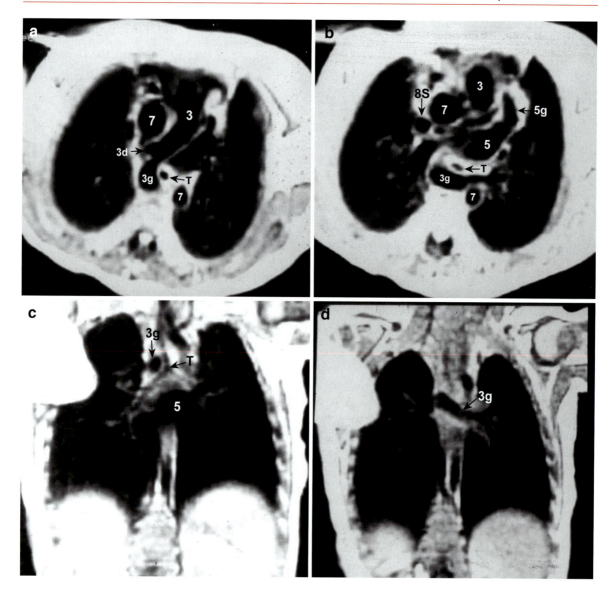

Fig. 5.17 (**a–e**) Anomalous left pulmonary artery. Four-month-old admitted to the intensive care unit with acute respiratory distress [53]. (**a**) Axial image demonstrating the origin of the left pulmonary artery (*3g*) from the right pulmonary artery with stenosis at this level (*3d*) (confirmed surgically), which encircles the trachea posteriorly (*T*); pulmonary artery trunk (*3*), aorta (*7*). (**b**) Axial image showing the retrotracheal course of the left pulmonary artery (*3g*), forming a vascular sling around the trachea (*T*); aorta (*7*), superior vena cava (*8s*), left atrium (*5*) and left atrial appendage (*5g*). (**c, d**) Coronal images. The left pulmonary artery (*3g*) arises to the right of the trachea and then has a retrotracheal course before rejoining the left hilum. Note the narrow trachea (*T*) and main bronchi (intrinsic stenosis due to complete cartilaginous rings). (**e**) Sagittal image demonstrating the vascular sling around the trachea (*T*) formed by the

anomalous left pulmonary artery: The pulmonary artery trunk (*3*) is pretracheal, while the anomalous left pulmonary artery has a retrotracheal course (*3g*); right ventricle (*2*), left ventricle (*6*). Also note (**c**) the right-left pulmonary asymmetry: Right main bronchus on the right which divides into right upper lobe bronchus and bronchus intermedius (trilobed lung) and horizontal left main bronchus on the left (bilobed lung). (**f, g**) Another case of anomalous left pulmonary artery in a newborn. Axial image demonstrates the vascular sling (*arrows*) around the trachea (*T*) formed by the pretracheal pulmonary artery trunk (*3*) and the retrotracheal anomalous left pulmonary artery (*white arrow*). Sagittal image demonstrates compression of trachea posteriorly by the anomalous left pulmonary artery; ascending aorta (*7a*), descending aorta (*7d*)

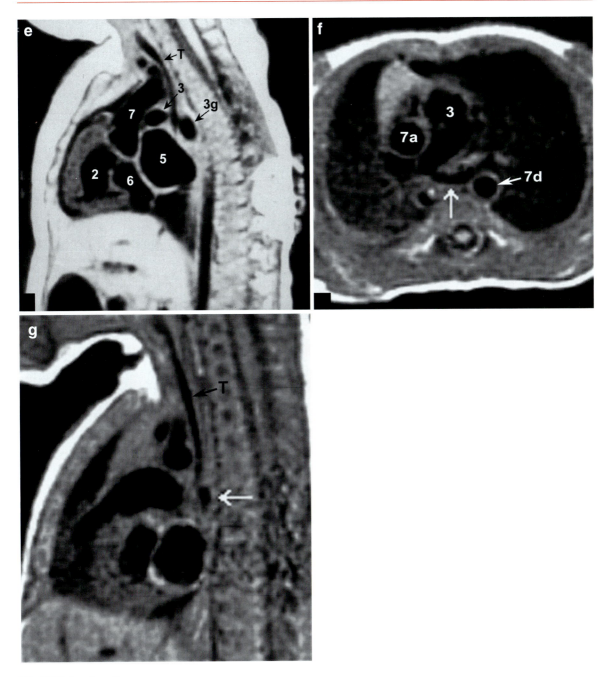

Fig. 5.17 (continued)

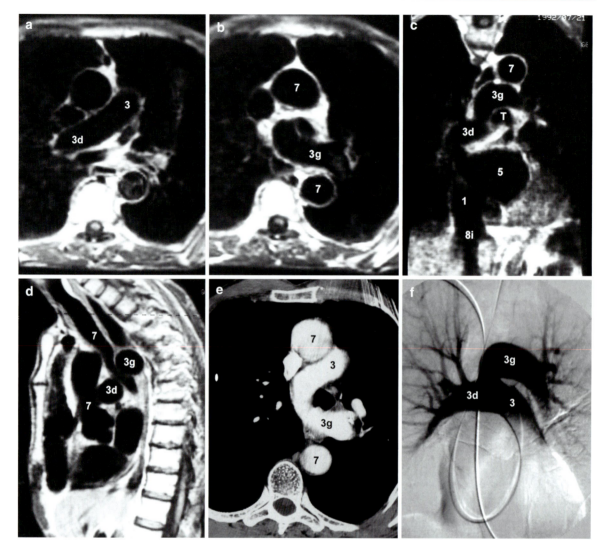

Fig. 5.18 Anomalous left pulmonary artery. Sixty-year-old patient with preoperative incidental discovery of anomalous left pulmonary artery [54]. (**a**, **b**) axial, (**c**) coronal and (**d**) sagittal MRI images; (**e**) axial CT scan and (**f**) pulmonary angiography, AP view. The left pulmonary artery (*3g*) arises from the right pulmonary artery (*3d*) to the right of the trachea (*T*); right atrium (*1*), left atrium (*5*), aorta (*7*), inferior vena cava (*8i*), pulmonary artery (*3*)

recurrent laryngeal nerve paralysis [66]. This anomaly, being benign in nature, does not require any treatment.

• Imaging

Radiography shows an abnormally high aortic arch causing widening of the mediastinum on the AP film and posterior indentation on the lateral film.

Echocardiography may suggest the diagnosis by visualizing an abnormally high aortic arch on a suprasternal view.

MRI and CT (Fig. 5.20) provide the same information, MRI being non-invasive and nonirradiating.

5.11 Isolated Subclavian Artery, Brachiocephalic Trunk (Innominate Artery) or Left Common Carotid Artery-Congenital Subclavian Steal Syndrome

Isolated subclavian artery is a rare malformation, which can be explained embryologically by double interruption between the descending aorta and left subclavian artery posteriorly to the left ligamentum arteriosum (site of involution 1) and between the subclavian artery and left common carotid artery (site of involution 3),

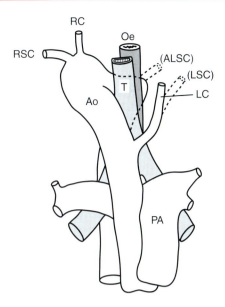

Fig. 5.19 Diagram of the cervical aorta showing the usual variant with right aortic arch. Cervical aorta is often associated with anomalies of the origins of the supra-aortic vessels, such as aberrant left subclavian artery (ALSC), or direct origin of subclavian arteries from the arch. Ascending aorta with cervical arch (Ao), pulmonary artery (PA) right common carotid artery (RC), right subclavian artery (RSC), left common carotid artery (LC), left subclavian artery (LSC), trachea (T), oesophagus (Oe)

resulting in isolation of the subclavian artery in the opposite side of the aortic arch. No vascular ring is thus present (see Fig. 5.9). This anomaly was first described by Ghon in 1908 [67] and the term "isolation" was first introduced by Steward in 1964 [68].

If the ductus arteriosus remains partly patent, the blood supply of the subclavian artery is ensured by the pulmonary arteries. Due to the lower pressure in the pulmonary arterial circulation, pulmonary steal can occur. Isolated left subclavian artery with a right aortic arch is far more common than isolated left subclavian artery [69]. It is frequently associated with conotruncal malformations [70]. If cardiac anomalies are not associated upper left (or right) limb cyanosis can be the only presentation.

Closure of the ductus arteriosus results in "truly" isolation of the subclavian artery with revascularization of the upper limb via the collateral circulation from descending aorta, or via the circle of Willis and the homolateral vertebral artery with retrograde circulation possibly resulting in subclavian steal syndrome) (Fig. 5.21). For this reason, this entity is also incorrectly called "congenital subclavian stenosis or atresia".

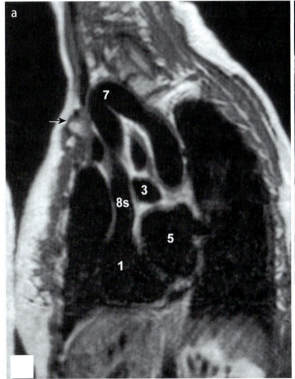

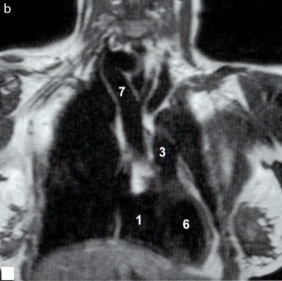

Fig. 5.20 Cervical aorta. (**a**) LAO spin-echo image in the plane of the arch. The aorta describes a hairpin arch (7) in an abnormally high position, well above the sternal (clavicles – *arrows*).

(**b**) Coronal image: the aorta describes a loop in the inferior cervical region on the right. Right atrium (*1*), left atrium (*5*), pulmonary artery (*3*), superior vena cava (*8s*), left ventricle (*6*)

The cerebral repercussions are not as severe as in acquired subclavian steal syndrome in adults and this anomaly is better tolerated in younger children [71]. Symptoms, when present, consist of dizziness, headache, visual disorders accentuated by movements of the arm supplied by the aberrant subclavian artery. Limb atrophy or CNS anomalies have also been described; treatment consists of restoring continuity between the aorta and the subclavian artery via a conduit.

By a similar mechanism, double interruption in 1 and 4 and 3 and 4 can lead to isolation of a BCT or left common carotid artery (see Fig. 5.9).

5.11.1 Persistent Fifth Aortic Arch

This malformation results in a normal aortic arch duplicated by a second aortic arch in the concavity (Fig. 5.22). The superior lumen, with a normal diameter, is derived from the fourth arch and the smaller inferior lumen corresponds to persistence of the fifth arch. This anomaly is very rare [72]; the angiographic features of

a case with double right aortic arch have been described [73]. This anomaly is usually associated with congenital heart disease (tricuspid atresia, cor triatriatum, tetralogy of Fallot, pulmonary atresia with VSD, single coronary artery, etc.) and discovered during assessment of the associated congenital heart disease. In a series of four cases recently published, CE-MRA confirmed persistent fifth aortic arch clarifying uncertain echocardiographic findings [74].

5.11.2 Anomalous Brachiocephalic Trunk (Innominate Artery)

This anomaly will be discussed below.

5.11.3 Pseudo-Coarctation or Kinking of the Aorta

This entity is discussed in Chap. 6 (coarctation).

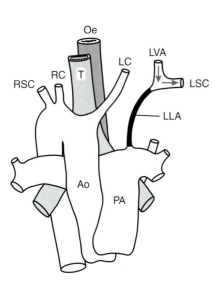

Fig. 5.21 Diagram of congenital subclavian artery stenosis with subclavian steal syndrome (on right aortic arch): Isolation of the subclavian artery results in vascularization of the upper limb by the collateral circulation and partly by retrograde flow from the homolateral vertebral artery (LVA) (subclavian steal – *arrows*) (see double involution at 1 and 3, Fig. 5.9 for an explanation of the mechanism). Ao (aorta), PA (pulmonary artery), right and left common carotid arteries (RC and LC), right and left subclavian arteries (RSC and LSC), oesophagus (Oe), trachea (T)

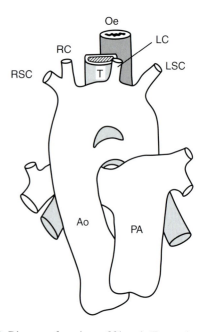

Fig. 5.22 Diagram of persistent fifth arch. Two arches are present on the same side: A normal aortic arch (derived from the fourth arch), with a second aortic arch in the concavity of the first (persistent fifth aortic arch). Ascending aorta (Ao), pulmonary artery (PA), right common carotid artery (RC), left common carotid artery (LC), left subclavian artery (LSC), trachea (T), oesophagus (Oe)

5.11.4 Tracheobronchial Compression Secondary to Cardiovascular Malformations

Some ventricular septal defects induce a large left-to-right shunt with high pulmonary blood flow and marked enlargement of the right ventricular outflow tract. This dilatation of the pulmonary arterial tree can induce compression of the bronchial tree, responsible for more or less early respiratory symptoms with recurrent bronchitis and/or obstructive emphysema of the left lung ("left main bronchus syndrome"[7]). Some cardiac malformations are accompanied by anomalies of the anatomical relations between the carina and pulmonary artery branches (Fig. 5.23), compromising, in particular, the patency of the left main bronchus (hyparterial bronchus – see Chap. 2). Finally, as mentioned above, in the case of combination with tetralogy of Fallot, a large right aortic arch can compress the right main bronchus that it crosses superiorly.

A large patent ductus arteriosus, due to its position, as well as pulmonary atresia can also induce respiratory symptoms.

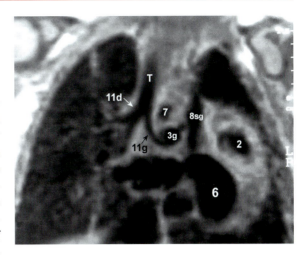

Fig. 5.23 MRI, coronal oblique image in a 2-month-old with emphysema of the left lung due to obstruction of the left main bronchus, as well as complex congenital heart disease with dominant left ventricle (*6*), malposition of the great vessels and tubular hypoplasia of the aorta (see Chap. 6, Fig. 6.9 and Chap. 4, Fig. 4.22). Double vena cava superior is present; here the left superior vena cava is displayed (*8sg*). Note compression of the bronchus by the left pulmonary artery (*3g*). Posteroinferior left dominant ventricle (*6*) and anterosuperior rudimentary right ventricle (*2*), aorta (*7*). Also note the right-left pulmonary asymmetry: Short, vertical, eparterial right main bronchus on the right (*11d*), which divides into the right upper lobe bronchus and right middle lobe bronchus (trilobed lung) and long, horizontal, hyparterial left main bronchus on the left (*11g*) (bilobed lung) (also see Fig. 5.19b, Chap. 2, Figs. 2.2 and 2.7 and Chap. 3, Fig. 3.2)

5.12 Intrinsic Tracheal Anomalies with Tracheal Compression by a Vessel in Normal Position

The tracheal wall can present functional anomalies inducing varying degrees of expiratory collapse. These features of airways dyskinesia can only be visualized by endoscopy. Dyskinesia may be confined to one or several tracheal rings, in which case it usually corresponds to a congenital malformation. It can be accompanied by vascular malformations (e.g. double aortic arch), or may induce tracheal compression by a vessel in a normal position; e.g. "anomalous origin" of the BCT (innominate artery). Lower airway dyskinesia sometimes involves the entire tracheobronchial tree and is then considered to be either "essential" or

secondary to raised intrapulmonary pressure in a context of various obstructive bronchial diseases.

The trachea or bronchi can also be the site of rigid stenoses due to complete cartilaginous rings. Congenital tracheal stenoses can be isolated or part of a more complex vascular malformation (particularly anomalous left pulmonary artery).

5.12.1 Anomalous Brachiocephalic Trunk (Innominate Artery)

In their initial description, Gross and Neuhauser considered this anomaly to be an abnormal origin of the BCT, situated too far to the left, and they classified it with aortic arch anomalies.

However, a number of subsequent studies have shown that the BCT arises to the left of the trachea in 95% of normal children and that it induces anterior

---

[7]Related to the intimate anatomical relations of the left pulmonary artery which crosses over the left main bronchus by describing a superolaterally convex arch (see Chap. 2).

indentation of the trachea in 30% of normal children. This appearance is only considered to be significant when the tracheal lumen is reduced by more than 50% or when it is accompanied by marked dyskinesia. Although this syndrome of tracheal compression by the BCT has been well described, it can no longer be considered to be a congenital aortic arch anomaly, but rather a functional anomaly causing clinical signs related to decreased rigidity of the trachea. The most severe symptomatic forms of this condition are usually observed in the context of associated oesophageal atresia, with or without tracheo-oesophageal fistula.

• Clinical Features

Depending on the degree of tracheal compression, clinical signs may range from simple stridor with barking cough to more severe respiratory involvement, such as chronic bacterial colonization of the lower airway, persistent dyspnoea with hyperextension of the head and neck, failure to thrive, and anoxic spells.

In children who have undergone surgical correction of oesophageal atresia, tracheal compression by the innominate artery is a classical cause of failure to extubate neonates after surgical repair of oesophageal atresia. Later on, choking episodes are particularly suggestive when they occur while swallowing solid foods. They usually indicate oesophageal anastomosis post-operative restenosis, the upper segment of which being overdistended by food and flattening the malacic trachea onto the innominate artery.

Most cases are not so severe and only require conservative management as the disorders generally improve during the first years of life. Surgery may only be discussed in children with poor tolerance or life-threatening events despite appropriate medical care, consisting of anterior aortopexy. An interesting alternative consists of endoscopic tracheal stenting (Figs. 5.25 and 5.26) for several months whilst the space between the BCT and the trachea enlarges physiologically with growth of the aortic arch.

The key examination is bronchoscopy, which usually shows pulsatile compression of the cervicothoracic segment of the trachea; the extrinsic indentation is classically right anterolateral (Fig. 5.25), but sometimes anteroposterior in major forms. Loss of the right radial and carotid pulses when applying pressure to the notch by a rigid bronchoscope is inconstantly observed [75]. Bronchoscopy also allows assessment of the degree of associated tracheal dyskinesia.

• Imaging

MRI axial images when performed, clearly visualize the horizontal BCT (innominate artery) passing from left to right and compressing the trachea anteriorly. Sagittal images show focal compression of the trachea and assess its severity (Fig. 5.24). Bright-blood Cine-MR sequences demonstrate the pulsatile nature of the tracheal compression.

5.12.2   Post-operative Vascular Malposition with Secondary Airway Compression

Some congenital heart diseases induce an anomaly of the anatomical relations between the great vessels and the trachea: Transposition of the great vessels (Fig. 5.23), tetralogy of Fallot, and double outlet right ventricle. Surgical correction of the cardiovascular anomaly can accentuate these abnormal anatomical relations, sometimes inducing significant tracheobronchial compression (Figs. 5.27 and 5.28). Surgical revision increases compressive phenomena due to mediastinal fibrosis induced by these successive operations. Calibration by endotracheal or endobronchial stent may be considered on the basis of comparison of endoscopic and MRI findings (Fig. 5.29).

In the absence of any primary cardiovascular anomaly, other congenital malformations can induce vascular compression of the airways after surgical correction, particularly in the presence of severe pulmonary hypoplasia responsible for side-to-side rocking of the heart and mediastinum. The trachea is then compressed between a vessel anteriorly and the vertebrae posteriorly ("vertebral compression" syndrome) (Fig. 5.30).

We have observed the following unusual case: Congenital aortic stenosis in a neonate, dilated by balloon catheter endovascular insertion during the neonatal period [76], which subsequently caused dilatation of the BCT (innominate artery) with major compression of the trachea (Fig. 5.31). Tracheal obstruction was relieved by surgical anterior aortopexy, and the respiratory symptoms dramatically improved.

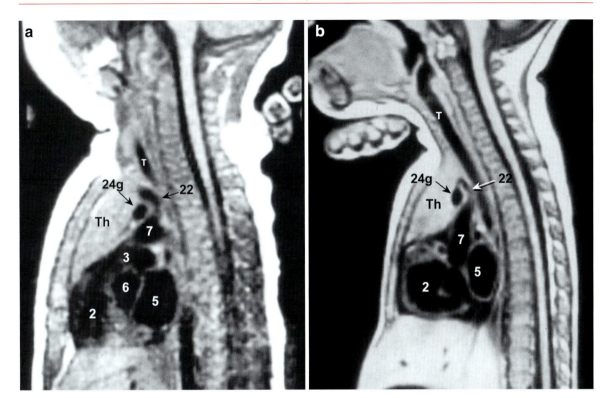

Fig. 5.24 Neonate presenting with severe hypoxic spells. Anteroposterior compression of the superior part of the intrathoracic trachea (*T*) by the brachiocephalic trunk (innominate artery BCT – *22*). MRI clearly demonstrates compression by the BCT on sagittal (**a**) image. Compare the sagittal image (**a**) with that of a normal case without tracheal compression (**b**). Sagittal (**d**) and axial (**e**) cine-MR image clearly demonstrate compression (*white arrows*) of the trachea (air filled – black signal), anteriorly by the BCT (circulating blood – bright signal) (*arrows*). Thymus (*Th*), aorta (*7*), right pulmonary artery (*3*), left atrium (*5*), left ventricle (*6*), right ventricle (*2*) and left brachiocephalic vein (*24g*). Also note, as in Fig. 5.23, the right-left pulmonary asymmetry: Short, vertical, eparterial right main bronchus on the right (*11d*), which divides into the right upper lobe bronchus and right middle lobe bronchus (trilobed lung) and long, horizontal, hyparterial left main bronchus on the left (*11g*) (bilobed lung) (also see Fig. 5.19b, Chap. 2, Figs. 2.2 and 2.7 and Chap. 3, Fig. 3.2)

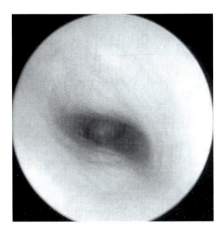

Fig. 5.25 Tracheal endoscopy in a neonate with failure to extubate after surgical correction of oesophageal atresia. Pulsatile right anterolateral compression of the intrathoracic trachea, with dynamic expiratory collapse

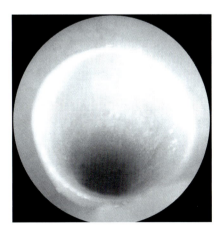

Fig. 5.26 Same patient as in Fig. 5.25 after insertion of a silicone stent with an outer diameter of 6 mm. Resolution of symptoms and successful extubation

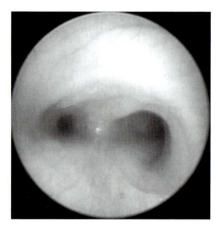

Fig. 5.27 Endoscopic view of the main carina in a one-month-old child after surgical correction of transposition of the great vessels (arterial switch, see Chap. 8, Figs. 8.13–817). Note the decreased calibre of the left main bronchus compared to the right main bronchus (extrinsic, pulsatile stenosis)

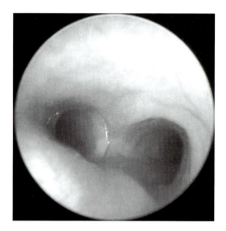

Fig. 5.29 Endoscopic view of the main carina in the same child after insertion of a silicone stent (outer diameter 5 mm) into the left main bronchus

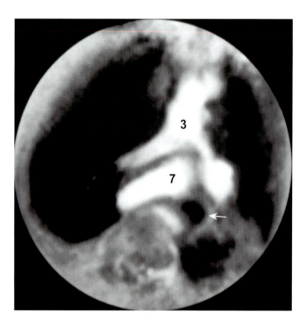

Fig. 5.28 MRI, axial bright-blood sequence of the main carina (right and left are reversed compared to the endoscopic image, same patient as in Fig.5.27). The right mainstem bronchus has a normal calibre (*arrow*); the left bronchus is almost virtual, compressed by the aortic arch (*7*). Note the anomalous position of the aorta (transposed) in relation to the pulmonary artery (*3*)

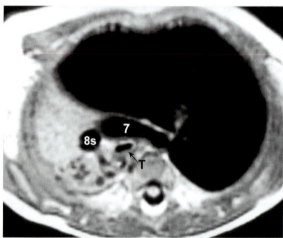

Fig. 5.30 MRI, axial image in a neonate after surgical reduction of congenital right diaphragmatic hernia, who could not be extubated post-operatively. Endoscopy showed major tracheal twisting. The marked right pulmonary hypoplasia induces a right-sided shift of the heart and tension on the aortic arch (*7*) with prevertebral compression of the trachea (*T*). This compression was relieved by insertion of an inflatable right intrathoracic prosthesis, which recentered the mediastinum and released the trachea; superior vena cava (*8s*)

5.12.3 *Tracheal Compression by a Non-Vascular Mediastinal Mass*

Although not related to an aortic arch anomaly, some dysembryoplastic tumours of the mediastinum may have a similar clinical and endoscopic presentation, the reason why they are discussed in this chapter. They are rare and difficult to diagnose, as they are masked by the opacity of the mediastinum; they are difficult to visualize on conventional radiology. Ultrasoud by a substernal view is contributive. Multi-slice contrast enhanced CT scan with its high spatial resolution and the inherent modern post-processing techniques (multiplanar and 3D image reconstruction, including volume-rendered imaging and virtual bronchoscopy [25–27]) is also a valuable tool in diagnosing mediastinal masses

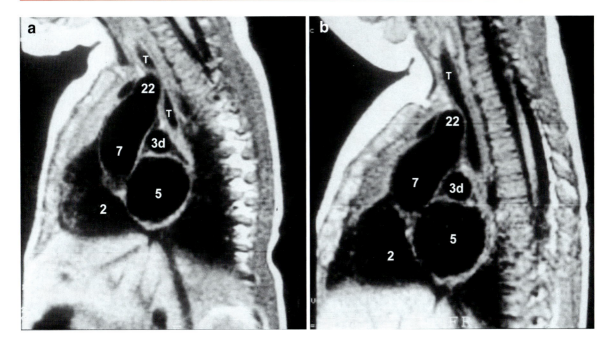

Fig. 5.31 Dilatation of the brachiocephalic trunk secondary to aortic stenosis (jet lesion) in a 1-month-old infant [64]. (**a**) Preoperative sagittal image: Severe compression of the trachea (*T*) by the dilated brachiocephalic trunk (innominate artery *22*). (**b**) Post-operative sagittal image at the same level. After aortopexy and anterior fixation onto the sternum, the indentation of the trachea is much less marked; aorta (*7*), right pulmonary artery (*3d*), left atrium (*5*), right ventricle (*2*)

compromising the airways [27, 28]. These tumours arise in the poorly distensible, narrow mediastinal space of young infants. They rapidly compress the airways and are classically responsible for asthma-like symptoms in infants. Failure to diagnose these tumours may lead to acute respiratory failure or pulmonary

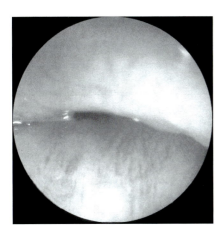

Fig. 5.32 Endoscopy in a 6-month-old child anteriorly diagnosed as asthmatic and admitted in the intensive care unit with acute respiratory distress. Complete and non-pulsatile extrinsic compression of the main carina

destruction. The endoscopic appearance is that of extrinsic tracheobronchial compression at a level corresponding to the site of the mass. The non-pulsatile nature of the compression may not always be apparent due to transmitted pulsations when the mass is in contact with the heart or aorta.

Two radiological forms are encountered:

- Solid tumours: teratomas and dysembryomas. Radiopaque structures (dental buds, calcifications) are sometimes visible on conventional radiology; MRI provides little information compared to computed tomography.
- Cystic tumours, usually with a liquid content. They can be difficult to distinguish from the surrounding mediastinal structures on computed tomography when the cyst content is thick. They include bronchogenic cysts (Figs. 5.32 and 5.33), neurenteric cysts and oesophageal duplication cysts.

The differential diagnosis of these dysembryoplastic tumours of the mediastinum of young children rarely includes lymphadenopathy (inflammatory, neoplastic), which generally has a very different clinical expression and clinical course.

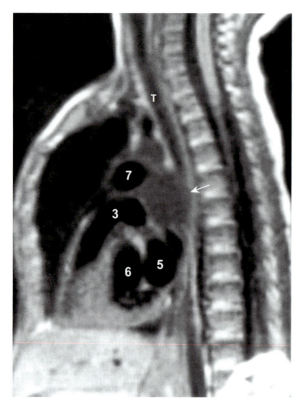

Fig. 5.33 MRI, sagittal image in the same child. Note the cystic image (*arrow*) which compresses the anterior surface of the carina; trachea (*T*). Histological examination: Bronchogenic cyst. Aorta (*7*), pulmonary artery (*3*), left atrium (*5*), left ventricle (*6*)

References

 1. Corone P, Vernant P. Anomalies des arcs aortiques. Encycl Med Chir, Coeur et vaisseaux. 1970:11040 M50, p. 8.
 2. Edwards JE. Anomalies of derivatives of aortic arch system. Med Clin North Am. 1948;32:925–49.
 3. Losay J, Binet JP. Diagnostic des anomalies des arcs aortiques. Encycl Med Chir, Radiodiagnostic III. 1991;32015: F60.
 4. Remy J, Beguery P, Brombart M. Anomalies des arcs aortiques. Traité de Radiodiagnostic: XIX (fasc.2) EI, 1978, Masson.
 5. Enderlein M, Silverman N, Stanger P, Heymann M. Usefulness of suprasternal notch echocardiography for diagnosis of double aortic arch. Am J Cardiol. 1986;57:359–61.
 6. Gomez A, Lois J, George B, Alpan G, Williams R. Congenital abnormalities of the aortic arch. MR imaging. Radiology. 1987;165:691–5.
 7. Wood RE, Postma D. Endoscopy of the airways in s and children. J Pediatr. 1988;112:1–6.
 8. Desnos J. L'endoscopie de diagnostic dans les malformations congénitales trachéo-bronchiques. Chir Pédiatr. 1984;25:202–6.
 9. Couvreur J, Grimfeld A, Tournier G, Autier CH, Le Moine G, Gaurtier CC, et al. La dyskinésie trachéale (trachéomalacie) chez l'enfant. Réflexions à propos de 127 cas reconnus par endoscopie. Sem Hop Paris. 1981;57:688–97.
10. Donato L, Livolsi A, Grimfeld A, Kastler B, Benoit M, Messer J. Sténoses trachéo-bronchiques congénitales: exploration par résonance magnétique. Med Infant (Paris). 1991;8:583–7.
11. Benjamin B. Endoscopy in congenital tracheal anomalies. J Pediatr Surg. 1980;15:164–71.
12. Kastler B, Livolsi A, Germain P, Zollner G, Willard D, Wackenheim A. Magnetic resonance imaging in congenital heart diseases of newborns: preliminary results in 23 patients. Eur J Radiol. 1990;10:109–17.
13. Soulen RL, Donner RM. Advances in non-invasive evaluation of congenital anomalies of the thoracic aorta. Radiol Clin North Am. 1985;23:727–36.
14. Fletcher BD, Darborn DG, Mulopulos GP. MR imaging in s with airway obstruction: preliminary observation. Radiology. 1986;160:245–9.
15. Julsrud PR, Ehman RL. Magnetic resonance imaging of vascular rings. Mayo Clin Proc. 1986;61:181–5.
16. Bisset III GS, Strife JL, Kirks DR, Bailey WW. Vascular rings: MR imaging. AJR Am J Roentgenol. 1987;149:251–6.
17. Kersting-Sommerhoff BA, Sechtem VP, Fisher MR, Higgins CB. MR imaging of congenital anomalies of the aortic arch. AJR Am J Roentgenol. 1987;149:9–13.
18. Kastler B, Livolsi A, Germain P, et al. Contribution of MRI in the evaluation of vascular rings in infants and newborns. RSNA, 76th Assembly and Annual Meeting, Chicago, 25–30 November 1990. Radiology 1990;177, abstract p. 99.
19. Sarbeu M, De Blic J, Le Bourgeois M, Mamou Mani T, Revillon Y. Approche diagnostique pratique des anomalies des arcs aortiques. Rev Mal Resp. 1990;7:51–7.
20. Lebras Y, Kastler B, Livolsi A, Germain P, et al. Intérêt de l'IRM dans les anomalies des arcs aortiques. Feuillets de Radiologie. 1992;32:347–54.
21. Berdon WE. Rings, slings, and other things: vascular compression of the infant trachea updated from the midcentury to the millennium – the legacy of Robert E. Gross, MD, and Edward B.D. Neuhauser, MD. Radiology. 2000;216:624–32.
22. Donnelly LF, Strife JL, Bisset III GS. The spectrum of extrinsic lower airway compression in children: MR imaging. AJR Am J Roentgenol. 1997;168:59–62.
23. Katz M, Konem E, Rozenman J, et al. Spiral CT and 3D image reconstruction of vascular rings and associated tracheobronchial anomalies. J Comput Assist Tomogr. 1995;19: 564–8.
24. Lowe GM, Donaldson JS, Backer CL. Vascular rings: 10-year review of imaging. Radiographics. 1991;11:637–46.
25. Haramati LB, Glickstein JS, Issenberg HJ, Haramati N, Crooke GA. MR imaging and CT of vascular anomalies and connections in patients with congenital heart disease: significance in surgical planning. Radiographics. 2002;22:337–49.
26. Berrocal T, Madrid C, Novo S, Gutierrez J, Arjonilla A, Gomez-Leon N. Congenital anomalies of the tracheobronchial tree, lung, and mediastinum: embryology, radiology, and pathology. Radiographics. 2004;24:e17. doi:10.1148/rg.e17.
27. Yenduduri S, Guillerman RP, Chung T, Braverman RM, Dishop MK, Giannoni CM, et al. Continuing medical education: multimodality imaging of tracheobronchial

disorders in children. Radiographics. 2008;28:e29. doi:10.1148/rg.e29.

28. Winters WD, Effmann EL. Congenital masses of the lung: prenatal and postnatal imaging evaluation. J Thorac Imaging. 2001;16:196–206.

29. Moodie D, Yiannikas J, Gill C, et al. Intravenous digital subtraction angiography in the evaluation of congenital abnormalities of the aorta and aortic arch. Am Heart J. 1982;104:628–34.

30. Chernin M, Pond G, Sahn D. Digital subtraction angiography of the aortic arch. Cardiovasc Intervent Radiol. 1984;7:196–203.

31. Tonkin I, Gold R, Moser D, Laster R. Evaluation of vascular rings with digital subtraction angiography. AJR Am J Roentgenol. 1984;42:1287–91.

32. Otero-Cagide M, Moodie D, Sterba D, et al. Digital subtraction angiography in the diagnosis of vascular rings. Am Heart J. 1986;112:1304–8.

33. Wolman I. Syndrome of constricting double aortic arch in infancy. J Pediatr. 1939;14:527–33.

34. Gross R, Ware P. The surgical significance of aortic arch anomalies. Surg Gynecol Obstet. 1946;83:435–48.

35. Shuford WH, Sybers G. The aortic arch and its malformations. With emphasis on its angiocardiographic features. Springfield: Charles C. Thomas Edition; 1973.

36. Kastler B, Livolsi A, Germain P, Daltroff G, Willard D. Diagnostic de double arc aortique en période néonatale: apport de l'imagerie par résonance magnétique. A propos d'une observation. J Radiol. 1988;69:625–8.

37. Bernard C, Galloy MA, Marcon F, Prevot J, Hoeppel JC, Pernot C, et al. Apport de l'IRM au diagnostic de double arc aortique. Arch Mal Coeur. 1988;81:1277–80.

38. Manou Mani T, Lallemand D, Brunelle F, Barth MO. IRM des anomalies des arcs aortiques chez l'enfant. Premiers résultats. J Radiol. 1988;69:751–7.

39. Simoneaux SF, Bank ER, Webber JB, Parks WJ. MR imaging of the pediatric airway. Radiographics. 1995;15:287–98.

40. Stark J, Roesler A, De Leval M. The diagnosis of airway obstruction in children. J Pediatr Surg. 1985;20:113–7.

41. Mc Faul R, Millard P, Nowicki E. Vascular rings necessitating right thoracotomy. J Thorac Cardiovasc Surg. 1981;82:306–9.

42. Molz G, Burri B. Aberrant subclavian artery (arteria lusoria): sex differences in the prevalence of various forms of the malformation. Virchows Arch A Pathol Anat Histol. 1978;380:303–15.

43. Hastreiter AR, D'cruz IA, Talat-Cantez E. Right sided aorta. Part I. Occurrence of right aortic arch in various types of congenital heart disease. Br Heart J. 1966;28:722.

44. Neuhauser E. The roentgen diagnosis of double aortic arch and other anomalies of the great vessels. Am J Roentgenol Radium Ther. 1946;56:1–12.

45. Vogl T, Wilimzig C, Hofmann U, Dresel S, Lissner J. MRI in tracheal stenosis by innominate artery in children. Padiatr Radiol. 1991;21:89–93.

46. Knight L, Edwards J. Right aortic arch: types and associated cardiac anomalies. Circulation. 1974;50:1047–51.

47. Garti I, Aygen M, Vidne B, et al. Right aortic arch with mirror-image branching causing vascular ring: a new classification of the right aortic arch patterns. Br J Radiol. 1973;46:115–9.

48. Schlesinger AE, Mendeloff E, Sharkey AM, Spray TL. MR of right aortic arch with mirror-image branching and a left ligamentum arteriosum: an unusual cause of a vascular ring. Pediatr Radiol. 1995;25:455–7.

49. Gidding S, Beekman R, Lebowitz E, et al. Airway compression by a right aortic arch in the absence of a vascular ring. Chest. 1984;85:703–5.

50. Fournial JF, Stanley P, Fouron JC, Guerin R, Davignon A. Les anomalies de l'arc aortique. A propos de 30 cas opérés chez l'enfant. Arch Mal Coeur. 1975;5:485–95.

51. Belarbi N, Sebag G, Holvoet P, Delagaussie P, Lupogazloff JM, et Hassan M. Arc aortique gauche avec aorte descendante droite et ligament artériel droit chez un nourrisson. J Radiol. 1998;79:61–3.

52. Fortier-Beaulieu M, Mozziconacci JG, Expert-Bezancon MC. Oesophage et pathologie respiratoire en pédiatrie. Technique et indication de l'examen radiologique. Ann Pédiatr. 1983;30:211–7.

53. Cohen S, Landing B. Tracheostenosis and bronchial abnormalities associated with pulmonary artery sling. Ann Otol Rhinol Laryngol. 1976;85:582–90.

54. Sade R, Rosenthal A, Fellows K, et al. Pulmonary artery sling. J Thorac Cardiovasc Surg. 1975;69:333–46.

55. Gumbier C, Mullins C, Mc Namara D. Pulmonary artery sling. Am J Cardiol. 1980;45:311–5.

56. Berdon WB, Baicer DH, Wung JT, Chrispin A, Kozlowski K, De Silva M, et al. Complete cartilage-ring tracheal stenosis associated with anomalous left pulmonary artery: the ring-sling complex. Radiology. 1984;152:57–64.

57. Contro S, Miller R, White H, Potts WJ. Bronchial obstruction due to pulmonary artery anomalies. I vascular sling. Circulation. 1958;17:418.

58. Capitanio MA, Ramos R, Kirkpatrick JA. Pulmonary sling: roentgen observation. Am J Roentgenol Radium Ther Nucl Med. 1971;112:28.

59. Malmgren N, Laurin S, Lundstron NR. Pulmonary artery sling: diagnosis by magnetic resonance imaging. Acta Radiol. 1988;529:7–9.

60. Livolsi A, Kastler B, Donato L, Willard D, Geissert J. Diagnostic par imagerie par résonance magnétique d'une artère pulmonaire rétrotrachéale. Ann Angiol Cardiol. 1991;40:29–32.

61. Jahn C, Kastler B, Gangi A, Allal R, Dumont P, Abbes A, Bourjat P, et al. Diagnostic d'une opacité médiastinale chez l'adulte. Imagerie d'aujourd'hui, avril. 1993.

62. Mullins CE, Gillette PC, Mc Namara DG. The complex of cervical aortic arch. Pediatrics. 1973;51:210.

63. Bourdon JL, Hoeffel JC, Worms AM, Picard L, Pernot C. L'aorte cervicale: aspects radiologiques, à propos d'un cas avec dysplasie artérielle diffuse. J Radiol Electrol. 1978;59(2):133–40.

64. Kennard DR, Spigos DG, Tan SS. Cervical aortic arch: correlation with conventional radiologic studies. AJR Am J Roentgenol. 1983;141:295–7.

65. Unal A, Baran U, Eyup H, Ergun S. Cervical aortic arch; a case report. Angiology. 1997;48:659.

66. Delabrousse E, Clair C, Couvreur M, Clergeot-Grelier ML, Kastler B. Crosse aortique cervicale révélée par une paralysie récurentielle droite. J Radiol. 2000;81:542–4.

67. Ghon A. Uber eine seltene Entwicklungsstorung des Gefasssystems. Verh Dtsch Ges Pathol. 1908;1(2):242–7.

68. Stewart JA, Kincaid OW, Edwards JE. An atlas of vascular rings and related malformations of the aortic arch system. Springfield: Thomas; 1964.
69. Baudet E, Roques XF, Guibaud JP, Laborde N, Choussat A. Isolation of the right subclavian artery. Ann Thorac Surg. 1992;53(3):501–3.
70. Nath PH, Castaneda-Zuniga W, Zollikofer C, Delany DJ, Fulton RE, Amplatz K, et al. Isolation of a subclavian artery. AJR Am J Roentgenol. 1981 Oct;137(4):683–8.
71. Becker AE, Becker MJ, Edwards JE. Congenital anatomic potentials for subclavian steal. Chest. 1971;60:4–13.
72. Gerlis LM, Dickinson DF, Wilson N, Gibbs JL. Persistent fifth aortic arch. A report about two new cases and a review of the literature. Int J Cardiol. 1987;16:185–92.

73. Boothryod E, Walsh KP. The fifth aortic arch: a missing link? Pediatr Radiol. 1999;29:52.
74. Zhon Y, Jaffe RB, Zhu M, Sun A, Li Y, Gao W. Contrast enhanced MRA of persistent fifth aortic arch in children. Pediatr Radiol. 2007;37(3):256–63.
75. Fearon B, Shortredd R. Tracheo-bronchial compression by congenital cardiovascular anomalies in children. Syndrome of apnea. Ann Otol Rhinol Laryngol. 1963;72:749–69.
76. Livolsi A, Donato L, Germain P, Kastler B, Bintner M, Casanova R, et al. Pre- and post-operative MRI study of an aneurysms of the right brachiocephalic artery with tracheal compression. Eur J Pediatr. 1993;152:457–60.

Malformations of the thoracic aorta are relatively frequent and are grouped into three different categories:

- Aortic arch anomalies, which have already been described in the previous chapter.
- Decreased caliber of the aorta with coarctation of the aortic isthmus responsible for left ventricular outflow tract obstruction and accounting for 95% of cases (together with rarer coarctation of the abdominal aorta and interrupted aortic arch).
- Dilatation of the aortic lumen, essentially in the context of Marfan disease.

Development of magnetic resonance imaging (MRI) and computed tomography (CT) have helped to overcome the limitations of echocardiography [1] and angiography [1, 2] for the depiction of extracardiac vascular structures.

CT is an effective and rapid imaging modality for the evaluation of aorta, determination of the degree of coarctation, and visualization of collateral vessels [3, 4]. However, in contrast to MRI, CT is limited by the inability to provide hemodynamic information [4, 5]. It has nevertheless the advantages of widespread availability and short acquisition times [4]. Moreover, it can be performed on patients with a pacemaker or an internal cardioverter-defibrillator [6]. Multislice CT allows for faster acquisition, higher spatial resolution, and simultaneous assessment of cardiovascular structures and lung parenchyma. It therefore represents a valuable tool for the evaluation of patients with aortic malformations[7]. When coupled with electrocardiographic (ECG) data, motion artifacts are reduced and CT accurately delineates rapidly moving cardiac and paracardiac structures. The various postprocessing techniques available (multiplanar reformation, maximum intensity projection (MIP), and volume rendering) are helpful for a better understanding of pathologies and three-dimensional visualization of complex anatomy. However, its drawbacks include exposure of the patient to ionizing radiation (which is particularly of concern in young women and in the pediatric population) and the risks inherent to iodinated contrast material. Moreover, the ability to perform ECG-gated CT is limited by the temporal resolution of the scanner. Imaging with this technique may not be feasible in patients with high heart rates (for example, young children, who may have a heart rate as high as 200 beats per minute) due to increased motion artifacts. Thus, these disadvantages must be kept in mind when considering the use of CT, particularly in pediatric patients [4].

Multiplanar, multislice MRI with its large field of view and spontaneous contrast (lumen/walls), allows examination of the entire thoracic and abdominal aorta, particularly on LAO images, in the plane of the aortic arch ("candy cane" sagittal oblique view). From the very beginnings of MRI in the early 1980s [8–12], exploration of the aorta already represented a targeted and promising application of cardiovascular MRI. Constant progress has been made since that time, and today MRI also offers important noninvasive flow-sensitive measurements. MRI has been further improved by the development of gadolinium-enhanced magnetic resonance angiography and phase-contrast MR velocity mapping techniques [13–16].

6.1 Examination Techniques

The investigation always begins with a preliminary series of ECG-gated axial black blood sequences (fast spin-echo or double IR sequences) (see Chap. 1). The second series of LAO images is acquired in the plane of the aortic arch.

B. Kastler, *MRI of Cardiovascular Malformations*,
DOI: 10.1007/978-3-540-30702-0_6, © Springer-Verlag Berlin Heidelberg 2011

The slice thickness is adapted to the size of the child: 3–5 mm in infants and 5–8 mm in older children and adults. Optimal visualization of small vascular structures, particularly the narrowed aortic isthmus, can be obtained by performing stacks of intertwined and overlapping images, 5 mm thick (i.e., slice interval of 2–3 mm, Fig. 2.14 and see Chap. 2).

The caliber of the aorta must be measured from edge to edge on LAO images (cursor perpendicular to the aortic walls) and not on axial images which, like CT, can overestimate the aortic diameter. The ascending and descending segments of the aorta are also clearly visualized on coronal images.

We also always perform LAO gradient-echo cine-MRI to detect increased flow in the coarctation (Figs. 6.15 and 6.16) and/or to confirm the presence of a false channel when dissection is suspected. In the case of dilatation of the aorta, the assessment is completed by gradient-echo cine-MRI with axial and coronal images through the aortic root and left ventricle to detect possible aortic incompetence (signal flow void jet) (Fig. 6.22c).

This time-consuming protocol can be completed with gadolinium-enhanced magnetic resonance angiography sequences. Their short acquisition time (less than 1 min to visualize the entire aorta) eliminates the need for ECG gating and allows visualization of the contrast agent's first pass, as in conventional aortography or spiral CT scan (without ionizing radiation and the adverse effects of iodinated contrast agents). The vascular signal is based on T1 shortening of arterial blood by the paramagnetic contrast agent. Consequently, it is less dependent on blood flow than cine-MRI, with fewer artifacts, and when the gadolinium bolus injection is performed correctly, ideally on breath-hold sequences, there is no venous contamination or respiratory movements [13–16]. However, the circulatory time is shorter in children, particularly in infants, and the interval between injection and the start of the sequence must be carefully adapted to obtain the maximum bolus effect.

Phase-contrast MR angiography, by allowing measurement of flow velocities at various levels of the aorta (velocity mapping), allows assessment of blood flow and pressure gradients [17–19].

6.2 Coarctation of the Aorta

It is difficult to provide a simple and complete definition of coarctation of the aorta. The word "coarctation" is derived from the Latin coarctatio, indicating the action of pressing or squeezing. Applied to the aortic arch, this term designates sufficient narrowing of the aortic lumen to constrict blood flow. It is a frequent malformation, with a remarkable variety of forms, which can induce serious complications.

The severity, as well as the site and extent of coarctation can vary considerably from one patient to another and according to the age of discovery of the disease. Bonnet [20] classically distinguished postductal coarctations of older children and adults from preductal coarctations of neonates and infants. A clinical distinction, not based only on two anatomical forms, appears to be more adapted to modern imaging modalities, as the diagnosis of coarctation is primarily clinical and is essentially established in two types of clinical settings:

- More than one half of cases present before the age of 1 year in a neonate or an infant presenting with life-threatening cardiac distress and suspected coarctation.
- The other forms may be discovered in young adults with a systolic murmur or arterial hypertension, often remain asymptomatic, and are discovered incidentally at any age (infants, children, or adults) with no criteria of immediate severity.

In both cases, and as for many other cardiovascular malformations, the objectives of complementary investigations are clearly defined: to confirm the diagnosis, to establish a sufficiently precise assessment of the lesions to guide the surgical procedure, and to follow the postoperative course.

The place of the various imaging modalities in this assessment has changed over recent years. Angiography is no longer performed. Although this used to be the most sensitive imaging technique, it is not devoid of risks, particularly in the first clinical situation of severe coarctation. Doppler echocardiography is simple to perform and is clearly the first-line examination [21, 22]. Transthoracic echocardiography is often sufficient to define the surgical indication in infants and young children [11], but is of more limited value in older children and adults [23]. MRI completes echocardiography, as it can be performed in both clinical settings. It provides a satisfactory morphological approach and allows evaluation of flow anomalies related to the stenosis.

Before discussing the two main clinical presentations, we first consider a classification of coarctation according to its site, the severity and length of the stenosis, and the presence of associated cardiac malformations.

6.3 Frequency

Coarctation of the aorta is a frequent congenital malformation, observed in 4–6 per 1,000 births and representing 4–10% of all congenital malformations [24, 25]. It is more frequent in boys than in girls (2/3: 1/3) [26].

Coarctation of the aorta was the third most frequent cardiovascular anomaly observed in an autopsy series of 1,000 subjects over the age of 2 years [27].

The frequency of coarctation of the aorta has been reported to be 0.06% in the general population [28], 18% in the siblings, and 27% in the descendants of a subject with coarctation.

6.4 Anatomical Forms

The various anatomical forms are shown schematically in Fig. 6.1.

6.4.1 Coarctation of the Aortic Isthmus

The region of the isthmus, that is, the segment of the aorta between the origin of the left subclavian artery and the site of implantation of the ligamentum arteriosum or ductus arteriosus, is by far the most frequent site of coarctation. Two anatomical forms of coarctation of the aortic isthmus, which represents more than 95% of all coarctations, are usually distinguished [20, 27]:

- Preductal form, in which the stenosis is situated before the site of insertion of the ductus arteriosus, which generally remains patent (Figs. 6.1a, b and 6.2). In addition to focal constriction, the transverse aorta may show a long segmental tubular hypoplasia. This form is often associated with other cardiac malformations, and subjects with this form usually present symptoms at birth with congestive heart failure.
- Postductal form, in which the stenosis is situated after the site of insertion of the ductus arteriosus, which is usually closed (Figs. 6.1a, c and 6.3). The anomaly, a shelf-like indentation of the posterolateral aortic wall is usually short and isolated. Significant aortic stenosis at the coarctation site is rarely encountered during infancy. Coarctation is

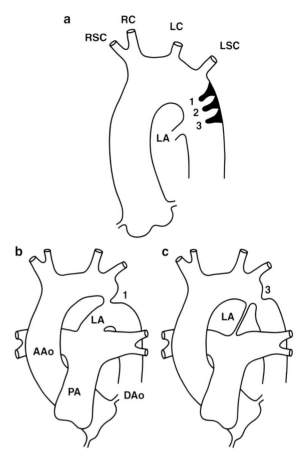

Fig. 6.1 Site of coarctation in relation to the ductus arteriosus (DA): preductal (1 image (**a**)), juxtaductal (2 image (**a**)) and postductal (3 image (**a**)). DA, ligamentum arteriosum (LA), and type of coarctation obtained: preductal form ("infantile") (**b**) and postductal form ("adult") (**c**). AAo, DAo, pulmonary artery (PA), right common carotid artery (RC), left common carotid artery (LC), right subclavian artery (RSC), LSC

thus discovered later in older patients. The obstruction of blood flow across the constriction area induces progressive formation of collateral circulation pathways to ensure proper downstream blood flow. Additional bicuspid aortic valves are common (70%) with possible aortic stenosis or regurgitation.

These two forms correspond to the classic infantile and adult types described by Bonnet [20], but his classification is no longer pertinent, as preductal coarctations can remain asymptomatic for a long time, while postductal coarctations are symptomatic during childhood. Furthermore, the ductus arteriosus can remain patent in some cases of postductal coarctation and may be closed in the preductal form [29].

Fig. 6.2 Preductal coarctation of the aorta in an infant.
Sagittal oblique (LAO)
spin-echo and gradient-echo
cine-MRI images in the plane
of the aortic arch (7).
(**a**) Anatomical spin-echo
image demonstrating the site
of the coarctation. The
following diameters were
determined: site of coarctation: 3.6 mm, proximal:
7.1 mm, and distal: 13.6 mm
(poststenotic dilatation);
PA (3). (**b, c**) Gradient-echo
cine-MRI during systole:
post-isthmic vertical jet of
signal void indicating
significant stenosis (*white
arrow*) and oblique jet (*black
arrowhead*) at the site of
insertion of ductus arteriosus
(DA) on the aorta (only seen
in **b**). (**d**) Axial spin-echo
image showing dilatation
of the PA (3) and double
superior vena cava (*right*
8sd, *left* 8sg) (see Chap. 4,
Fig. 4.4)

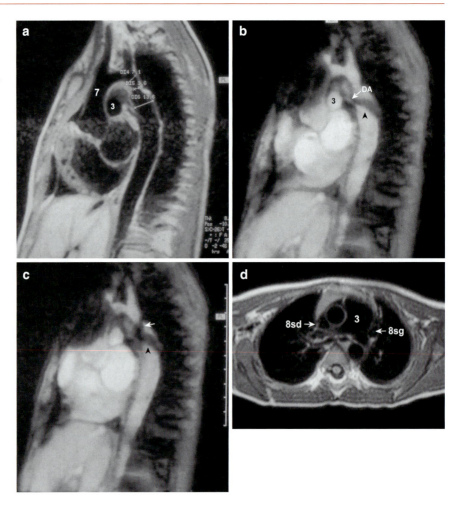

Some authors distinguish a third juxtaductal form, similar to the postductal form, but often associated with a partially patent ductus arteriosus [30].

6.4.2 Atypical Sites

Coarctations situated proximally or distally to the isthmus represent only 0.5–4% of all coarctations. Coarctations situated proximally to the isthmus are exceptional and often correspond to aortic arch anomalies with segmental atresia (Fig. 6.4) [31].

Most atypical sites involve the abdominal aorta. About 300 cases have been reported in the literature. Although hypertension in the upper limbs is the dominant sign common to all forms of coarctation, abdominal coarctations constitute a distinct anatomical and pathophysiological entity. Imaging and the resulting

surgical management especially are very different [32] and are discussed below (Figs. 6.17 and 6.19). Classically, abdominal coarctations are not associated with coarctation of the aortic isthmus, although this combination can exist (Fig. 6.18).

6.5 Forms According to the Type of Stenosis

The stenosis can vary in severity and length; two main types are observed:

6.5.1 Typical Form: Localized Coarctation

The aortic lumen is abruptly narrowed (Figs. 6.3 and 6.5). The diaphragm within the aorta is generally

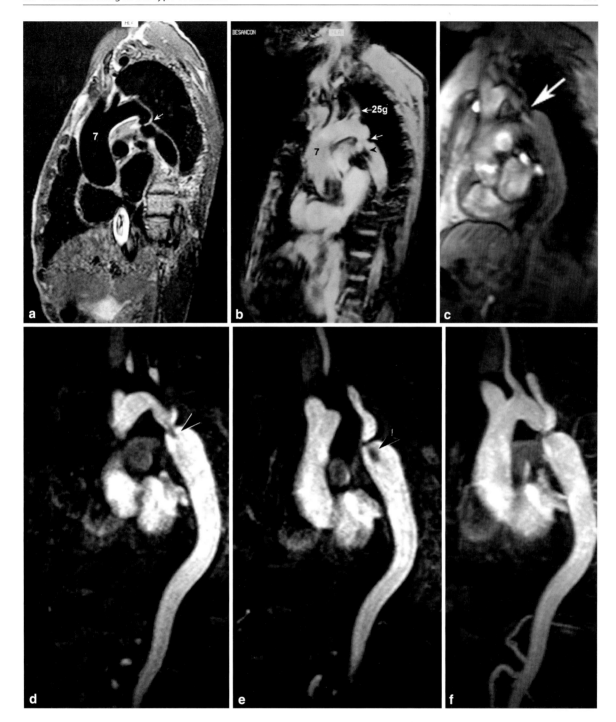

Fig. 6.3 (**a** and **b**) Postductal coarctation of the aorta in an adult [42]. Sagittal oblique (LAO) spin-echo and gradient-echo cine-MRI images in the plane of the aortic arch. (**a**) Anatomical spin-echo image: coarctation of the aortic isthmus (7) forming a diaphragm (hour glass image – *arrow*). (**b**) Gradient-echo cine-MRI during systole in the same plane: signal void (*black – arrowhead*) over the narrowed orifice left subclavian artery 25g.

(**c–f**) When the aortic coarctation is severe, as in this second case, the flow void jet (*arrow*) seen on sagittal oblique (LAO) gradient-echo cine-MRI images (**c**) can thus also be present on the contrast-enhanced MRA images (Dota-Gd, Guerbet, France), as is clearly seen (*arrowheads*) on both native maximum intensity projection (MIP) images (**d** and **e**) (also see Fig. 6.13b)

Fig. 6.4 Coarctation of the horizontal segment of a right aortic arch. The coarctation (*arrows*) is situated on the horizontal segment of the aorta (7). (**a**) LAO spin-echo image. (**b**) Gradient-echo cine-MRI. The jet effect of this coarctation has induced aneurysmal dilatation (**a**) of the RSC (25d). (**c**) The aneurysm (**a**) compresses the inferior cervical ganglion (*arrowhead*) situated immediately posteriorly, causing Horner syndrome, which led to discovery of the anomaly. (**d**) The aortic arch courses to the right of the trachea (T)

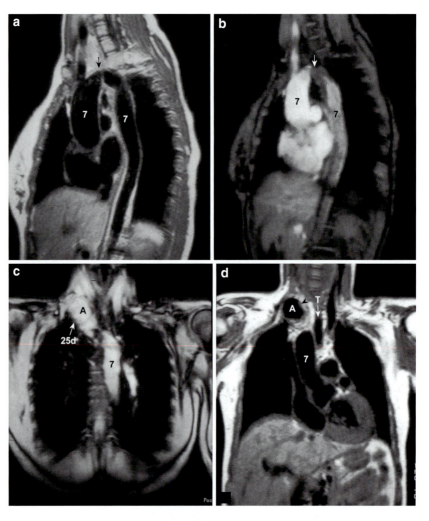

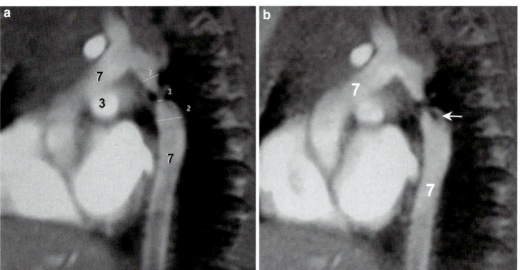

Fig. 6.5 Preductal coarctation of the aorta. Sagittal oblique (LAO) gradient-echo cine-MRI images in the plane of the aortic arch (7) before (**a**) and after (**b**) angioplasty. (**a**) The following diameters were determined: site of coarctation: 2 mm, proximal: 6 mm, and distal: 9 mm; PA (3). (**b**) Severe coarctation persists despite attempted balloon catheter dilatation. Note the presence of a poststenotic jet of signal void (in systole – *arrow*)

not circumferential, but often directed from left to right, leaving an eccentric passage for blood flow, at the level of insertion of ligamentum arteriosum. The degree of stenosis can range from complete atresia to slight narrowing.

Moderate stenosis raises the differential diagnosis with pseudocoarctation of the aorta, characterized by elongation of the aortic arch in the first segment of the descending aorta, resulting in kinking just over the ligamentum arteriosum (Figs. 6.6 and 6.7). Apart from this elongation, pseudocoarctation [33, 34] can be distinguished from coarctation by the less severe narrowing of the aorta and the absence of significant hemodynamic repercussions (flow void jets) (Fig. 6.6). The absence of collateral circulation also constitutes an additional argument (Fig. 6.7).

6.5.2 Atypical Form: Tubular Coarctation

In this rare form, the stenotic segment is longer, corresponding to hypoplasia of a segment of the aortic isthmus (Figs. 6.8 and 6.10) sometimes replaced by a portion of fibrous tissue (patent or obstructed) (Fig. 6.9). In this case, the differential diagnosis concerns interrupted aortic arch (discussed below), which is characterized by disruption, classically well demarcated, between two aortic segments, which can be connected by a fibrous cord. Interrupted aortic arch, particularly type A (see Figs. 6.19 and 6.20), can be considered to be an extreme form of tubular coarctation [21]. Contrast-enhanced MRA displaying the significant segmental narrowing on a large Fov is useful in this context to differentiate tubular coarctation from interruption (Fig. 6.10). In practice, emergency surgery is required in both cases.

6.6 Associated Malformations

Although the incidence of congenital heart disease in the general population is estimated to be 0.6%, this incidence ranges between 10 and 72% in subjects with coarctation [26, 35].

6.6.1 Cardiovascular Malformations

Other malformations also situated on the aortic arch are the most frequent associated anomalies. Bicuspid aortic valve is very frequently associated, in 27–46% of cases of coarctation, depending on the series. In practice, coarctation exclusively associated with bicuspid aortic valve is considered to be an isolated form. In about 10% of cases, coarctation is associated with stenosis of the aortic orifice, corresponding to aortic stenosis and subaortic stenosis. Aortic regurgitation and premature degeneration of the aortic media can be responsible for aneurysms and possible rupture.

Two-thirds of coarctations in neonates and infants are associated with varying degrees of tubular hypoplasia of the aortic arch, ventricular septal defect, and patent ductus arteriosus (Fig. 6.8). This entity, classified into five main groups by Becker et al. [36], corresponds to coarctation syndrome or complex coarctation.

Other associated cardiac malformations — ventricular septal defect, persistent left superior vena cava (Fig. 6.2), transposition of the great vessels, double outlet right ventricle, and single ventricle — are observed more rarely. Associated mitral anomalies, with a frequency of between 2 and 8%, can be missed [37]. Intracranial aneurysms are also frequently observed.

6.6.2 Noncardiovascular Malformations

Noncardiovascular congenital malformations, especially gonadal dysgenesis, are associated in 8% of cases of coarctation [26]. Between 1/4 and 1/8 of subjects with Turner syndrome also present coarctation [38, 39]. Other malformations — club foot, hypospadias, mental retardation, and congenital cataract — are reported more rarely.

6.7 Clinical Forms

6.7.1 Minimally Symptomatic or Asymptomatic Forms

These forms are more likely to be discovered later (early detection being possible by an early clinical diagnosis or even by fetal echocardiography). Diaphragmatic narrowing of the aortic lumen is generally situated adjacent (juxtaductal form) or slightly distal (postductal form) to the site of insertion of the ligamentum arteriosum

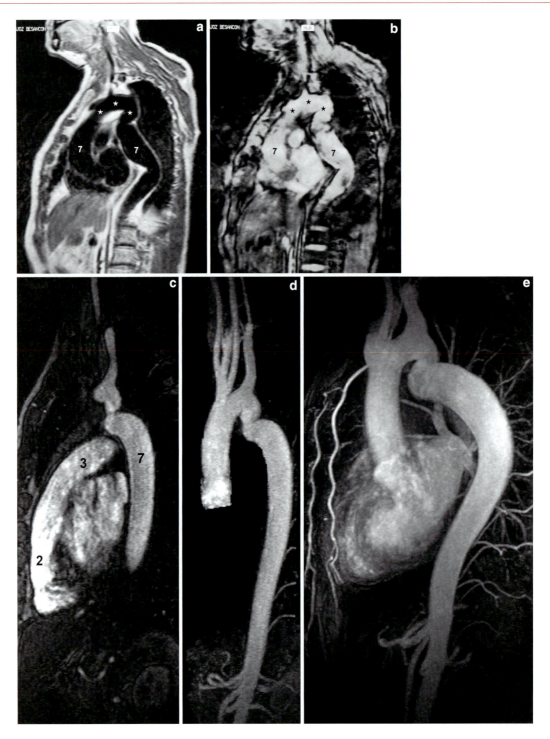

Fig. 6.6 (**a** and **b**) Pseudocoarctation of the aorta in an adult. Sagittal oblique (LAO) spin-echo (**a**) and gradient-echo cine-MRI (**b**) images in the plane of the aortic arch. Elongated supra-isthmic aorta (*stars-7*) followed by a kinking appearance; no severe turbulence (dephasing) distal to the kinking on cine-MRI. This criterion is however not discriminative: a tortuous aorta without significant stenosis can present dephasing due to turbu-lent flow, however with no significant hemodynamic obstruction (presence of a true jet of signal void). (**c–e**) Other case of pseudocoarctation of the aorta, MRA LAO native image (**c**) and MIP and 3D reconstructions (**d** and **e**) show the significant kink-ing of the aorta (7) in the isthmic region with no significant col-lateral circulation (internal thoracic (mammary) arteries and intercostals arteries); right ventricle (2) PA (3)

Fig. 6.7 Pseudocoarctation in a 19-year-old-man. (**a**, **b**) Sagittal oblique (LAO) spin-echo images in the plane of the aortic arch (7) (7 mm thick with a gap of 5 mm from (**a**) to (**b**)). Hairpin elongation of the aorta in the region of the isthmus (*stars*) with kinking, but no real stenosis. (**c**) Axial image. No increase of caliber of the internal thoracic (mammary) arteries (*arrows*); PA (3). Note that, as the aortic arch extends cranially beyond the manubrium sternae, we have here an authentic additional cervical aorta (these two entities can be linked from the embryological point of view) (also see Fig. 5.20 Chap. 5)

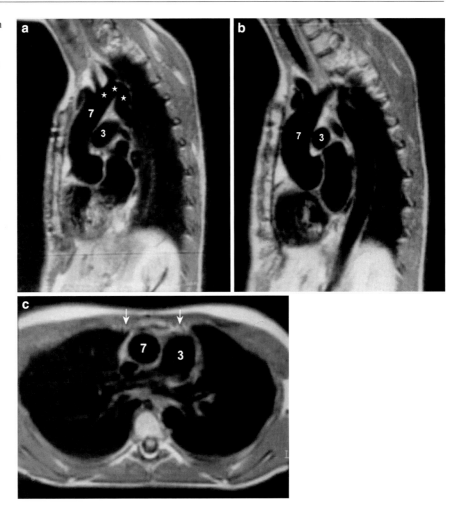

Fig. 6.8 Coarctation of the aorta with hypoplasia of the horizontal segment in a newborn. (**a**) Sagittal oblique (LAO) image in the plane of the aortic arch demonstrating segmental stenosis of the aortic isthmus (7 – *arrow*), posteriorly to a hypoplastic horizontal segment (*arrowheads*). (**b**) Axial image through the aortic arch demonstrating hypoplasia of the horizontal segment of the aorta (*arrowheads*)

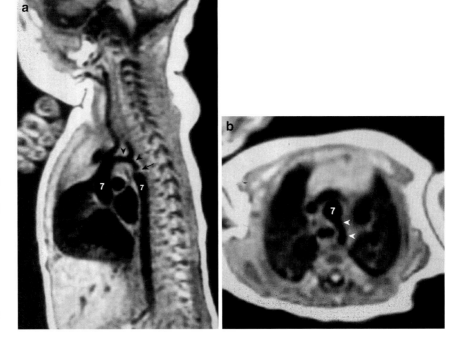

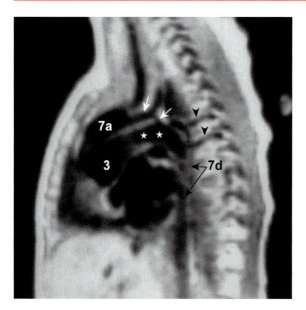

Fig. 6.9 Extreme form of coarctation with tubular hypoplasia of the aorta. Complex congenital heart disease with dominant left ventricle and transposition of the great vessels (see Chap. 7) and common venous confluence (see Chap. 5, Fig. 5.23 and Chap. 4, Fig. 4.22). The AAo (7a) is situated anteriorly to the PA trunk (3), its horizontal segment is hypoplastic (*arrows*), and the descending thoracic aorta (7d) is supplied by a large patent DA (*stars*). Also note the presence of a collateral circulation (*arrowheads*) (also see Fig. 6.21)

(residual ductus arteriosus) (Figs. 6.1 and 6.3). The distal aortic segment is generally dilated (poststenotic dilatation). The collateral circulation gradually develops to reenter the aorta beyond the obstruction, especially via the scapular, internal mammary, and intercostal vessels (Figs. 6.11–6.13, and 6.18). Rib notching, caused by dilated, tortuous intercostal arteries that can be observed on chest radiographs at the age of about 11 years, are now observed much less frequently as a result of early surgical management. The coarctation is generally isolated by apart from bicuspid aortic valve, observed in 27–46% of cases (or sometimes aberrant subclavian artery (see Chap. 8, Fig. 8.25)).

Pseudocoarctation [33, 34], an uncommon aortic developmental anomaly, occurs when the third and seventh aortic dorsal segments fail to fuse. It consists of elongation and kinking of a tortuous aortic arch and can be difficult to distinguish from true coarctation. The narrowing of the aorta is less severe, with no significant hemodynamic obstruction (turbulences, but no true flow void jet) and absence of a pressure gradient on phase-contrast MR. Thus, no abnormal development of collateral circulation appears (Figs. 6.6 and 6.7).

MR phase velocity mapping displays no significant accelerated flow and increased pressure gradient [40].

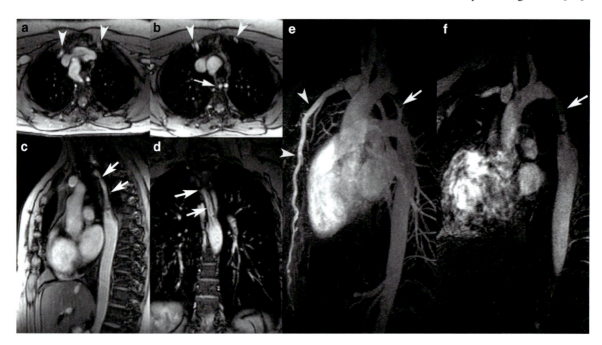

Fig. 6.10 Extensive coarctation-hypoplasia of the thoracic aorta in an adolescent. Contrast-enhanced MRA (Dota-Gd, Guerbet, France) multiplanar axial (**a**, **b**), LAO (**c**) coronal (**d**) native image and MIP reconstructions (**e**, **f**) show the significant segmental narrowing on the proximal DAo (*arrows*). Note also the extensive collateral circulation: markedly enlarged internal thoracic (mammary) (*arrowheads*) and intercostal arteries which are partly superimposed on the PA system (also see Fig. 13 and postoperative evaluation, Chap. 8, Fig. 8.26)

Fig. 6.11 Collateral pathways in coarctation of the aorta: precoarctation aorta (1); postcoarctation aorta (2); subclavian artery (3); axillary artery (4); internal thoracic (mammary) artery (5); external iliac artery (6); vertebral artery (7); anterior spinal artery (8); superior intercostal artery (9); intercostal arteries (10); perforating arteries (anastomosing with posterior intercostal arteries) (11); inferior epigastric artery (12); lumbar arteries (13); thyrocervical trunk (14); transverse cervical artery (15); transverse scapular artery (16); subscapular artery (17)

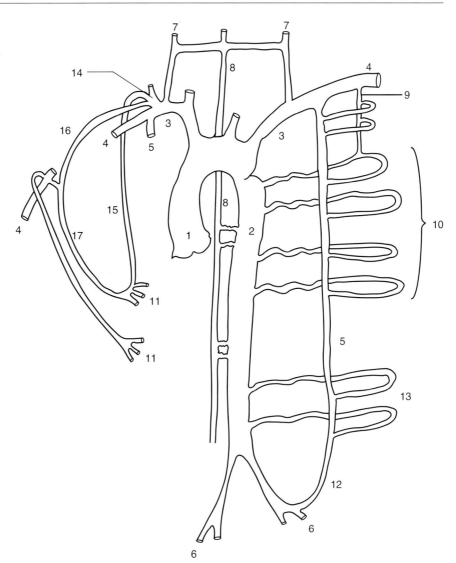

6.7.2 Symptomatic Forms

Symptomatic forms present with features of neonatal or infantile heart failure. In two-thirds of cases, symptomatic forms correspond to coarctation syndrome associated with varying degrees of coarctation (usually preductal), tubular hypoplasia of the aortic arch[1], ventricular septal defect, and patent ductus arteriosus [41, 42] (Figs. 6.8 and 6.9). The lesion, which ranges from simple hourglass stenosis to a circular diaphragm (more frequent, Fig. 6.5), is continuous with muscle fibers of the ductus arteriosus. It is usually situated slightly proximally to the insertion of ductus arteriosus. Its position (over or more rarely distal

to the ductus arteriosus) determines the direction of flow in the ductus arteriosus (proximally to the aortic arch or distally to the descending aorta). Apart from tubular hypoplasia of the horizontal segment, hypoplasia of the proximal segment of the descending aorta may also be observed more rarely (Fig. 6.10). The remaining one-third of symptomatic cases presents an isolated but severe form of coarctation.

Assessment of coarctation of the aorta must precisely determine its site, severity, and extent, and must also evaluate the caliber of the subclavian artery (which can be narrowed or widened[2]), define the degree of left ventricular hypertrophy, and assess the collateral circulation

---

[1]If it is isolated and significant, it corresponds to a transitional form with an interrupted aortic arch, which can be considered to be an extreme form of hypoplasia.

[2]Evaluation of the calibre of the subclavian artery is important as some correction techniques use the proximal segment of this artery in the surgical procedure (Walhausen procedure, see Figs. 6.23d and 6.25).

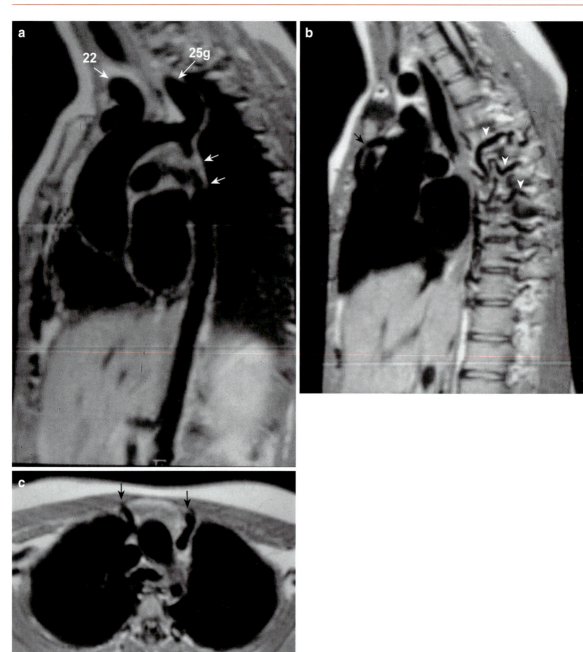

Fig. 6.12 Incidental late discovery of coarctation in a 17-year-old-boy (assessment of hypertension, impalpable femoral pulses). (**a**) Sagittal oblique (LAO) image in the plane of the aortic arch showing stenosis of the isthmus (*arrows*) * with dilatation of the supraaortic vessels (LSC – 25 g, BCT – 22). (**b**) LAO image. (**c**) Axial image. Note the extensive collateral circulation: markedly enlarged intercostal (*arrowheads*) and internal thoracic (mammary) arteries (*arrows*) (compare with Fig. 6.7). *A second series of overlapping and intertwined LAO images is needed to clearly demonstrate patency of the zone of stenosis

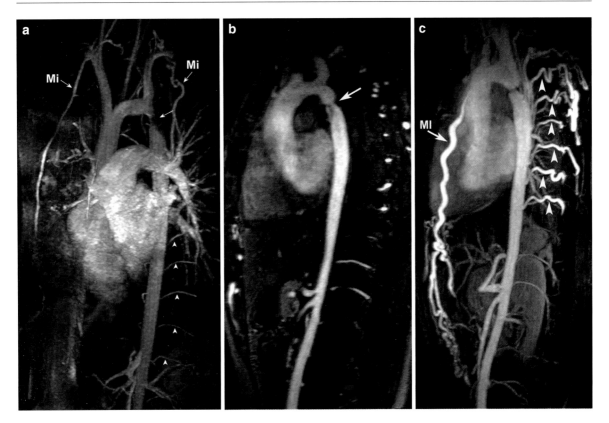

Fig. 6.13 Coarctation of the aorta and collateral circulation (in two adolescents): value of gadolinium injection (Dota-Gd, Guerbet, France). The coarctation site (isthmus-*arrows*) is clearly visible in both cases (**a–c**). Note the extensive collateral circulation: markedly enlarged internal thoracic (mammary – Mi) and intercostal arteries (*arrowheads*) more significant on the second case (**b**), Also note on (**b**) the presence of a severe coarctation confirmed by the presence of a flow void jet at the coarctation site on the Contrast-enhanced MR image (also see Fig. 6.3d, e)

(Figs. 6.12, 6.13, and 6.18) and the presence of a bicuspid aortic valve usually detected by echography.

In experienced hands, Doppler echocardiography is generally a reliable method for assessment of coarctation of the aorta in young children and infants or even antenatally [43]. However, the small caliber of the aorta during the fetal and neonatal period can be misleading (as most of the fetal blood flow passes via a sometimes large ductus arteriosus). Echocardiographic access to the aortic isthmus is not always easy in older children or postoperatively and this modality is of limited value in this setting (Fig. 6.14), as clearly demonstrated by a comparative study with MRI on 23 infants with suspected coarctation [44], in which MRI clarified seven cases that could not be completely evaluated by echocardiography.

Axial anatomical black blood sequences (fast spin-echo or double IR sequences), completed by oblique images in the plane of the aortic arch (LAO), are particularly suitable for examination of the entire thoracic aorta. These sequences generally provide good visualization of the zone of coarctation and its extent, the poststenotic dilatation at the origin of the descending aorta (Figs. 6.2–6.5, and 6.8), and the collateral circulation (Figs. 6.12, 6.13, and 6.18) [45]. However, when the aorta is tortuous or very narrow (particularly in the aortic isthmus), which is frequent in patients with coarctation, all of the aorta cannot be visualized on a single imaging plane and it is not always easy to evaluate the zone of coarctation[3]. In this situation, thin 5 mm (or less) intertwined and overlapping images (gap of 2–3 mm, see Chap. 2, Fig. 2.14) must be acquired. In addition to LAO images, axial and particularly coronal images are also useful in these cases to optimally visualize the zone of coarctation, which is evaluated by comparing the results on all imaging planes (Fig. 6.15).

---

[3]Which must be distinguished from simple physiological narrowing and pseudocoarctation.

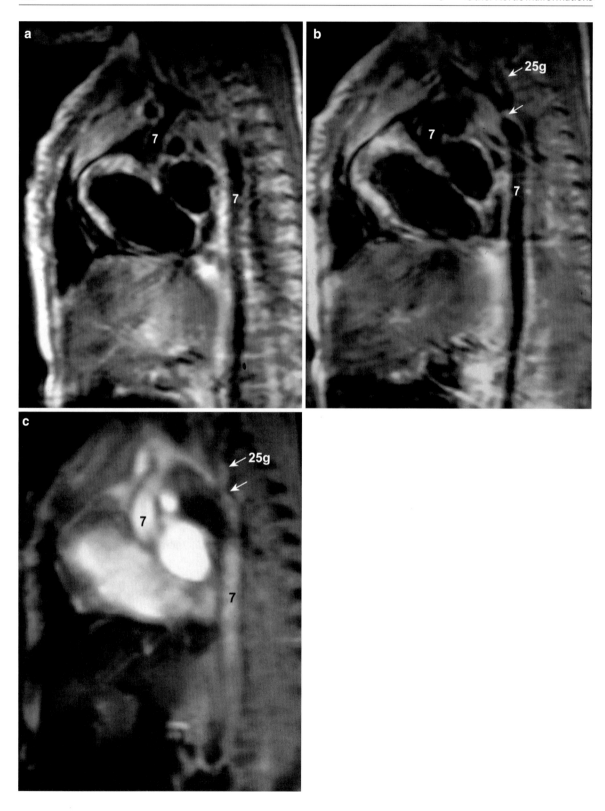

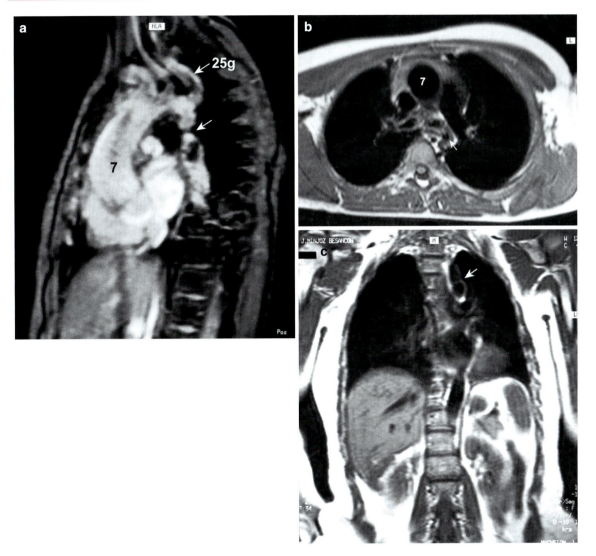

Fig. 6.15 Postductal coarctation of the aorta in a young adult. (**a**) Gradient-echo cine-MRI during systole showing the site of coarctation (*arrow*) and postisthmus signal flow void jet. Stenosis of the aortic lumen (*arrows* – compare with the caliber of the ascending aorta (AAo) – 7a) is confirmed on the axial (**b**) and coronal (**c**) images. Comparison with other imaging planes can be very useful when coarctation is not obvious on the LAO view. Left subclavian artery (LSC) (25 g)

Fig. 6.14 Preductal coarctation of the aorta in a newborn (echocardiography was inconclusive). A stack of 5 mm thick intertwined and overlapping images must be acquired to optimally visualize the narrowed aortic isthmus. (**a, b**) Anatomical LAO spin-echo images in the plane of the aortic arch (5 mm thick with a gap of 3 mm from (**a**) to (**b**)). The site of coarctation (*arrow*), behind the origin of the slightly dilated subclavian artery (25 g), is clearly visualized in (**b**) and is confirmed by presence of a flow void jet at the coarctation site on the gradient-echo cine-MR image (**c**); aorta (7)

Although not always obvious, the presence of a zone of signal void in the isthmus on gradient-echo cine-MRI sequence during systole generally indicates significant stenosis [46, 47][4] (Figs. 6.2, 6.3, 6.5, 6.15, and 6.16). To optimize the display of flow void, conventional gradient-echo cine-MRI sequences (with optimized long TE) rather than balanced-SSFP sequences (Fiesta/GE, True/FISP-Siemens, Balanced-FFE/Philips) should be used, the latter being (as mentioned in Chaps. 1 and 2) less sensitive to abnormal flow void jets. Left ventricular function and mass can also be evaluated on gradient-echo cine-MRI sequences. By displaying a flow void, gradient-echo cine-MRI is useful to evaluate a coarctation poorly visualized on fast spin-echo images (Fig. 6.16).

Gadolinium-enhanced magnetic resonance angiography is also a valuable adjunct in difficult cases. After image acquisition, reconstructions can be performed in all planes and visualization of the 3D cine-MRI loop can facilitate assessment of the zone of coarctation (Figs. 6.3, 6.5, 6.10, and 6.13). Due to its high resolution, CE-MRA has also become the mainstay in evaluating collateral circulation; it can also visualize small lesions of the aortic wall (such as formation of an aneurysm or dissection in operated coarctation [48]).

When the coarctation is severe, the flow jet seen on oblique (LAO) gradient-echo cine-MRI images (C) can also be present on the MRA images (Figs. 6.3d, e, and 6.13b).

MR phase velocity mapping across the stenosis can be used to assess the pressure gradient by means of a modified Bernoulli equation [49, 50]. The difference of flow between the proximal descending aorta (just distal to the coarctation) and distal descending aorta can also be calculated by this technique. As this difference corresponds to the blood inflow derived from the collateral circulation, this method is useful in cases of moderate stenosis, and also when deterioration is observed after surgery [51, 52]. Analysis of flow patterns in the descending aorta allows estimation of the severity of aortic stenosis [49, 53, 54]. The collateral circulation can also be assessed qualitatively by phase-contrast cine-MRI [51, 55].

MRI has totally superseded cardiac catheterization and angiography for the preoperative assessment of coarctation when the echocardiographic assessment is incomplete [56]. Compared to CT-scan, it is nonionizing

(a desirable feature in young patients) and gives access to functional information; thus, MRI appears to be the best suited for both diagnosis of coarctation and postsurgical follow-up [48, 52, 57, 58].

Postoperatively or after percutaneous transluminal angioplasty [59], MRI is also complementary to echocardiography in evaluating the results and detecting possible complications such as restenosis (Fig. 6.5), aneurysm (see Chap. 8, Figs. 8.24 and 8.25), or hematoma. [45, 57–62]. About one quarter of patients develop hypertension, which is more frequent in the case of delayed surgery. Recurrent hypertension sometime after the operation is suggestive of restenosis. The geometry of the aortic arch plays an important role in the long-term prognosis. Gothic shaped-arches have been incriminated in residual or recurrence of hypertension and developing left ventricular hypertrophy [63–66].

6.8 Coarctation of the Abdominal Aorta

Coarctation of the abdominal aorta is a rare anomaly. It is a distinct entity requiring different management to that of coarctation of the isthmus. It is due to an anomaly of fusion of the primitive dorsal aortic arches during the fourth week of embryonic life [67–69]. It often extends to involve the descending thoracic aorta. Clinically, it resembles coarctation, as proximal hypertension is observed in the upper limbs while hypotension is observed in the lower limbs, which present barely palpable pulses. There is usually, but not always, no anomaly of the proximal thoracic aorta, particularly the isthmus (Fig. 6.18). When all portions of the thoracic and abdominal aorta are concerned the term hypoplasia is used. Aortic hypoplasia, an exceedingly rare cardiovascular anomaly, has been described [70].

Conventional angiography used to be the only imaging modality that was able to diagnose this anomaly, but we have used MRI to precisely document several cases of coarctation of the abdominal aorta [71] (Figs. 6.17–6.19). It confirms the diagnosis, defines its severity and its extent (thoracic segment), verifies whether or not renal arteries are involved, and visualizes the kidneys. Useful imaging planes for the abdominal segment are coronal (renal arteries) and sagittal images (coeliac trunk and inferior and superior mesenteric arteries). Gadolinium-enhanced magnetic resonance angiography sequences, displaying the aorta on a large Fov, are also essential in this context (Fig. 6.19).

---

[4]N.B.: turbulent flow and/or acceleration has a black signal, while normal flow has a white signal, see Chaps. 1 and 2.

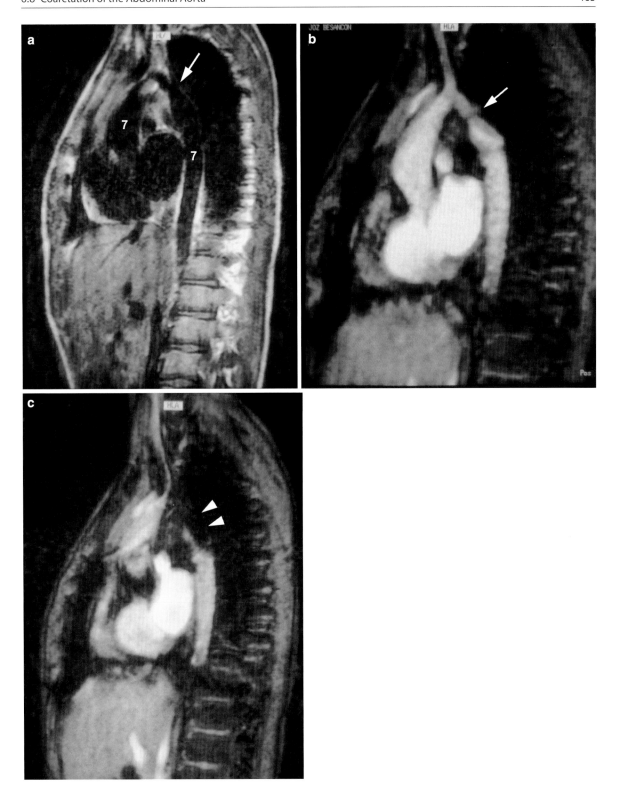

Fig. 6.16 Coarctation of the aorta. Sagittal oblique (LAO) spin-echo and gradient-echo cine-MRI images in the plane of the aortic arch. (**a**) Anatomical spin-echo image: the horizontal segment and aortic isthmus (7), corresponding to the site of coarctation (*arrow*), are not clearly visualized. (**b**) Gradient-echo cine-MRI during dias-tole: good filling (*white* signal) of the aorta allowing assessment of its caliber, especially in the stenotic zone (*arrow*). (**c**) Gradient-echo cine-MRI during systole: signal void jet throughout the postisthmus region (*arrowheads*), another feature indicating significant stenosis

Fig. 6.17 Coarctation- hypoplasia of the abdominal aorta in a small-for-dates neonate. (**a, b**) Coronal spin-echo images in the plane of the abdominal aorta: very severe narrowing of the infrarenal abdominal aorta (7i); compare with the thoracic aorta normal size (7d) (MRI performed in 1989 [50])

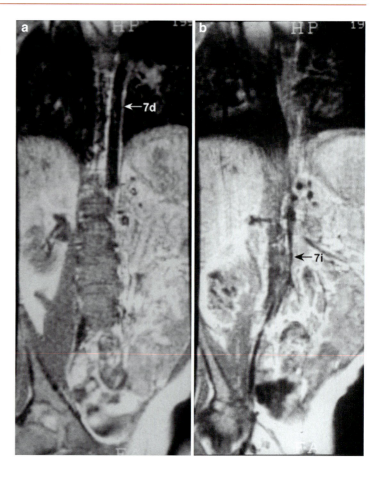

6.8.1 Interrupted Aortic Arch

This is a rare anomaly, characterized by complete interruption of the aortic lumen between the ascending aorta and the descending aorta. It resembles severe forms of coarctation of the aorta (Fig. 6.9) and is almost always associated with ventricular septal defect and patent ductus arteriosus [72]. Three types of interrupted aortic arch are distinguished according to the site of interruption in relation to the brachiocephalic vessels (Fig. 6.20):

- Type A: interruption between left subclavian artery and ductus arteriosus

- Type B: interruption between left common carotid and left subclavian arteries
- Type C: interruption between brachiocephalic trunk and left common carotid artery.

Each type is divided into two subtypes according to the presence or absence of aberrant (retro-esophageal) left subclavian artery.

Type B is the most frequent type and is often associated with DiGeorge syndrome [73, 74]. Type C is rare [75]. Interrupted aortic arch is rarely isolated [76–78] and, apart from ventricular septal defect, can be associated with truncus arteriosus, double outlet right ventricle, and D- or L-transposition of the great vessels [79].

Fig. 6.18 Coarctation of the aorta in an 18-year-old-man with hypertension. Doppler echocardiography was not contributive. (**a**) Axial spin-echo image: hypertrophied internal thoracic (mammary) arteries (*arrows*). (**b**) LAO spin-echo image in the plane of the aortic arch: diaphragm coarctation (*arrow*) 15 mm posteriorly to the origin of the LSC. (**c**) Coronal spin-echo image: hypertrophied intercostal arteries (*arrowheads*). Note the hypoplasia of the abdominal aorta (7i). (**d, e**) Sagittal oblique (LAO) spin-echo and gradient-echo cine-MRI images: postoperative appearance after resection and end-to-end anastomosis of the two aortic segments (Crawford procedure): slight narrowing (*arrows*) with no significant flow disturbances on gradient-echo cine-MRI (also see Chap. 5 Figs. 5.8d and 5.18d, (**e**) and Chap. 8, Figs. 8.23b and 8.24 for the Crawford procedure)

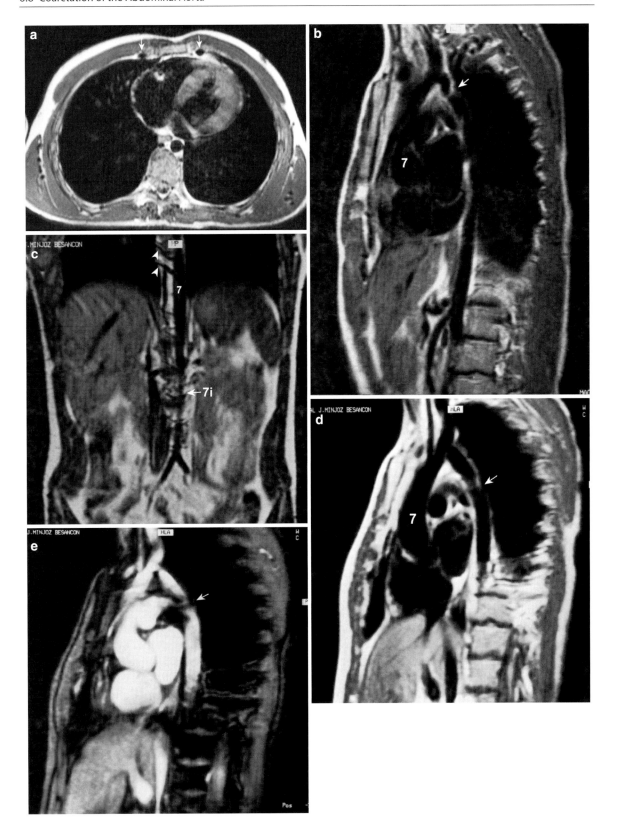

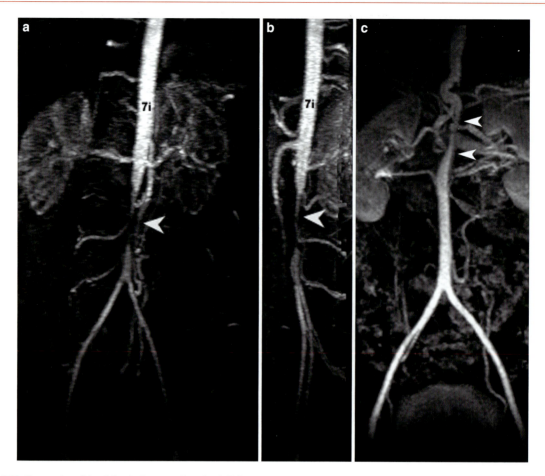

Fig. 6.19 Coarctation of the abdominal aorta: value of gadolinium-enhanced MRA. MIP projections for reliable analysis of the lumen of the entire abdominal aorta (7i) (Dota-Gd, Guerbet, France). The zone of coarctation is clearly demonstrated (*arrowheads*) in these two cases: (**a**) and (**b**) infrarenal abdominal aorta coarctation (sagittal and coronal MIP projections), and (**c**) suprarenal segmental coarctation (*arrowheads*) displayed on a coronal MIP projection

Echocardiography is not always able to visualize the anomaly due to its very high position in the mediastinum (particularly in the case of right aortic arch); a suprasternal approach is the most appropriate. Interrupted aortic arch is often a diagnosis of exclusion, suspected in a context of severe clinical features with hypoplasia of the ascending aorta, discontinuity between the ascending aorta and descending aorta and presence of a patent ductus arteriosus supplying the descending aorta (Fig. 6.21) [80–82]. Extreme dilatation of the pulmonary artery, entirely masking the aortic isthmus, may prevent a definitive diagnosis on echocardiography.

MRI is particularly useful in this setting, avoiding the need for angiography. LAO images show a straight hypoplastic ascending aorta, giving rise to the various neck vessels and interruption of the arch with specific determination of its site and extent (Fig. 6.21). An image shifted to the right in the same imaging plane shows the ductus arteriosus arising from the pulmonary artery and supplying the descending aorta ("pseudo-arch" appearance). Axial and coronal images show disruption of the aortic arch. MRI is also useful for assessment of associated anomalies: site and severity of VSD, presence of subaortic obstruction, and possible compression of adjacent organs (tracheobronchial tree).

This anomaly is treated surgically. Angiography is no longer necessary when good quality MR images can be obtained.

6.8.2 Dilatations of the Ascending Aorta

Dilatations of the ascending aorta essentially correspond to Marfan syndrome characterized by idiopathic

Fig. 6.20 Diagram showing the three possible sites of interrupted aortic arch. Type (**a**): interruption between LSC and DA. Type (**b**): interruption between left common carotid (LC) and left subclavian arteries. Type (**c**): interruption between brachiocephalic trunk (BCT) and left common carotid artery. RC, AAo, DAo, PA, RC, RSC

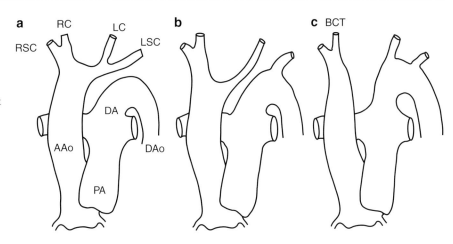

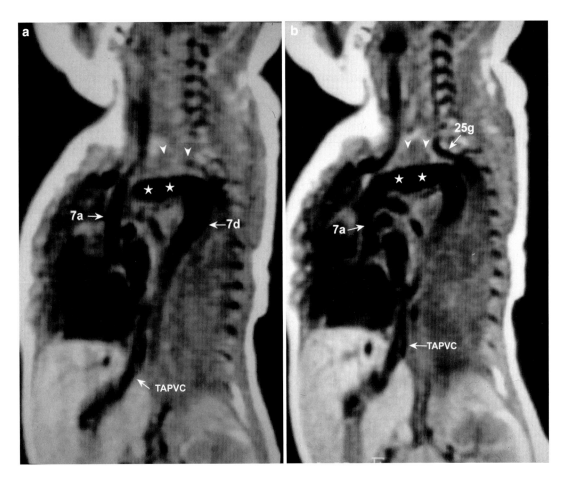

Fig. 6.21 Interrupted aortic arch with infradiaphragmatic total anomalous pulmonary venous connection (not demonstrated by echocardiography) [59]. One-day-old neonate presenting features of cardiorespiratory distress. MRI performed as an emergency. (**a**, **b**) LAO images. The narrowed ascending aorta (7a) gives rise to the BCT. The descending aorta (7d) has a normal caliber. The aortic arch is interrupted (*arrowheads*) between the left common carotid artery anteriorly and the LSC (25 g) posteriorly (type B).

Do not confuse the aortic arch with the "pseudo-arch" formed by a large patent ductus arteriosus (*star* – no supraaortic vessels!) anastomosing with the descending aorta. Also note infradiaphragmatic total anomalous pulmonary venous connection (TAPVC – *arrowheads*) (see Fig. 15 – coarctation with extreme hypoplasia of the horizontal segment and also see Chap. 4, Fig. 4.11 and Chap. 8, Fig. 8.27 for the postoperative appearance) cystic degeneration of the media with aortoannular ectasia [79, 83], which can be isolated. In its complete form, in addition to the anomaly of the ascending aorta, Marfan syndrome comprises cardiac involvement with myxomatous transformation of the aortic and mitral valves, as well as bone and joint anomalies, resulting in a typical morphotype: tall stature, long, thin limbs, arachnodactyly, joint hypermobility, low muscle mass, pectus excavatum or pectus carinatum and ophthalmological lesions with lens dislocation. Degeneration of the media is more severe in the aortic root, with typical localized dilatation of the sinus of Valsalva ("tulip bulb" appearance) (Figs. 6.22 and 6.24) or fusiform dilatation of the ascending aorta with restoration of a normal diameter before the origin of the supraaortic vessels (Fig. 6.23). These children require regular and prolonged surveillance; dilatation of the aorta or its branches can occur early with severe aortic regurgitation (sometimes the only clinical sign) with a risk of rupture [84]. Aortic dissection (Fig. 6.25) is quite a frequent complication [85].

MRI is very useful (particularly in the case of chest deformity interfering with echocardiography) to precisely study the degree of dilatation of the aortic root, and MR measurements are reliable and reproducible [86, 87]. MRI allows noninvasive follow-up of the course of the aneurysm and can be used to guide the indication for surgery. LAO, coronal and sagittal images are used to analyze the ascending aorta (Figs. 6.22 and 6.23). Dilatation of the ascending aorta and coarctation may coexist (Fig. 6.25). Although MRI, as compared to CT, is not the primary diagnostic tool for detecting complications such as dissection, it can reliably visualize the intimal flap between the true and false channel (Fig. 6.26), and the presence of thrombosis [88–90]. MRI and cine-MRI visualize the repercussions on cardiac chambers, the presence of aortic regurgitation (Figs. 6.22c and 6.23c), and anomalies of the mitral and tricuspid valves. MRI is also useful for postoperative follow-up to detect hematoma, a periprosthetic circulating pocket, or an aneurysmal complication. Conventional angiography has been abandoned for the diagnosis and long-term surveillance, as gadolinium-enhanced MRI provides excellent quality angiography (Fig. 6.25).

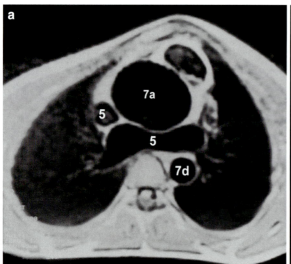

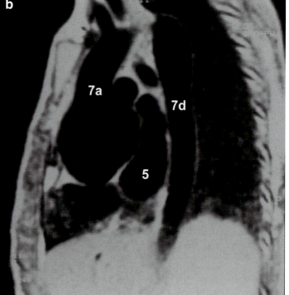

Fig. 6.22 Marfan syndrome. (a) Axial image demonstrating the difference in caliber between the dilated root of the aorta (7a) and the descending aorta (DAo) (7d). Also note the pectus carinatus deformity. (b) Sagittal oblique (LAO) image in the plane of the aortic arch, demonstrating significant "tulip bulb" dilatation of the aortic root (compare with the caliber of the AAo – 7a); left atrium (5). (c) Long-axis gradient-echo cine-MRI through the aortic root (7a) and left ventricle (6). There is slight eccentric aortic regurgitation (jet of signal void – *arrow*). Note that the posterior semilunar valve (*arrowhead*) – posterior wall of the aorta – is continuous inferiorly with the anterior leaflet of the mitral valve (gv); posterior leaflet of the mitral valve (pv) (also see Chap. 2, Fig. 2.9).

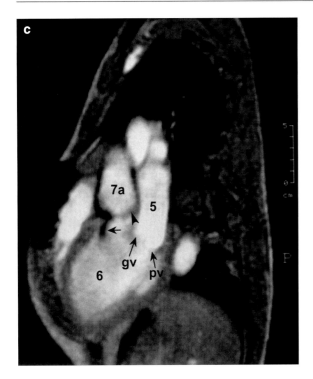

Fig. 6.22 (continued)

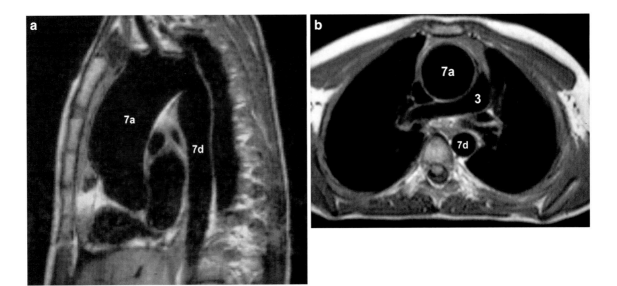

Fig. 6.23 Marfan syndrome. (**a**) Sagittal oblique (LAO) image in the plane of the aortic arch showing fusiform dilatation of the AAo (7a). Unlike the classical appearance, dilatation of the origin of the aorta in the sinus of Valsalva is more limited and the supraaortic vessels are not affected. (**b**) Axial image demonstrating the difference in caliber between the dilated ascending aorta (7a) and the descending aorta (7d). Also note the difference in caliber with the PA trunk (3), which usually has a similar caliber*. (**c**) Coronal gradient-echo cine-MR image through the aortic root (7a) and left ventricle (6), demonstrating slight aortic regurgitation (jet of signal void – *arrow*, whose summit or conus is situated at the site of coarctation of the aortic valves); right atrium (1). Also see Chap. 8, Fig. 8.15. * In adults, the diameter of the PA at its origin is usually equal to around 0.85 times that of the aorta

Fig. 6.23 (continued)

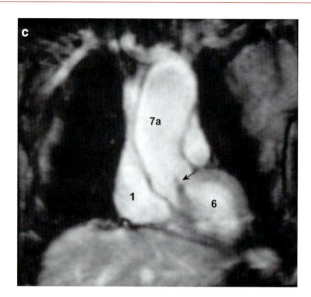

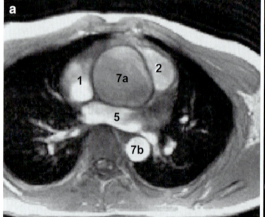

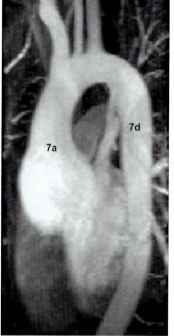

Fig. 6.24 Marfan syndrome. (**a**) Native axial image demonstrating the difference in caliber between the severely dilated aortic root (7a) and the DAo (7d); right atrium (1), left atrium (5), right ventricle – pulmonary infundibulum (2). (**b**) MIP reconstruction demonstrating significant "tulip bulb" dilatation of the aortic root

Fig. 6.25 Marfan syndrome and aortic coarctation. (**a**) Sagittal oblique (LAO) gradient-echo cine-MR image in the plane of the aortic arch showing dilatation of the proximal aorta and typical flow void at coarctation site (*arrow*). (**b**) MIP reconstruction confirms the findings

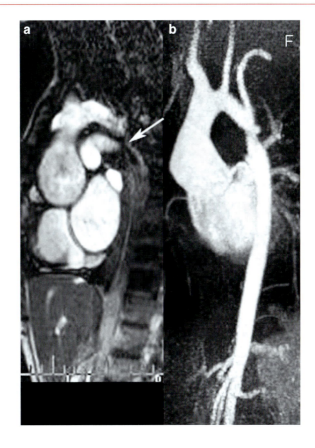

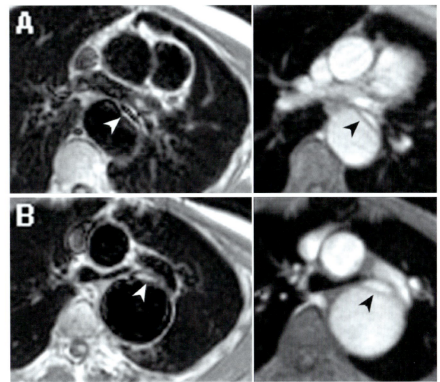

Fig. 6.26 Type A aortic dissection in Marfan syndrome: the intimal flap (*arrowhead*) and the two channels are visible on sequential black blood (*left*) and bright blood cine-MRI (*right*) images

Fig. 6.26 (continued)

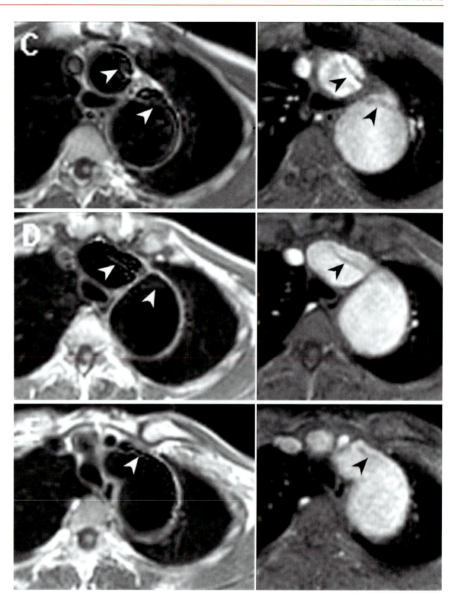

6.9 Conclusion

MRI clearly contributes both in the pre and postoperative assessment of coarctation and other malformations of the aorta by completing the echocardiographic investigation. Significant advances have recently been achieved contributing further to the important place of MRI, a nonionizing anatomical and functional imaging technique particularly useful in evaluating the pediatric population [91–93].

References

1. Haramati LB, Glickstein JS, Issenberg HJ, et al. MR imaging and CT of vascular anomalies and connections in patients with congenital heart disease: significance in surgical planning. Radiographics. 2002;22:337–47; discussion 348–9.
2. Goo HW, Park IS, Ko JK, et al. CT of congenital heart disease: normal anatomy and typical pathologic conditions. Radiographics. 2003;23(Spec Issue):S147–65.
3. Sebastia C, Quiroga S, Boye R, et al. Aortic stenosis: spectrum of diseases depicted at multisection CT. Radiographics. 2003;23 Spec No:S79–91. Review.

4. Leschka S, Oechslin E, Husmann L, et al. Pre- and postoperative evaluation of congenital heart disease in children and adults with 64-section CT. Radiographics. 2007;27(3):829–46. Review.

5. Gutberlet M, Hosten N, Vogel M, et al. Quantification of morphologic and hemodynamic severity of coarctation of the aorta by magnetic resonance imaging. Cardiol Young. 2001;11:512–20.

6. Kaemmerer H, Stern H, Fratz S, et al. Imaging in adults with congenital cardiac disease (ACCD). Thorac Cardiovasc Surg. 2000;48:328–35.

7. Flohr T, Stierstorfer K, Raupach R, et al. Performance evaluation of a 64-slice CT system with z-flying focal spot. Rofo. 2004;176:1803–10.

8. AMPARO EG, Higgins CB, Hoddick W, et al. Magnetic resonance imaging of aortic disease: preliminary results. AJR. 1984;143:1203–9.

9. Herfkens RJ, Higgins CB, Hricak H, et al. Nuclear magnetic resonance imaging of the cardiovascular system: normal and pathologic findings. Radiology. 1983;147:749–59.

10. Higgins CB, Stark D, Mc Namara M, et al. Multiplane magnetic resonance imaging of the heart and major vessels: studies in normal volunteers. AJR. 1984;142:661–7.

11. Soulen RL, Donner RM. Advances in noninvasive evaluation of congenital anomalies of the thoracic aorta. Radiol Clin North Am. 1985;23:727–36.

12. Fletcher BD, Jacobstein MD, Nelson AD, et al. Gated magnetic resonance imaging of congenital cardiac malformations. Radiology. 1984;150:137–40.

13. Prince MR. Gadolinium-enhanced MR aortography. Radiology. 1994;191:155–64.

14. Prince MR, Narasimham DL, Jacoby WT, Williams DM, Kyung JC, Marx MV. Three-dimensional gadolinium-enhanced MR angiography of the thoracic aorta. AJR. 1996;166:1387–97.

15. Ho VB, Prince MR. Thoracic MR aortography: imaging techniques and strategies. Radiographics. 1998; 18: 287–309.

16. Krinsky GA, Rofsky NM, Decorato DR, Weinreb JC, Earls JP, Flyer MA. Thoracic aorta: comparaison of gadolinium-enhanced three-dimentional MR angiography with conventional MR imaging. Radiology. 1997;202:183–93.

17. Mostbeck GH, Caputo GR, Higgins CB. MR measurement of blood flow in the cariovascular system. AJR. 1992; 159:453–61.

18. Reddy GP, Higgins CB. Congenital heart disease: measuring physiology with MRI. Semin Roentgenol. 1998;33:228–38.

19. Pelc LR, Pelc NJ, Rayhill SC, Castro LJ, Glover GH, Herfkens RJ. Arterial and venous blood flow: noninvasive quantification with MR imaging. Radiology. 1992; 185: 809–12.

20. Bonnet LM. Sur la lésion dite sténose congénitale de l'aorte dans la région de l'isthme. Rev Med Paris. 1903; 23: 108–26.

21. Didier F, Cloez JL. Syndrome d'hypoplasie du coeur gauche. Syndrome de coarctation. E.M.C., Radiodiagnostic. Coeurpoumon, 32-015-D-40; 1994.

22. Huhta JC, Gutgesell HP, Latson LA, Huffines FD. Two-dimensional echocardiographic assessment of the area in s and children with congenital heart disease. Circulation. 1984;70:417–24.

23. Kastler B, Livolsi A, Bernard Y, Germain P, Allal R, Clair C. Intérêt de l'IRM dans le l'IRM dans l'exploration des cardiopathies congénitales chez l'enfant et le nouveau-né. La coarctation de l'aorte. In: Brunotte F, Wolf JE. Résonance Magnétique nucléaire en cardiologie. Médicorama. 1997;309:108–9.

24. Hoffman JIE. Incidence, mortality and natural history. In: Anderson RH, Macartney FJ, Shinebourne EA, Tynan M, editors. Paediatric cardiology, vol. 1. Edinburgh: Churchill Livingstone; 1987. p. 3–14.

25. Keith JD. Coarctation of the aorta. In: Keith JD, Rowe RD, Vlad P, editors. Heart disease in infancy and childbood. New York: Macmillan; 1978. p. 736–60.

26. Campbell M, Polani PE. The aetiology of coarcation of the aorta. Lancet. 1961;1(7175):463–468..

27. Abbott ME. Coarctation of the aorta of the adult type. II. A statistical and histological retrospect of 200 recorded cases with autopsy of stenosis or obliteration of the descending arch in subjects above the age of two years. Am Heart J. 1928;3:392–421; 574–617.

28. Nora JJ, Nora AU. Recurrence risks in children having one parent with congenital heart disease. Circulation. 1976; 53:701.

29. Soulie P. Coarctation aortique. In: Soulie P, editor. Les cardiopathies congénitales. Flammarion Médecine sciences; 1978. p. 433–74.

30. Petracek MR, Hammon JW Jr. Thoracic aortic (isthmic) coarctation. In: Dean RH, O'Neill JA Jr, editors. Vascular disorders of childhood. Lea and Febiger, Philadelphia; 1983. p. 36–50.

31. Delabrousse E, Kastler B, Couvreur M, Clair C, Bernard Y. MR Diagnosis of a congenital abnormality of the thoracic aorta with an aneurysm of the right subclavian artery presenting as a Horner's syndrome in an adult. Eur Radiol. 2000;10:650–2.

32. Moresco KP et al. Abdominal aortic coarctation: CT, MRI, and angiographic correlation. Comput Med Imaging Graph. 1995;19:427–30.

33. Limet R. Coarctations et pseudo-coarctations de l'isthme aortique. In: Kieffer E, Godeau P, editors. Maladies artéri-'elles non athéromateuses de l'adulte. Edts AERCV; 1994. p. 31–44.

34. Wang WB, Lin GM. Pseudocoarctation and coarctation. Int J Cardiol. 2009;133(2):e62–4.

35. Hutchins GM. Coarctation of the aorta explained as a branch point of the ductus arteriosus. Am J Pathol. 1971; 63(2):203–9.

36. Becker AE, Becker MJ, Edwards JE, et al. Anomalies associated with coarctation of the aorta. Particular reference to infancy. Circulation. 1970;41:1067–75.

37. Bouhour JB, Lefevre N, Nicolas G. Etude de l'association coarctation de l'aorte-insuffisance mitrale congénitale. Arch mal Cœur. 1977;70:337.

38. Dawson-Falk KL, Wright AM, Bakker B, Pitlick PT, Rosenfeld RG. Cardiovascular evaluation in turner syndrome: utility of MR imaging. Austr. Radiol. 1992; 36:204–9.

39. Nora JJ, Tores FG, Sinha AK, Mc Namara DG. Characteristic cardiovascular anomalies of XO Turner syndrome, XX and XY phenotype and XO/XX Turner mosaic. Am J Cardiol. 1970;25:639–41.

40. Hope MD, Levin JM, Markl M, Draney MT, Alley M, Herfkens RJ. Images in cardiovascular medicine. Four-dimensional magnetic resonance velocity mapping in a healthy volunteer with pseudocoarctation of the thoracic aorta. Circulation. 2004;109(25):3221–2.

41. Wielenga G, Dankmeijer J. Coarctation of the aorta. J Pathol Bacteriol. 1968;95:265–74.

42. Ho SY, Anderson RH. Coarctation, tubular hypoplasia and the ductus arteriosus: a histological study of 35 specimens. Br Heart J. 1979;41:268–74.

43. Allan LD, Chita SK, Andersonrh RH, et al. Coarctation of the aorta in prenatal life: an echocardiographic, anatomical and funcitonal study. Br Heart J. 1988;59:356–60.

44. Parson JM, Baker EJ, Hayes A, et al. MRI of the great arteries in infants. Intern J Cardiol. 1990;28:73–85.

45. Von Schulthess GK, Higashimo SM, Higgins CB, et al. Coarctation of the aorta: MR imaging. Radiology. 1986;158:469–74.

46. Eichenberger AC, Jenni R, von Schulthess GK. Aortic valve pressure gradients in patients with aortic valve stenosis: quantification with velocity-encoded cine MR imaging. AJR. 1993;160:971–7.

47. Sechtem U, Pflugfelder PW, White RD, et al. Cine MR imaging: potential for the evaluation of cardiovascular function. AJR. 1987;148:239–46.

48. Bogaert J, Kuzo R, Dymarkowski S, Janssen L, Celis I, Budts W, et al. Follow-up of patients with previous treatment for coarctation of the thoracic aorta: comparison between contrast-enhanced MR angiography and fast spin-echo MR imaging. Eur Radiol. 2000;10(12):1847–54.

49. Mohiaddin RH, Kilner PJ, Rees S, Longmore DB. Magnetic resonance volume flow and jet velocity mapping in aortic coarctation. J Am Coll Cardiol. 1993;22(5):1515–21.

50. Oshinski JC, Parks WJ, Markou CP, Bergman HL, Larson BE, Ku DN. Improved measurement of pressure gradients in aortic coarctation by magnetic resonance imaging. J Am Coll Cardiol. 1996;28:1818–26.

51. Steffens JC, Bourne MW, Sakuma H, O'Sullivan M, Higgins CB. Quantification of collateral blood flow in coarctation of the aorta by velocity encoded cine magnetic resonance imaging. Circulation. 1994;90:937–43.

52. Eichhorn JG, Fink C, Delorme S, Hagl S, Kauczor HU, Ulmer HE. Magnetic resonance blood flow measurements in the follow-up of pediatric patients with aortic coarctation - a re-evaluation. Int J Cardiol. 2006;113(3):291–8. Epub 27 Dec 2005.

53. Mühler EG, Neuerburg JM, Rüben A, Grabitz RG, Günther RW, Messmer BJ, et al. Evaluation of aortic coarctation after surgical repair: role of magnetic resonance imaging and Doppler ultrasound. Br Heart J. 1993;70(3):285–90.

54. Nielsen JC, Powell AJ, Gauvreau K, Marcus EN, Prakash A, Geva T. Magnetic resonance imaging predictors of coarctation severity. Circulation. 2005;111(5):622–8.

55. Julsrud PR, Breen JF, Felmlee JP, Warnes CA, Connolly HM, Schaff HV. Coarctation of the aorta: collateral flow assessment with phase-contrast MR Angiography. AJR. 1997;169:1735–42.

56. Papavero R, Kastler B, Clair C, Litzler JF, Delabrousse E, Livolsi A, et al. Coarctation de l'aorte thoracique: évaluation et suivi en IRM. J Radiol. 2001;82:555–61.

57. Didier D, Saint-Martin C, Lapierre C, Trindade PT, Lahlaidi N, Vallee JP, et al. Coarctation of the aorta: pre and postoperative evaluation with MRI and MR angiography; correlation with echocardiography and surgery. Int J Cardiovasc Imaging. 2006;22(3–4):457–75.

58. Shih MC, Tholpady A, Kramer CM, Sydnor MK, Hagspiel KD. Surgical and endovascular repair of aortic coarctation: normal findings and appearance of complications on CT angiography and MR angiography. AJR Am J Roentgenol. 2006;187(3):W302–12.

59. Bank ER, Aisen AM, Rocchini AP, et al. Coarctation of the aorta in children undergoing angioplasty: pretreatment and posttreatment MR imaging. Radiology. 1987;162:235–40.

60. Riquelme C, Laissy JP, Menegazzo D, Debray MP, Cinqualbre A, Langlois J. MR Imaging of coarctation of the aorta and its postopeartive complications in adults: assesment witn spin-echo and Cine-MR imaging. Magn Reson Imaging. 1999;17:37–46.

61. oxer RA, La Corte MA, Singh S, et al. Nuclear magnetic resonance imaging in evaluation and follow up of children treated for coarctation of the aorta. J Am Coll Cardiol. 1986;7:1095–8.

62. Rees S, Somerville J, Ward C, et al. Coarctation of the aorta: MR imaging in late postoperative assessment. Radiology. 1989;173:499–502.

63. Ou P, Bonnet D, Auriacombe L, Pedroni E, Balleux F, Sidi D, et al. Late systemic hypertension and aortic arch geometry after successful repair of coarctation of the aorta. Eur Heart J. 2004;25(20):1853–9.

64. Ou P, Mousseaux E, Celermajer DS, Pedroni E, Vouhe P, Sidi D, et al. Aortic arch shape deformation after coarctation surgery: effect on blood pressure response. J Thorac Cardiovasc Surg. 2006;132(5):1105–11.

65. Ou P, Celermajer DS, Mousseaux E, Giron A, Aggoun Y, Szezepanski I, Sidi D, Bonnet D. Vascular remodeling after "successful" repair of coarctation: impact of aortic arch geometry. J Am Coll Cardiol. 2007;49(8):883–90. Epub 8 Feb 2007.

66. Ou P, Celermajer DS, Raisky O, Jolivet O, Buyens F, Herment A, et al. Angular (Gothic) aortic arch leads to enhanced systolic wave reflection, central aortic stiffness, and increased left ventricular mass late after aortic coarctation repair: evaluation with magnetic resonance flow mapping. J Thorac Cardiovasc Surg. 2008;135(1):62–8.

67. Onat T, Zeren E. Coarctation of the abdominal aorta: review of 91 cases. Cardiologia (Basel). 1969;54:140.

68. Riemenschneider TA, Emmanouilides GC, Hirose F, Linde LM. Coarctation of the abdominal aorta: report of the three cases and review of the literature. Pediatrics. 1969;44:716.

69. Ben-Shoshan M, Rossi NP, Korns ME. Coarctation of the abdominal aorta. Arch Pathol. 1973;95:221.

70. Celik T, Kursaklioglu H, Iyisoy A, Turhan H, Amasyali B, Kocaoglu M, et al. Hypoplasia of the descending thoracic and abdominal aorta: a case report and review of literature. J Thorac Imaging. 2006;21(4):296–9.

71. Livolsi A, Germain P, Kastler B. Etude d'une hypoplasie de l'aorte abdominale par IRM chez un nourrisson. Ann Cardiol Angiol. 1990;32:99–101.

72. Van Praagh R, Bernhard WF, Rosenthal A, Parisi LF, Fyler DC. Interrupted aortic arch; surgical treatment. Am J Cardiol. 1971;27:200–11.

73. Roberts WC, Morrow AG, Braunwald E. Complete interruption of the aortic arch. Circulation. 1962;26:39–59.

74. Vanmierop LHS, Kutsche LM. Interruption of the aortic arch and coarcation of the aorta: pathologenetic relations. Am J Cardiol. 1984;54:829–34.

75. Moller JH, Edwards JE. Interruption of aortic arch. Anatomic patterns and associated cardiac malformations. Am J Roentgenol. 1965;95:557–72.

76. Dische MR, Tsai M, Baltaxe HA. Solitary interruption of the arch of the aorta. Clinicopathologic review of eight cases. Am J Cardiol. 1975;345:271–7.

77. Higgins CB, French JW, Silverman JR, Wexler L. Interruption of the aortic arch: preoperative and postoperative clinical, hemodynamic and angiographic features. Am J Cardiol. 1977;39:563–71.

78. Milo S, Massini C, Goor DA. Isolated atresia of the aortic arch in a 65-year-old man. Surgical treatment and review of published reports. Br Heart J. 1982;47:294–7.

79. Riggs TW, Berry TE, Aziz KU, Paul MH. Two-dimensial echocardiographic features of interruption of the aortic arch. Am J Cardiol. 1982;50:1385–90.

80. Smallhorn JF, Anderson RH, Macartney FJ. Cross-sectional echocardiographic recognition of interruption of aortic arch between left carotid and subclavian arteries. Br Heart J. 1982;48:229–35.

81. Livolsi A, Kastler B, Marcellin L, Casanova R, Bintner M, Haddad J. MR diagnosis of subdiaphragmatic anomalous pulmonary venous drainage in a newborn. J Comput Assist Tomogr. 1991;15:1051–3.

82. Wagenvoort CA, Neufeld HN, Edwards JE. Cardiovascular system in Marfan's syndrome and idiopathic dilatation of the ascending aorta. Am J Cardiol. 1962;9:496.

83. Lemon DK, White CK. Anulaortic ectasia: angiographic, hemodynamic and clinical comparison with aortic valve insufficiency. Am J Cardiol. 1978;41:482.

84. Murdock JL, Walker BA, Halpern BL, Kuzma JW, Mckusick VA. Life expectancy and causes of death in the Marfan syndrome. N Engl J Med. 1972;286:804.

85. Robert WC. The aorta: its acquired diseases and their consequences as viewed from a morphologic perspective. In: Lindsay I Jr, Hurst JW, editors. The aorta. Grune and Stratton: New York; 1979. p. 51 (30 references).

86. Kersting-Sommerhoff BA, Sechtem UP, Schiller NB, et al. MRI of the thoracic aorta in Marfan patients. J Comp Assist Tomogr. 1987;11:633–9.

87. Schaefer S, Peshock RM, Malloy CR, et al. Nuclear magnetic resonance imaging in Marfan's syndrome. J Am Coll Cardiol. 1987;9:70–4.

88. Glazer HS, Gutierrez FR, Levitt RG, et al. The thoracic aorta studied by MR imaging. Radiology. 1985;157:149–55.

89. Kersting-Sommerhoff BA, Higgins CB, White RD, et al. Aortic dissection: sensitivity and specificity using ROC curve analysis. Radiology. 1988;166:651–5.

90. Amparo EG, Higgins CB, Hricak H, Sollitto R. Aortic dissection: magnetic resonance imaging. Radiology. 1985;155:399–406.

91. François CJ, Carr JC. MRI of the thoracic aorta. Magn Reson Imaging Clin N Am. 2007;15(4):639–51.

92. Lohan DG, Krishnam M, Saleh R, Tomasia A, Finn JP. MR imaging of the thoracic aorta. Magn Reson Imaging Clin N Am. 2008;16(2):213–34.

93. Lohan DG, Krishnam M, Saleh R, Tomasian A, Finn JP. Time-resolved MR angiography of the thorax. Magn Reson Imaging Clin N Am. 2008;16(2):235–48.

MRI is very useful for visualization of the right ventricular outflow tract, pulmonary artery (PA) trunk (retrosternal), and left and right branches (situated more posteriorly) due to its multislice (sagittal, axial, oblique, etc.) approach, its large field of view, and the absence of gas or bone artifacts which hinder US examination.

Echocardiography is unreliable for assessment of the pulmonary arteries beyond their proximal segment. Conventional X-ray angiography was also unreliable, especially in the absence of ventriculopulmonary connection (difficulties of opacification of the PA).

Evaluation of the right ventricular outflow tract, including the pulmonary arteries, is an essential part of the preoperative and postoperative assessment of certain forms of cyanotic heart disease. In pulmonary atresia, double outlet right ventricle (DORV) or other malformations responsible for decreased pulmonary blood flow, it is essential to identify the intrapericardial segment of the PA and the quality of distal runoff preoperatively. On echocardiography, it may be difficult to distinguish the intrapericardial PA from its branches and/or pericardial folds [1], especially when trying to visualize small nonconfluent pulmonary branches in the preoperative assessment of pulmonary atresia with VSD or other complex cyanotic congenital heart diseases. MRI is very useful in the assessment of the pulmonary circulation [2–5] and at present avoids the need for angiography [6], which was not very reliable in this field.[1]

In this chapter, we initially discuss malformations of the PA, followed by a brief review of the main anomalies affecting the right ventricular outflow tract (cyanotic heart disease), in which MRI is essentially useful to evaluate the pulmonary circulation. Postoperative evaluation, one of the formally demonstrated advantages of MRI, is discussed in detail in Chap. 8.

7.1 Examination Technique

The examination starts with a series of mediastinal axial ECG-gated black blood sequences (fast spin-echo or double IR sequences) that must always be completed in this type of disease by sagittal and coronal images (see Chap. 2) to ensure optimal visualization of the right ventricular outflow tract and pulmonary arteries.

The slice thickness is adapted to the size of the patient: 3–5 mm in newborn and young children, and 5–8 mm in older children and adults. Optimal visualization of small vascular structures and the tracheobronchial tree can be obtained by performing stacks of intertwined and overlapping images, 3–5 mm thick (i.e., slice interval of 2–3 mm, see Chap. 2, Examination technique).

Serial MRI images in the sagittal plane are perfectly adapted to visualize the entire right ventricular outflow tract on a single imaging plane: the right ventricle continuous with the pulmonary infundibulum, the PA trunk, and the left PA (see Chap. 2, atlas S4). Supravalvular or subvalvular stenoses are also easily identified on this view.

The right PA is clearly visualized on coronal images (see Chap. 2, atlas F8 and F9).

The PA trunk and its right and left branches are well visualized on axial images (Figs. 7.8–7.10 and see Chap. 2, Fig. 2.8 and atlas A4, A6).

---

[1]Particularly in the case of pulmonary artery atresia or nonconfluence of the right and left branches.

B. Kastler, *MRI of Cardiovascular Malformations*,
DOI: 10.1007/978-3-540-30702-0_7, © Springer-Verlag Berlin Heidelberg 2011

Bright-blood cine-MR imaging [7–16] and velocity mapping techniques [16–24] are useful to analyze stenosis on proximal pulmonary arteries, and CE-MRA [10, 11, 25] to confirm the patency of hypoplastic pulmonary vessels [26].

7.2 Pulmonary Artery Malformations

7.2.1 Unilateral Absence of Pulmonary Artery (UAPA)

This anomaly is defined as complete absence of one of the two branches of the PA and involves the sixth aortic arch or pulmonary arch. It is a rare anomaly accounting for 0.54–1.4% of all cases of congenital heart disease according to various authors [27, 28]. It is not hereditary, affects boys and girls with equal frequency, and involves both the right and the left PA.

7.2.1.1 Pathology

Right-sided unilateral absence of pulmonary artery (UAPA) is more common and is usually isolated. Left-sided absence can be associated [29–31] with various types of congenital heart disease, particularly tetralogy of Fallot, right aortic arch, pulmonary stenosis, VSD, or anomalous venous connection. It can be associated with pulmonary atresia with complete absence of bronchi and lung tissue (type I of Schneider's classification) or persistence of a bronchial stump (Schneider type II – Fig. 7.1).

The homolateral lung, when present, is generally hypoplastic, but presents normal segmentation; it is well differentiated in isolated UAPA. The association with pulmonary malformations has been clearly described [32] and depends on the embryological stage at which arrested development occurred and the malformations induced by this arrested development. The bronchial tree can be either normal or may present signs of bronchiectasis.

The pulmonary circulation on the affected side is ensured by systemic vessels derived from the aorta via the subclavian artery, bronchial arteries, abdominal aorta, or via transpleural collaterals [33–36] (see Fig. 7.2 and also Fig. 7.12).

7.2.1.2 Clinicopathological Forms

UAPA causes anatomical changes similar to those of pneumonectomy or PA thrombosis. Pulmonary artery hypertension occurs more or less rapidly, depending on the associated malformations [28, 30, 31, 37–39].

Isolated UAPA is well supported, as 30% of patients are asymptomatic and the anomaly is discovered incidentally on routine radiological examination, or following a complication (hemoptysis or, more rarely, acute pulmonary edema).

Left UAPA is often associated with tetralogy of Fallot. Other complex malformations, such as DORV, are frequently associated with left or right UAPA (Fig. 7.2). (Also refer to case presented in Fig. 7.5). UAPA associated with other malformations is usually diagnosed early in a context of PA hypertension and possibly asystolie. They present with respiratory symptoms: recurrent respiratory tract infections, hemoptysis, chest pain, and dyspnea.

7.2.1.3 Conventional Complementary Investigations

Chest radiograph may visualize a small unilateral lung with rib notching, unilateral reduction, or absence of hilar vascular opacities [28, 40–48]. Other signs include elevation of the homolateral hemidiaphragm and mediastinal shift.

Echocardiography is not always informative. It is sometimes difficult to confirm the absence of the left PA [49].

Chest CT [50, 51] can demonstrate a small lung with mediastinal shift and pleural thickening, and contrast-enhanced acquisition reveal complete absence of one of the two branches of the PA [96].

The diagnosis was classically demonstrated by conventional angiography [48, 52, 53], which demonstrated progressive interruption of the column of contrast agent with no opacification of the affected PA, and opacification of pulmonary veins on both sides during the venous phase [54]. It also visualized the systemic blood supply of the small lung.

7.2.1.4 MRI

The most contributive images are transverse images (Figs. 7.1 and 7.2), which confirm the absence of the right or left PA and the associated pulmonary hypoplasia

[33–37, 55, 96, 97, 98]. The other views are less reliable for the diagnosis of UAPA, but are useful for the assessment of associated anomalies. Gadolinium-enhanced magnetic resonance angiography sequences are well suited for displaying the unique PA with its branching vessels on a large FOV (Fig. 7.2c, d) [51].

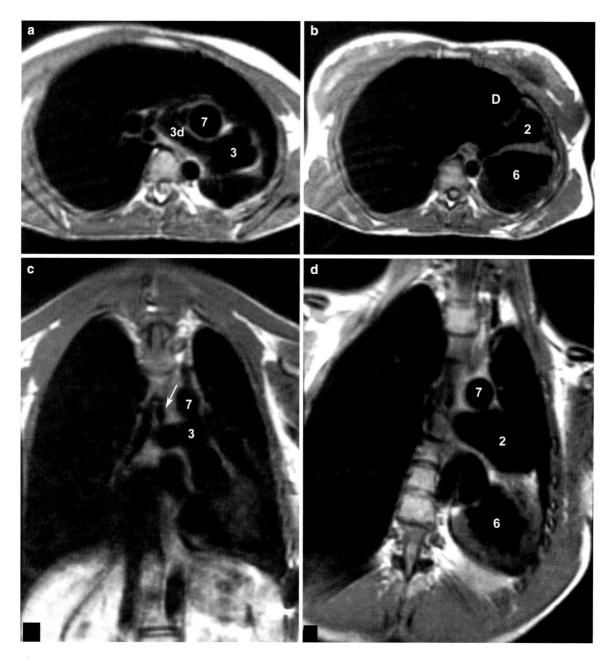

Fig. 7.1 (**a–d**) Absence of the left pulmonary artery (PA) with homolateral pulmonary atresia. (**a, b**) Axial spin-echo images: the PA trunk (3) gives rise to a single right branch (3d) with complete atresia of the left lung and significant left-sided mediastinal shift. The heart occupies the left lung field and is in contact with the chest wall. The pulmonary structure visible on the left side (D) actually corresponds to transmediastinal hernia of the right lung to the left; aorta (7), right ventricle (RV) (2) and left ventricle (LV) (6). (**c, d**) Coronal spin-echo images: the image through the tracheal bifurcation (**c**) shows a single bronchial stump on the left (*arrow*). (**e, f**) Absence of the right PA in a young adult female. Note on these axial cine-MRI images, a unique prominent left PA (3d), right ventricular hypertrophy (RVH) (2), and dilated right atrium (RA) (1); left atrium (LA) (5) LV (6), aorta (7)

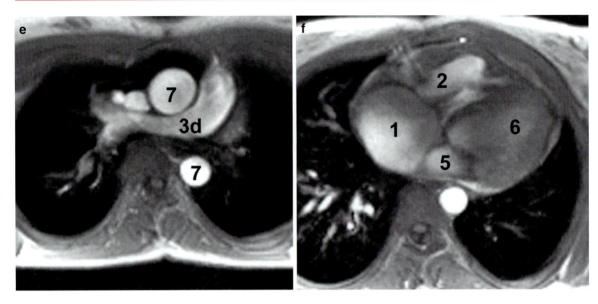

Fig. 7.1 (continued)

7.2.2 Anomalous Origin of Left Pulmonary Artery

This entity is described in Chap. 5.

7.2.3 Truncus Arteriosus

This anomaly accounts for 1% of all cases of congenital heart disease and corresponds to a single arterial trunk arising from the base of the heart over a single arterial valve (Figs. 7.3–7.5, also see Fig. 3.26, Chap. 3) [56, 57]. This truncus arteriosus gives rise to the coronary arteries, aorta, and pulmonary arteries.

7.2.3.1 Pathology

- Intracardiac anomalies: Truncus arteriosus is usually associated with a large ventricular septal defect (Fig. 7.5).
- Anomalies of the truncal valve: The truncal valve is bicuspid in 8% of cases, tricuspid in 66% of cases, and quadricuspid in 25% of cases. The presence of six semilunar leaflets is exceptional. The leaflets are often abnormal and thickened, leading to valve stenosis or regurgitation.
- Coronary arteries: Coronary arteries frequently have an anomalous origin, in 30–45% of cases, which can reliably by depicted by MRI [58–60]. The left orifice is often very high, close to the

origin of the PA branches (representing a risk during surgery).
- Aortic arch: The aortic arch is generally single with a large caliber, but a double aortic arch may sometimes be observed. The horizontal aorta can be atresic or hypoplastic in 10–20% of cases.
- Pulmonary branches: A large number of anatomical variants of the origin of pulmonary branches can be observed. Four types are defined according to the slightly modified classification of Van Praagh (Fig. 7.4) [56]:

  - Type I represents 60–70% of cases. The pulmonary trunk arises from the truncus arteriosus over the truncal valve and coronary arteries before giving rise to its two branches.
  - Type II represents 20–30% of cases. The two PA branches arise from two distinct orifices on the posterior surface of the truncus arteriosus. Pulmonary arteries can also arise from the lateral surfaces of the truncus arteriosus.
  - Type III is very rare. The truncus arteriosus gives a right PA and the artery considered to be the left PA is a collateral of the descending thoracic aorta.
  - Type IV corresponds to type I with interruption of the aortic arch or coarctation.

7.2.3.2 Clinicopathological Forms

Truncus arteriosus is a serious malformation because of the risk of early heart failure or pulmonary outflow

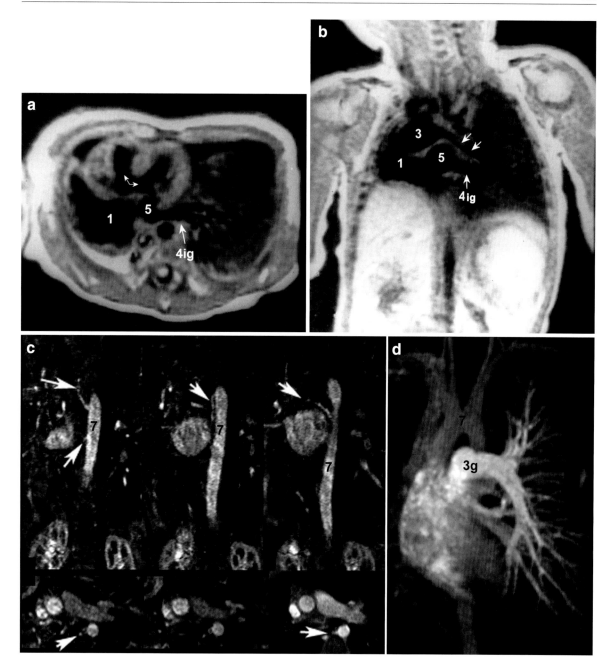

Fig. 7.2 (**a**, **b**) Absence of the right PA in a small-for-dates neonate with a complex multiple malformation syndrome (atresia of the right external ear, hypoplasia of the right mandible, coloboma of right upper eyelid and cleft palate). The chest radiograph shows complete absence of the right lung, and echocardiography demonstrates double outlet right ventricle (DORV) with transposition of the great vessels and ventricular septal defect, but cannot visualize the pulmonary arteries. (**a**) Axial spin-echo image showing complete atresia of the right lung with significant mediastinal shift to the right; the heart occupies the right lung field and is in contact with the chest wall; RA (1), LA (5), and left inferior pulmonary vein (4ig), ventricular septal defect (*double arrow*). (**b**) Coronal image through the two atria. The RA is very large. The right lung is absent and the heart is shifted to the right. The PA trunk (3) and a small left PA (*arrows*) are visible, but not the right PA. (**c**, **d**) In this second case of absence of the left PA, the right pulmonary lung blood supply is ensured by a network of aorto-pulmonary collateral vessels (bronchial vessels) derived from the descending thoracic aorta (7), visible (*arrows*) on the contrast-enhanced MRA (Dota-Gd, Guerbet, France) multiplanar coronal and axial reconstructions (**c**). The unique prominent left PA (3g) and left lung blood supply is well depicted on the MIP reconstruction (**d**); aorta (7)

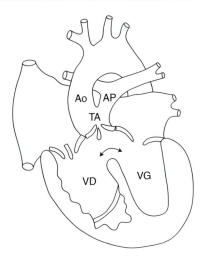

Fig. 7.3 Diagram of type I truncus arteriosus (TA) (the most frequent form): the aorta (Ao) and PA arise from a common trunk (TA) above the truncal valve, which generally comprises three valves; RV and LV, ventricular septal defect (*double arrow*), RA and LA

obstruction. It is usually an isolated finding; however, it can be associated with other anomalies like DiGeorge syndrome (20% of cases), which must be taken into account in the indication for surgery [57], or right aortic arch with mirror branching.

7.2.3.3 Hemitruncus Arteriosus

In this type of anomaly, one PA (usually the right) arises from the main PA and the opposite PA from the ascending aorta.

7.2.4 *Valvular Pulmonary Atresia*

Isolated valvular pulmonary atresia is a rare malformation and is usually associated with stenosis of the annulus, aneurysmal dilatation of the PA, and other malformations such as VSD, tetralogy of Fallot, DORV, tricuspid atresia, and aortic arch anomalies.

7.2.4.1 Clinical Features

Isolated valvular pulmonary atresia is well tolerated, but an associated VSD or other more complex cardiac

malformations are accompanied by early onset of severe heart failure. The severity of the malformation is determined by the aneurysmal dilatation of the PA which is responsable of ventilatory disorders by compression. This form must be distinguished from classical tetralogy of Fallot, as it has a much poorer prognosis with a mortality of 75%.

Echocardiography visualizes dilatation of the PA, but absence of the pulmonary valve and hypoplasia of the annulus are not always clearly identified. Pulsed Doppler echocardiography shows accelerated systolic flow across the stenosis and diastolic regurgitation.

Angiography provides a precise diagnosis of the anomaly.

MRI

MRI has the dual advantage of allowing morphological analysis of the anomaly and assessment of the effects on the tracheobronchial tree. Anteroposterior and lateral views visualize the aneurysmal dilatation of the PA and absence of the pulmonary valve. Postoperatively, MRI allows assessment of the quality of correction and decompression of the tracheobronchial tree.

7.2.5 *Valvular Pulmonary Stenosis*

Valvular pulmonary stenosis (Fig. 7.7a, b) can be isolated or associated with more complex diseases such as tetralogy of Fallot, transposition of the great vessels, etc. MRI is of little value in isolated pulmonary stenosis, as echocardiography allows a precise diagnosis and angiography constitutes the first stage of a pulmonary valvuloplasty procedure.

7.2.6 *Pulmonary Artery Stenosis and Atresia*

MRI [61], although it can diagnose subvalvular and proximal PA, is a key examination for the detection of peripheral PA stenosis (Figs. 7.7e, f and 7.9c, and Chap. 8, Fig. 8.2e and f for postoperative pulmonary stenosis), segmental hypoplasia or atresia (Figs. 7.6

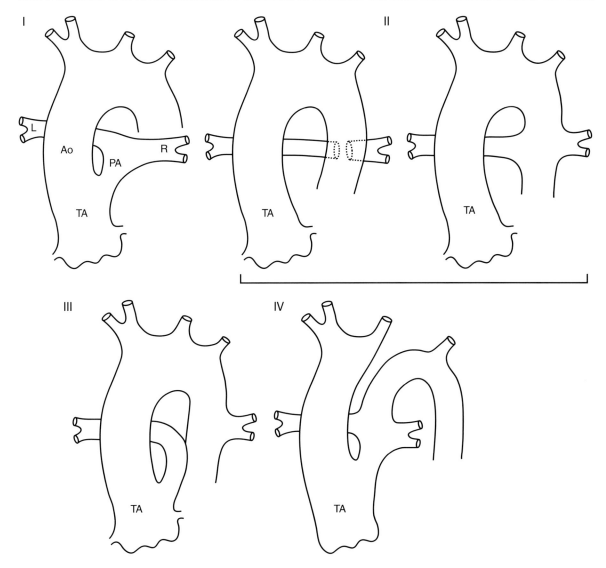

Fig. 7.4 Diagram of TA variants (types I–IV): see text. Aorta (Ao), pulmonary trunk (PA), right PA (d) and left PA (g), TA (also see Chap. 3, Fig. 3.26)

and 7.12) or nonconfluence of PA branches (Fig. 7.11 and see Chap. 8, Fig. 8.5), as these anomalies are poorly visualized on echocardiography. The same applies to tetralogy of Fallot with pulmonary atresia (pseudotruncus arteriosus), in which the atresic segment is generally situated proximally on the PA trunk, but can involve the entire trunk as far as the bifurcation. In this situation, it is important to determine the caliber, the confluent or nonconfluent nature of pulmonary arteries, and the quality of the collateral circulation via the bronchial artery network prior to revascularization surgery (Figs. 7.6 and 7.12).

MRI provides a complete assessment of the anomalies. MRI identifies the mechanism responsible when the anomalies are secondary to compression, shift, and deviation related to postoperative changes. Postoperative PA stenosis can occur at zones of insertion of reimplanted pulmonary arteries in correction of transpositions by arterial switch (see Chap. 8, Figs. 8.15 and 8.16) and on the inferior pulmonary insertion of the shunt in Blalock-Taussig shunts (see Chap. 8, Fig. 8.2).

Axial and coronal (oblique) views are used to visualize the right PA and sagittal (oblique) views are used to visualize the left PA (see Fig. 2.8, Chap. 2). CE-enhanced magnetic resonance angiography sequences can display the stenosis of the PA and major branching arteries on a large Fov (see Fig. 7.7e–h and also refer to Figs. 7.9 and 7.25 and Chap. 8, Fig. 8.2e, f for postoperative pulmonary stenosis)

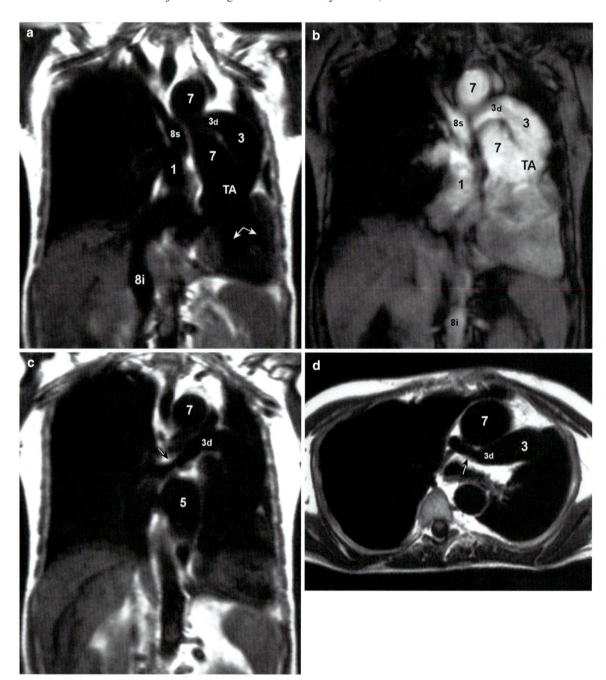

Fig. 7.5 TA type I and absence of the left PA (unique right PA) in a 43-year-old male. MRI coronal spin-echo (**a, b**) and cine-MRI (**c**) and axial spin-echo (**d, e** and **f**) images show the TA giving rise to both the aorta (7) and the pulmonary trunk and right unique PA (3 and 3d). The patient survived because, the stenosis on the right PA (*arrows*), by reducing the pulmonary blood flow, has protected the lungs. Secondary hypertension was thus prevented as would PA banding; ventricular septal defect (*double arrow*); RA (5), superior vena cava (8s), inferior vena cava (8i) (For TA also see Chap. 3, Fig. 3.26 and for PA banding see Fig. 7.23 and Chap. 8, Figs. 8.31 and 8.32.)

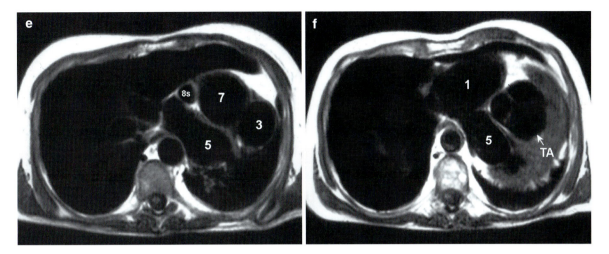

Fig. 7.5 (continued)

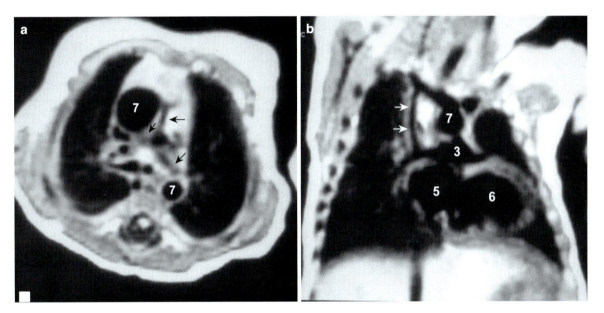

Fig. 7.6 Infant presenting with tetralogy of Fallot with severe hypoplasia of the PA trunk and branches (**a**, axial image, *black arrows*) not visualized by echocardiography. Revascularization of the pulmonary arteries was performed by Blalock-Taussig shunt between the right subclavian artery and right PA (**b**, coronal oblique image, *white arrows* – also see Chap. 8, Figs. 8.2e, f for postoperative complications); PA (3), aorta (7), LA (5), LV (6)

7.3 Cyanotic Heart Disease

7.3.1 Cyanosis

Cyanosis is the essential clinical feature with a variable expression according to the disease.

Cyanosis is a clinical concept corresponding to a bluish color of the skin and mucous membranes, observed whenever there is more than 5 g of reduced hemoglobin per 100 mL of blood in the capillary network [62]. It generally corresponds to an oxygen saturation of 85%.

It is, in this context, secondary to the presence of a right–left shunt [63]. This cyanosis is more marked in the extremities (fingers, lips, and ears) and disappears on pressure with a glass slide, confirming its circulatory nature.

Dyspnea, in the form of shallow, rapid breathing, is variable; it is observed on exertion, but also in response to emotions. These infants predominantly present delayed growth, in contrast with infants with a left–right shunt, who present poorer weight gain. Squatting, generally after exertion, is virtually observed only in tetralogy of Fallot. Nonspecific clubbing is also observed in cyanotic heart diseases, together with gingival hyperplasia, reflecting chronic hypoxia. Polycythemia can induce specific complications and is generally secondary to chronic hypoxia. Neurological effects mainly consist of hypoxic spells, usually observed in tetralogy of Fallot. Cerebrovascular accidents and brain abscess are observed more rarely.

Cardiac auscultation [64, 65] may detect murmurs, added heart sounds, or modification of normal heart sounds.

Fig. 7.7 (**a, b**) Severe valvular pulmonary stenosis in a small-for-dates neonate. Sagittal and coronal cine-MR images. The stenosis of the valves is seen as a signal-void turbulent jet (*arrows*) located above the site of pulmonary annulus. (Compare to (**c, d**)) RV (2), LV (6), LA (5), RA (1), aorta (7). (**c, d**) Infundibular stenosis in a newborn. The hypertrophic RV continuous with the funnel-shaped narrowed pulmonary infundibulum (muscular stenosis – *arrows*) is well depicted on these sagittal cine-MR images; RV (2), LV (6), LA (5). (**e–h**) Severe proximal stenosis of the left PA (3g) in a newborn with dextrocardia and major dilatation of the right heart chambers. The stenosis (*arrows*) visible on the sagittal balanced-SSFP image (Fiesta). Note the enlargement of the RA (1), dilatation and hypertrophy of the RV (2), and enlargement of the inferior vena cava (8i) (also refer to Figs. 7.9 and 7.25 and Chap. 8, Figs. 8.2e, f for postoperative pulmonary stenosis and Chap. 3 Fig. 3.28 for dextrocardia)

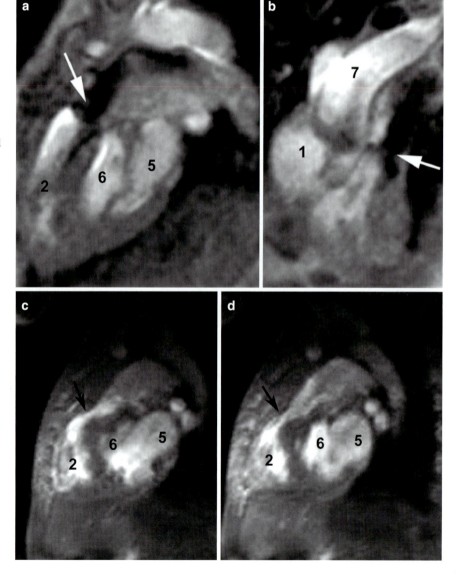

Fig. 7.7 (continued)

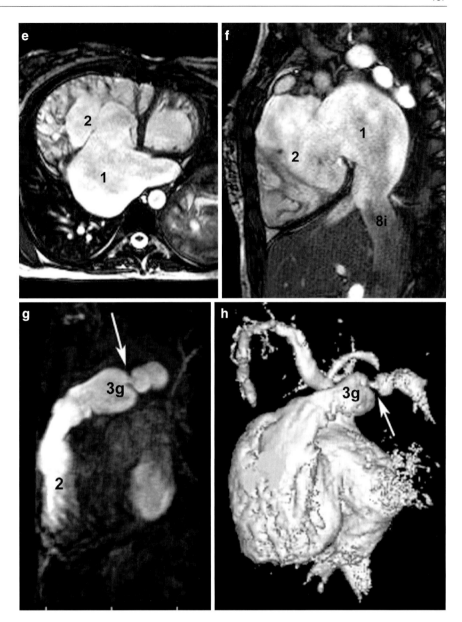

7.3.2 Tetralogy of Fallot

The four components of this anomaly were described by Antoine Fallot in 1888 [66] (Fig. 7.8): right ventricular infundibular stenosis (and often pulmonary stenosis), aortic valve (aortic root) overriding the two ventricles associated with a large subaortic ventricular septal defect, and right ventricular hypertrophy. The degree of right ventricular outflow tract obstruction is variable, but may comprise pulmonary atresia.

Tetralogy of Fallot is the most frequent form of cyanotic heart disease, representing 5–8% of all cases of congenital heart disease [67]. Considerable progress has been made in the surgical treatment of this serious malformation, which requires a complete preoperative anatomical assessment.

Fig. 7.8 Diagram of the four components of tetralogy of Fallot. (**a**) infundibular pulmonary stenosis (PSt), the aorta overrides the two ventricles over a large ventricular septal defect (*double arrow*) with RVH. (**b**) The aortic arch is situated on the *right* in about 30% of cases

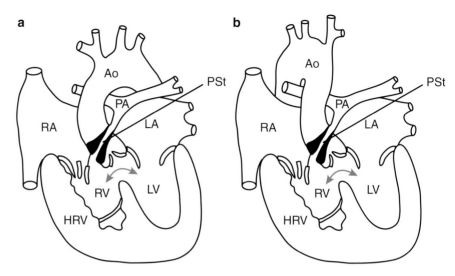

7.3.2.1 Pathology

The four anomalies result from anterior and right-sided displacement of the infundibular septum inducing unequal development of the right and left ventricles [68].

- Pulmonary stenosis

Infundibular stenosis (Fig. 7.7c, d): it is a constant and fundamental feature of this disease and is due to under-development of the subpulmonary conus. It is usually severe (tunnel-shaped), essentially muscular and tends to deteriorate with age [69]. A bicuspid (or even uni-cuspid) pulmonary valve is observed in two-thirds of cases, with PA hypoplasia resulting in subvalvular, valvular, and supravalvular stenosis.

The right ventricular outflow tract typically presents thin walls and a slightly narrowed lumen, but it can also be stenotic either at the bifurcation, or on distal branches. Proximal atresia of the pulmonary trunk, usually at the valvular level, is observed more rarely, corresponding to pseudotruncus arteriosus. The branch pulmonary arteries may be nonconfluent or completely absent. Nonconfluence, size, and number of the branch pulmonary arteries are critical to management of tetralogy of Fallot. A branch PA, usually the left, can originate from a patent ductus arteriosus.

- Ventricular septal defect

The subaortic VSD (Fig. 7.9a, e) is large with an area approximately equal to that of the aortic orifice, situated

Fig. 7.9 (**a**) Infant presenting with tetralogy of Fallot. Cranial to caudal axial fast spin-echo images. The significant infundibular muscular stenosis (tunnel-shaped) (*arrow*) and RVH (*arrow-head*) are well depicted at the level of the subpulmonary conus, as well as the ventricular septal defect (*double arrow*). The aortic root (7a) overrides the two ventricles and the interventricular septum. Note the dextroposition of the aorta (7d) (also refer to Fig. 7.7c, d); RA (1), PA (3), LA (5), LV (6). (**b, c**) Infant presenting with tetralogy of Fallot. The RVH (*arrowheads*) and tunnel-shape infundibular muscular stenosis (*arrows*) are well depicted at the level of the subpulmonary conus on these axial (**b**), sagittal axial (**c**) images. The descending aorta is in its normal position on the *left* (also refer to Fig. 7.7c, d) RA (1), RV (2), LV (6). (**d, e**) Infant presenting with tetralogy of Fallot diagnosed by echocardiography. (**c**) Axial image through the PA bifurcation (3). Distal pulmonary stenosis in the proximity of the bifurcation is also present (*arrows*). (**d**) Axial image through the cardiac chambers demonstrating the ventricular septal defect (*double arrow*). The aortic root (7) overrides the two ventricles and the interventricular septum. The descending aorta is located on the *left* (also refer to Fig. 7.7c, d). (**f, g**) Infant presenting with tetralogy of Fallot diagnosed by echocardiography (double superior vena cava also not seen). Spin-echo axial images. The tunnel-shaped infundibular muscular is well depicted on the image at the level of the subpulmonary conus (**f**). An additional PA hypoplasia resulting here in subvalvular, valvular, and supravalvular stenosis is clearly visible (*arrows*) on images through the pulmonary bifurcation (**g**). Note the right aortic arch (7) and double superior vena cava (*right* 8sd, *left* 8sg); RV (2) (also refer to Fig. 7.7c, d)

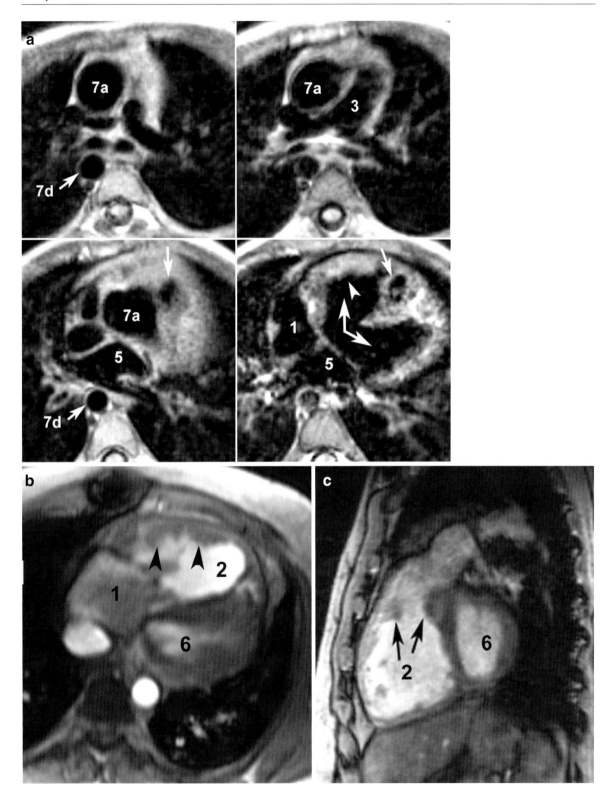

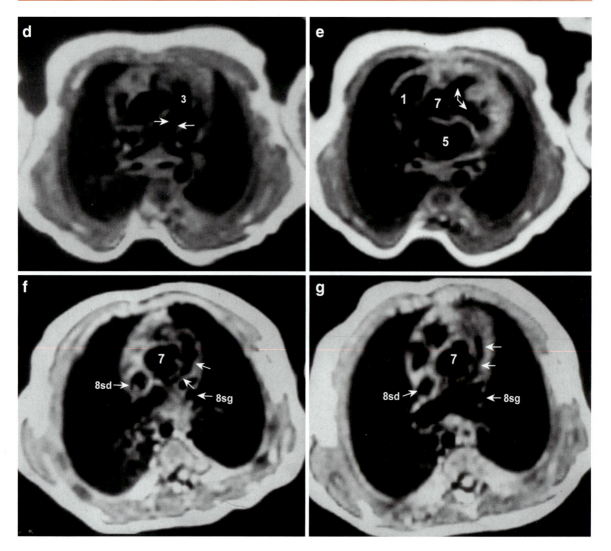

Fig. 7.9 (continued)

just above the defect, and is usually perimembranous or infundibular.

- Dextroposition of the aorta

The aorta overrides the two ventricular chambers over the interventricular septum (and the VSD) (Fig. 7.9a, e). It is enlarged (inversely proportional to the diameter of the PA). Usually, two-thirds of the aorta override the left ventricle and one-third overrides the right ventricle. There are extreme forms ranging from minimal dextroposition to an aorta arising from the right ventricle [70]. A fibrous mitro-aortic continuity is nevertheless preserved.

- Right ventricular hypertrophy

Right ventricular hypertrophy is secondary to right ventricular outflow tract obstruction (Figs. 7.7c, d and 7.9a–c, for right ventricular hypertrophy also refer to Fig. 7.7c, d).

- Associated anomalies

In about 30% of cases, the aortic arch is situated on the right (Fig. 7.9a, f, and g) [71]. It is important to identify associated anomalies of coronary arteries, present in one-third of cases [72], as a coronary branch can cross in front of the infundibular stenosis, for example, when the left anterior descending artery arises from the right coronary artery (5% of cases – or in the case of single right or left coronary artery[2] [58]).

Multiple ventricular septal defects or patent ductus arteriosus are rarely associated. The presence of aorto-pulmonary collateral vessels is less frequent than in pulmonary atresia (in which they constitute the only means of pulmonary revascularization, Fig. 7.12).

7.3.2.2 Clinical Features

The fundamental sign is cyanosis, the severity of which depends on the degree of stenosis. Other signs such as clubbing, squatting on exertion, dyspnea, and hypoxic spells are observed later.

• Echocardiography

Echocardiography easily confirms the diagnosis of tetralogy of Fallot, identifies the infundibular stenosis, VSD, and the degree of overriding of the aorta. Dextroposition of the aorta and PA stenosis are more difficult to visualize. Echocardiography cannot evaluate pulmonary blood flow or the caliber of the branch pulmonary arteries, the aorto-pulmonary collaterals, and proximal course of coronary arteries. MRI is required in the preoperative assessment of these features.

MRI

Serial MRI images in the sagittal plane are perfectly adapted to visualize all of the right ventricular outflow tract on a single imaging plane [73] (Figs. 7.7 and 7.9e, f): the right ventricle continuous with the narrowed pulmonary infundibulum, the PA trunk with a more or less abnormal valve and the left PA, and possibly ductus arteriosus (Fig. 7.12c, e). Supravalvular and subvalvular stenoses, and ductus arteriosus are at best displayed, (or optimally displayed) on this view (Figs. 7.7 and 7.9e, f). Coronal images are best suited to visualize the right pulmonary artery. Axial images are also useful for assessment of the PA trunk and left and right branches (Figs. 7.6, 7.8, 7.9, and 7.11), and to visualize the VSD (Figs. 7.8 and 7.9).

---

[2]A major coronary branch crossing anteriorly over the pulmonary infundibulum can be situated in the zone of incision during enlargement of the right ventricular outflow tract (for infundibular stenosis) (see Chap. 8, Fig. 8.29).

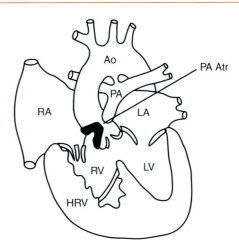

Fig. 7.10 Diagram of pulmonary atresia (PA Atr) with ventricular septal defect (extreme form of tetralogy of Fallot): the pulmonary circulation (PA) is exclusively derived from the systemic circulation via a patent ductus arteriosus (DA); aorta (Ao) overriding the right (RV) and left (LV) ventricles, ventricular septal defect (*double arrow*) and RVH, RA and LA

Aorto-pulmonary collaterals visible on black-blood images (Fig. 7.12a–c) are best depicted on Gd-enhanced MRA [74]. MR Imaging of coronary arteries is improving [58–60] (see Chap. 1, Fig. 1.10). To detect an abnormal course of the coronary arteries coronary angiography is not required any more (see Chap. 7).

7.3.3 Pulmonary Atresia with Ventricular Septal Defect

This congenital heart disease comprises complete right ventricular outflow tract obstruction and ventricular septal defect. Assessment of the right ventricular outflow tract is essential to determine the most appropriate surgical treatment. This entity is not rare, as it accounts for 2% of all cases of congenital heart disease.

7.3.3.1 Pathology

This is an extreme form of tetralogy of Fallot. In three-quarters of cases, pulmonary atresia corresponds to an elastic cord involving a segment of the PA (Fig. 7.11). The pulmonary valve and the proximal portion of the pulmonary trunk are usually involved. More rarely, only the pulmonary valve is imperforate. The ventricular septal defect may be either membranous or infundibular.

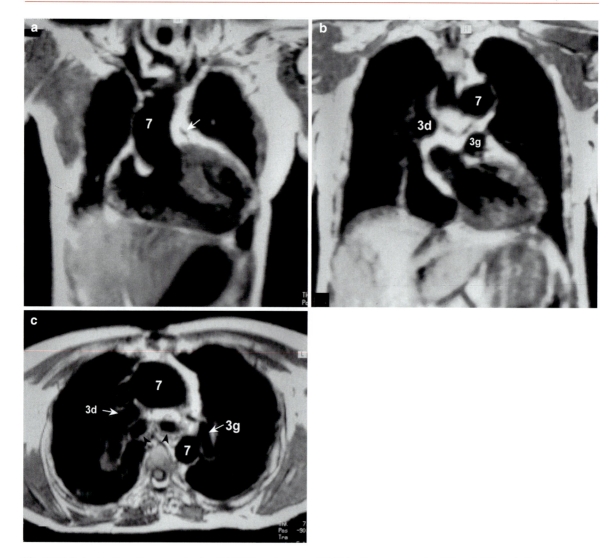

Fig. 7.11 Patient with pulmonary atresia with VSD and non-confluent pulmonary circulation, which cannot be visualized by echocardiography. (**a**) Coronal image clearly visualizing the pulmonary atresia (*arrow*); aorta (7). (**b**) Coronal image and (**c**) axial image. Note the absence of confluence of the *right* (3d) and *left* (3g) pulmonary arteries; left and right main bronchi (*arrowheads*). Nonconfluent branch pulmonary arteries require bilateral palliative shunts. A Blalock-Taussig shunt was performed on the left PA and a Waterston shunt was performed on the right PA (see same patient Chap. 8, Fig. 8.5)

7.3.3.2 Clinicopathological Forms

In severe forms, hypoplasia can involve the right and left pulmonary arteries (Fig. 7.6 and see Chap. 8, Fig. 8.4), while, in other cases, only one branch is stenotic (Fig. 7.25). In extreme cases, atresia extends beyond the bifurcation, corresponding to a nonconfluent form which may require bilateral palliative shunts (Fig. 7.11 and see Chap. 8, Fig. 8.5). In this case, the pulmonary circulation is supplied by systemic arteries: patent ductus arteriosus and bronchial and pleural arteries [75, 76] (Fig. 7.12).

When the ductus arteriosus is narrow or closes at birth, PA hypoplasia is very marked and associated with severe clinical symptoms.

In the absence of a patent ductus arteriosus, the pulmonary circulation is ensured by a network of collateral vessels derived from the descending thoracic aorta

(Fig. 7.12a–c), or more rarely, from the subclavian artery and exceptionally, the abdominal aorta. Shunts are observed at the hilum or on lobar or intraparenchymal branches.

The aorta generally overrides the interventricular septum by more than 50%. Associated cardiac anomalies are similar to those observed in tetralogy of Fallot.

7.3.4 Pulmonary Atresia with Intact Interventricular Septum

This very serious congenital heart disease is almost exclusively observed in neonates and has a very poor prognosis. By definition, it comprises a combination of right ventricular outflow tract atresia and intact interventricular septum.

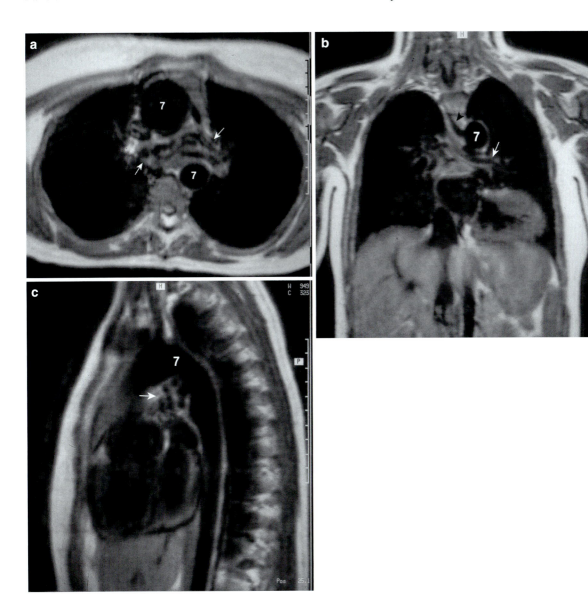

Fig. 7.12 (**a–c**) Extreme form of tetralogy of Fallot with pulmonary atresia extending to the pulmonary arteries. In this adolescent patient, the pulmonary blood supply is ensured by a network of collateral vessels derived from the descending thoracic aorta, clearly visible (*arrows*), anterior to bronchial tree, on axial (**a**), coronal (**b**), and sagittal (**c**) spin-echo images (also see Fig. 7.23). The PA itself is not visualized; note the presence of arteria lusoria (*black arrowhead*); aorta (7). (**d–f**) Pulmonary atresia in a neonate. The pulmonary blood supply is ensured by a patent DA visible (*arrows*) on sagittal fast spin-echo (**d**), sagittal gradient-echo (**e**), and axial gradient-echo (**f**) images; left PA (3g), aorta (7), RV (2), LV (6)

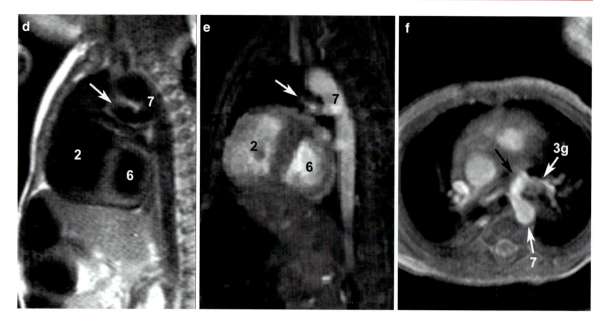

Fig. 7.12 (continued)

7.3.4.1 Pathology

Pulmonary atresia is a constant feature with fusion of two or three valve leaflets. Hypoplasia of the right ventricle may result in an almost absent ventricle. All components of the tricuspid valve are almost always abnormal, resulting in tricuspid stenosis and/or regurgitation [77]. An ostium secundum atrial septal defect is usually present. The pulmonary circulation is usually composed of two hypoplastic but confluent branches and a descending trunk in contact with the atresic orifice. The very abnormal coronary circulation is due to anomalous connection or adventitial fibrosis.

7.3.4.2 Clinicopathological Forms

The various clinicopathological forms are classified into three types of decreasing severity:

- Right ventricle reduced to its inlet chamber with atresia of the trabeculated chamber and subpulmonary infundibulum.
- Ventricle comprising the first two segments, but not the infundibulum.
- Right ventricle composed of three parts.

7.4   Transposition of the Great Vessels

The reader is also referred to Chap. 3.

This type of anomaly comprises a ventriculoarterial discordance: the aorta arises from the right ventricle, while the PA arises from the left ventricle. There are two main variants with very different pathophysiology and prognosis (see Chap. 3).

7.4.1   Complete transposition of the great vessels (Dextro-transposition or D-transposition)

- Pathology

D-transposition results from failed spiraling of the aortico-pulmonary septum. It represents about 9% of all cases of congenital heart disease. This form presents ventriculoarterial discordance but atrioventricular concordance (ventricles are in a normal position) (Fig. 7.13).

In the majority of cases, the atria are in situs solitus and, due to the atrioventricular concordance, the right ventricle is in a normal position, that is, to the right of the left ventricle (D-loop).

Fig. 7.13 Ventriculoarterial discordance with atrioventricular concordance in complete transposition of the great vessels (D-transposition – D-loop). (**a**) Simple form associated with foramen ovale or patent DA. (**b**) Complex forms associated with ventricular septal defect (*double arrow*) and/or subpulmonary stenosis (PSt). Aorta (Ao), PA, RA and LA, RV and LV (also see Figs. 7.14 and 7.15, Chap. 3, Figs. 3.16–3.20 and Chap. 8, Figs. 8.14, 8.15, and 8.22)

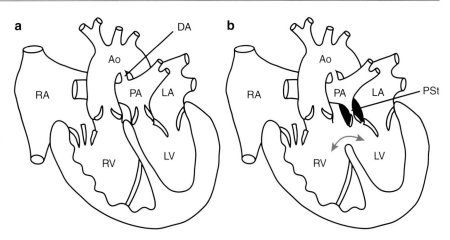

Ventriculoarterial discordance (the aorta arises from the right ventricle and the PA arises from the left ventricle) is associated with an abnormal spatial configuration of the great vessels: the aortic valve is situated on the right and slightly anteriorly (D-transposition) to the pulmonary valve (Figs. 7.14 and 7.15, also see Chap. 3, Figs. 3.17–3.20 and Chap. 8, Figs. 8.14, 8.15, and 8.22) with fibrous mitro-pulmonary continuity.

The term simple transposition is used when this malformation is isolated or associated with foramen ovale or patent ductus arteriosus. Right aortic arch and mirror branching are common associated anomalies. Complex transposition is associated with either ventricular septal defect or subpulmonary obstruction (Fig. 7.13b).

- Simple forms

There are no significant cardiac anomalies apart from patent foramen ovale (or ostium secundum ASD) and patent ductus arteriosus [78].

Anatomical variants of the origins of the coronary arteries may be observed and are classified into five types [79].

Pathophysiologically, this anomaly results in two parallel independent circulations: systemic and pulmonary.[3] The exchanges necessary for survival occur via the patent ductus arteriosus and foramen ovale, which is an essential element.

The ductus arteriosus normally closes at birth; the foramen ovale becomes insufficient leading to cyanosis and furthermore, severe hypoxia and the development of life-threatening metabolic acidosis [80] requiring urgent medical and surgical management (by balloon atrial septostomy "Rashkind procedure" [81] – see Treatment).

- Forms with ventricular septal defect

A large ventricular septal defect with a variable location is observed in one-third of cases. It often corresponds to an infundibular defect due to poor alignment of the outlet septum relative to the muscular septum [82]. Severe left shift of the outlet septum results in subpulmonary obstruction and aortic overriding, corresponding to transposition with VSD and pulmonary stenosis [83]. This variant resembles tetralogy of Fallot.

- Complex forms with pulmonary stenosis

These forms essentially consist of subvalvular stenosis rather than isolated valvular stenosis.

7.4.2 Corrected Transposition of the Great Vessels (Levo-Transposition or L-Transposition)

L-transposition[4] accounts for less than 1% of all cases of congenital heart disease.

---

[3]Superior vena cava and inferior vena cava → morphologically right atrium → morphologically right ventricle → aorta → systemic circulation → superior vena cava and inferior vena cava Pulmonary veins → morphologically left atrium → morphologically left ventricle → pulmonary artery → pulmonary circulation → lung → pulmonary veins.

---

[4]The term "double discordance" is now preferred to "corrected transposition."

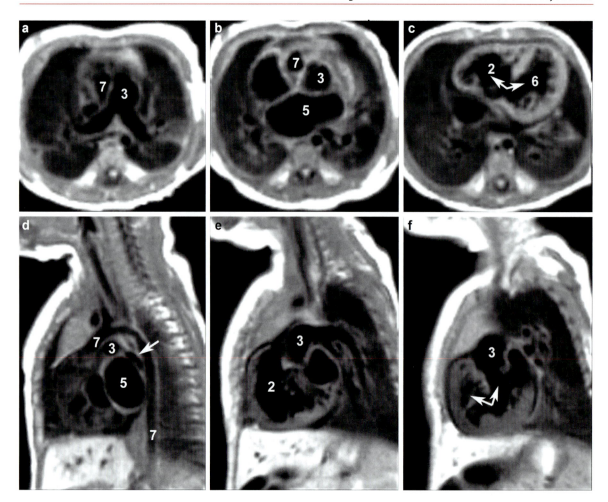

Fig. 7.14 (**a–f**) Complete transposition of the great vessels (D-transposition). (**a, b**) Axial fast spin-echo images through the origin of the aorta and the PA: the great vessels are transposed: the aorta (7) is situated anteriorly and to the *right* (D-transposition) of the PA (3). (**c**) Axial fast spin-echo image through the ventricles. (**d**) Fast spin-echo image in the plane of the aortic arch and (**e**) and (**f**) subsequent slices: the ascending aorta (7)

situated anteriorly (and on the *left*) and the PA (3) situated posteriorly (and on the *right*) run side by side without crossing over ("gun barrel" appearance). The aorta emerges from the RV (2) and the PA emerges from the LV (6). The patent DA (*arrow*) and the ventricular septal defect (*double arrow*) are also depicted; LA (5) (also see Fig. 7.14, Chap. 3, Figs. 3.17–3.20 and Chap. 8, Figs. 8.14 and 8.22)

Fig. 7.15 (**a, b**) Complete transposition of the great vessels (D-transposition) in a neonate (12 hrs age). (**a**) Sagittal oblique spin-echo image in the axis of the aortic arch: the aorta (7) situated anteriorly and the PA (3) situated posteriorly run side by side without crossing over ("gun barrel" appearance). The aorta emerges from the RV (2) and the PA emerges from the LV (6). The patent DA (*arrows*) is clearly visualized; LA (5). (**b**) Axial spin-echo image through the ventricles: the morphologically RV (2) is on the *right* (right loop) and is identified by the tricuspid valve (*arrowhead*) situated on the *right* and more anteriorly (and inferiorly towards the apex of the heart) compared to the mitral valve (*arrow*) which is situated more posteriorly and on the *left*, which identifies the morphologically LV (6) (also see Fig. 7.15, Chap.

1, Fig. 1.8, Chap. 3, Figs. 3.17–3.20 and Chap. 8, Figs. 8.14, 8.15, and 8.22). (**c, d**) Complete transposition of the great vessels (D-transposition). Contrast-enhanced MRA images (Dota-Gd, Guerbet, France). Multiplanar sagittal oblique reconstructions display the "gun barrel" aspect of the two vessels: the aorta (7) situated anteriorly (arising from the RV – 6), and the PA (3) situated posteriorly (arising from the LV – 2), run side by side. Adequate dynamic time-resolved MRA sequences allow confident separation of the pulmonary circulation (right and left PA – respect. *upper left and middle images*) and systemic circulation (aorta – *lower* images); note the patent DA (*arrow*) (also see Fig. 7.15, Chap. 1, Fig. 1.8, Chap. 3, Figs. 3.17–3.20, and Chap. 8, Figs. 8.14, 8.15, and 8.22)

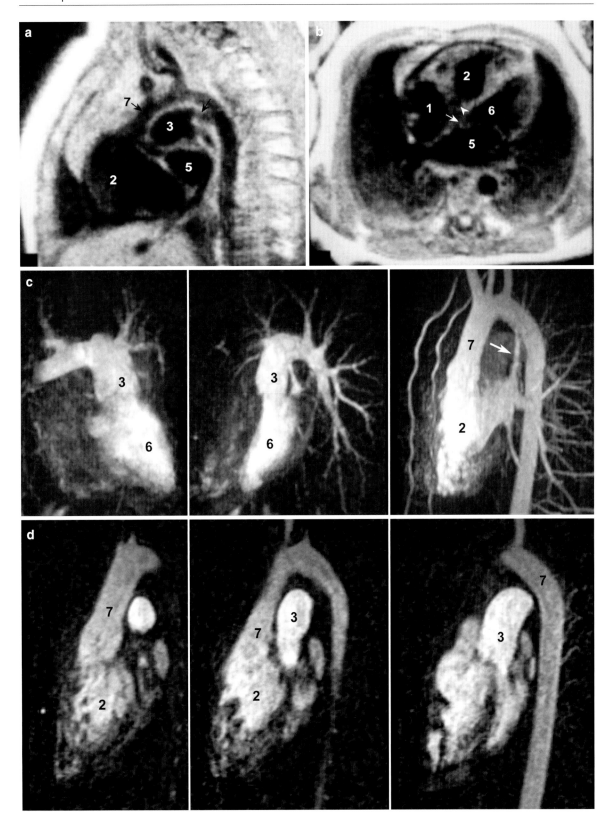

Fig. 7.16 Double ventriculoarterial and atrioventricular
discordance in corrected
transposition of the great
vessels (L-transposition,
L-loop). (**a**) Viable isolated
form with systemic RV which
is consequently hypertrophied
(RVH). (**b**) Complex form
associated with ventricular
septal defect (VSD) (observed
in 95% of cases) and/or
subpulmonary stenosis (PSt).
Aorta (Ao), PA, RA, LA, LV,
ventricular septal defect
(*double arrow*) (also see
Chap. 3, Fig. 3.16)

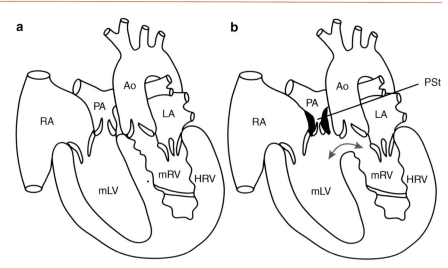

- Pathology

L-transposition results from malrotation of the bulboven-
tricular loop which in an opposite direction from normal
twist to the left. This form comprises double ventriculoarterial and atrioventricular discordance. The aortic
annulus is situated on the left and anteriorly (L-transposition) and the aorta arises from the morphologically right
ventricle situated on the left (L-loop), while the PA (on
the right and posteriorly) arises from the morphologically
left ventricle situated on the right. This is described as
corrected transposition of the great vessels (Fig. 7.16).

Ventricular inversion is associated with inversion of
the atrioventricular valves and coronary arteries: the
morphologically left atrioventricular valve (mitral) is
on the right and presents a fibrous continuity with the
pulmonary valve (mitro-pulmonary continuity), while

the morphologically right atrioventricular valve (tricuspid) is on the left with tricuspido-aortic discontinuity [84]. The tricuspid valve on the left is situated more
anteriorly (and inferiorly towards the apex of the heart)
than the mitral valve, which is situated more posteriorly (offset AV valves clearly visible on axial images,
Fig. 7.17 and Chaps. 2 and 3 Figs. 17–20 and Chap. 8,
Figs. 8.14, 8.15, and 8.22).

The coronary artery situated on the right gives rise
to the left anterior descending artery and circumflex
artery, while the coronary artery situated on the left
travels in the left atrioventricular groove and gives rise
to the posterior descending artery.

- Clinicopathological forms

When the anomaly is isolated, the circulation can be
considered to be normal as the systemic and pulmonary

Fig. 7.17 (**a**) Corrected transposition of the great vessels
(L-transposition, L-loop) in an adolescent. Axial and small-axis
subsequent slices. *Upper row middle image*: Axial spin-echo
image through the origin of the aorta and the PA: the great vessels are transposed: the ascending aorta (7a) is situated anteriorly and to the left (L-transposition) of the PA (3). *Lower row left
image*: Axial spin-echo image through the ventricles: the morphologically RV (2′) is on the *left* (L-loop) and is identified by
the tricuspid valve (*white arrowhead*) on the *left* and situated
more anteriorly (and inferiorly towards the apex of the heart)
than the mitral valve (*white arrow*), which is situated more posteriorly and on the *right*, identifying the morphologically LV
(6′). The trabeculated RV is hypertrophied, as it is connected to
the aorta and the systemic circulation (the RV is the systemic
ventricle). Note the presence of a moderator band (between
white arrowheads), another criterion for identification of the

morphologically RV; descending aorta (7), RA (1), LA (5) (also
see Chap. 3, Figs. 3.17, 3.21, and 3.22). (**b**) Another case of corrected transposition of the great vessels (L-transposition, L-loop)
which can be identified with the same criteria as case (**a**). There
is a pulmonary stenosis, which is depicted on the white coronal
blood gradient-echo cine-MR images as a flow void originating
at the narrowed site (*arrows* on PA 3); RA (1), RV (2′), PA (3),
LA (5), aorta (7) (also see Chap. 3, Figs. 3.17, 3.21, and 3.22).
(**c**) In this case of corrected transposition of the great vessels
(L-transposition, L-loop, see (**a**) for identification criteria), as in
(**b**), there is an additional pulmonary stenosis which is depicted
on the white blood gradient-echo cine-MR images (on the *right*)
as a flow void originating at the narrowed site (*arrows* on PA 3);
RA (1), RV (2′), LA (5), LV (6′), aorta (7) (also see Chap. 3,
Figs. 3.17, 3.21, and 3.22)

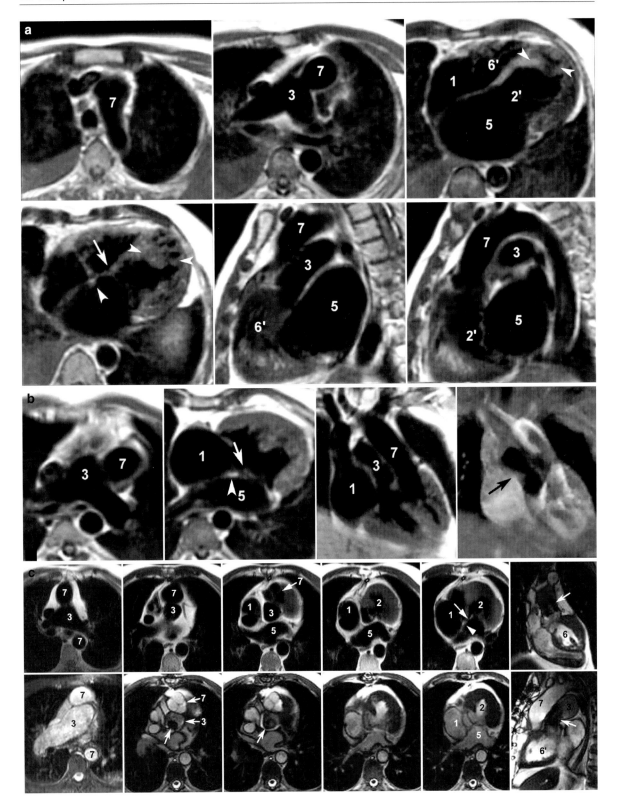

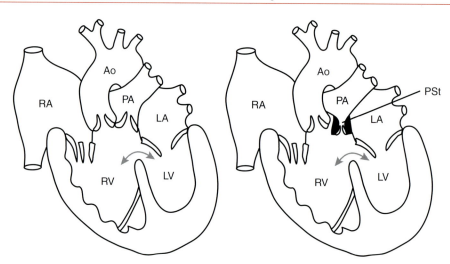

Fig. 7.18 Diagram of DORV: (**a**) DORV without infundibular pulmonary stenosis. The aorta (Ao) and PA emerge from the RV and are situated side by side (the aorta is generally to the right of the PA, D-malposition). The ventricular septal defect (*double arrow*) may be subaortic, subpulmonary (Taussig-Bing disease), or both subaortic and subpulmonary. (**b**) DORV with infundibular pulmonary stenosis (PSt – 30% of cases). RA, LA, LV (when the VSD is subaortic, this form is almost identical to tetralogy to Fallot, see Chap. 7, Fig. 7.7a)

circulations are in series and this anomaly may run undetected until adulthood. However, the right ventricle plays the role of the systemic ventricle as it is connected to the aorta and the systemic circulation.[5]

However, more than 95% of patients present associated anomalies including dextrocardia (25 %), large ventricular septal defect or single ventricle, malformation of the morphologically atrioventricular right valve (tricuspid) with regurgitation, resembling Ebstein anomaly, pulmonary atresia or stenosis (Fig. 7.17c–f) with intact interventricular septum, also presenting with cyanotic heart disease resembling tetralogy of Fallot.

7.5 Double Outlet Right Ventricle

7.5.1 Pathology

DORV is a rare malformation (1.5% of all cases of congenital heart disease) characterized by emergence of the aorta and PA from the morphologically right ventricle (Figs. 7.18 and 7.19, also see Chap. 3, Fig. 3.23), usually associated with situs solitus and right ventricular loop. The PA is in a normal position arising from a right ventricular conus, while the aorta also arises from the right ventricle via a second conus, usually to the right of the PA (D-malposition) and the two vessels travel side by side. Less frequently, the aorta is situated anteriorly, and even more rarely, it is situated on the left (L-malposition).

7.5.2 Clinical Features

The clinical presentation depends on the associated anomalies. The only possible left ventricular outflow tract is via a ventricular septal defect (Fig. 7.19c), a constant feature that is situated, in decreasing order of frequency, in subaortic, subpulmonary (Taussig-Bing disease), and both subaortic and subpulmonary positions. The site of the VSD is important, as it determines the direction of flow: the circulation is relatively normal in the case of subaortic VSD, while the circulation is comparable to that of transposition of the great vessels in the case of subpulmonary VSD.

Systemic obstruction at the subaortic conus or coarctation is observed in 50% of cases (Fig. 7.19d–f).

---

[5]Superior vena cava and inferior vena cava → morphologically right atrium → morphologically left ventricle → pulmonary artery → pulmonary circulation → lung → pulmonary vein → morphologically left atrium → morphologically right ventricle → aorta → systemic circulation → superior vena cava and inferior vena cava.

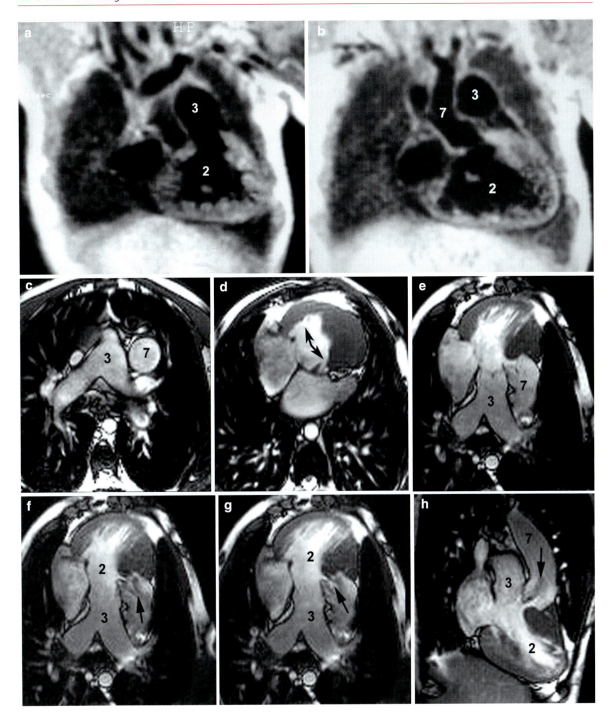

Fig. 7.19 (**a, b**) DORV in an infant. (**a**) Coronal spin-echo image through the origin of the PA (3), which arises from the trabeculated RV (2) via a (right subpulmonary) ventricular conus. (**b**) Coronal spin-echo image through the origin of the aorta (7), which also arises from the trabeculated RV (2) via a second (right subaortic) ventricular conus. The PA and aorta (here as usual located to the right of the PA) both emerge from the RV and run side by side on axial images (see Chap. 3, Fig. 3.24 and Chap. 8, Fig. 8.32 for the postoperative appearance).

(**c–h**) Another case of DORV with obstruction of subaortic conus. Axial gradient-echo (**c–g**) and coronal (**h**) images with balanced-SSFP (Fiesta). The PA is in the normal position while the aorta which also arises from the RV is located on the *left* (L-malposition – less usual). The two vessels travel side by side. The systemic obstruction at the subaortic conus or coarctation, observed in 50% of cases, is depicted as a flow void jet at stenosis site (*arrows*); RV (2), PA (3), aorta (7). Note the VSD (*double-headed arrow*)

Pulmonary stenosis, generally infundibular, is present in 20% of cases, particularly in the case of subaortic VSD.

DORV associated with pulmonary stenosis and subaortic ventricular septal defect is very similar to tetralogy of Fallot, and is even associated with right aortic arch in 30% of cases.

DORV without pulmonary stenosis associated with subpulmonary ventricular septal defect (Taussig-Bing disease) is very similar to transposition of the great vessels with large ventricular septal defect without pulmonary stenosis, but the presence of an extremely dilated PA situated alongside the aorta rather than posteriorly is an argument in favor of DORV (Fig. 7.19).

7.6 Double Outlet Left Ventricle

In double outlet left ventricle (DOLV), the two great vessels emerge from the morphologically left ventricle (Fig. 7.20, also see Chap. 3, Fig. 3.23). The aorta is situated either on the left or on the right of the PA. A ventricular septal defect and pulmonary stenosis are usually present. This anomaly is extremely rare and has a similar clinical presentation to that of tricuspid atresia, tetralogy of Fallot, or transposition of the great vessels with ventricular septal defect.

This entity must not be confused with the more frequent DORV associated with situs inversus, in which the two great vessels emerge from a left-sided morphologically right ventricle.

7.7 Single Ventricle

7.7.1 Pathology

Single ventricle is a rare malformation (1.5% of all cases of congenital heart disease) characterized by the fact that blood flow derived from the atria via the atrio-ventricular valves enters a single ventricle or largely dominant ventricle (Figs. 7.21–7.23, also see Chap. 3, Fig. 3.9c, Chap. 4, Fig. 4.22, and Chap. 5, Fig. 5.23). In 80% of cases, the large chamber corresponds to a morphologically left ventricle (with an infundibulum representing a rudimentary right ventricle) and, in 5% of cases, it corresponds to a morphologically right ventricle. However, the single ventricle can also be undifferentiated. The rudimentary right ventricle is generally situated anterosuperiorly and the rudimentary left ventricle is generally situated posteroinferiorly.

7.7.2 Clinicopathological Forms

Pulmonary stenosis or atresia is usually present with a similar clinical presentation to that of tetralogy of Fallot. D- or L-malposition of the great vessels is present in 80% of cases and the aorta always arises from the infundibulum when it is present. Single ventricle may be associated with asplenia, sometimes in combination with other cardiovascular anomalies (see Chap. 3, Fig. 3.6).

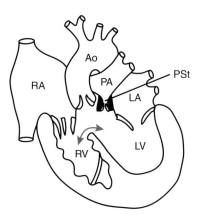

Fig. 7.20 Diagram of DOLV, usually comprising infundibular pulmonary stenosis (PS) (also see Chap. 3, Fig. 3.23b). Aorta (Ao), PA, RA and LA, RV and LV, ventricular septal defect (*double arrow*)

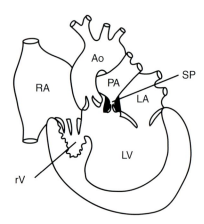

Fig. 7.21 Diagram of single left ventricle (SLV) with rudimentary RV (80% of cases), D-malposition of large vessels, and infundibular pulmonary stenosis (PSt). Rudimentary right ventricle (rV), aorta (Ao), pulmonary artery, (PA), RA, LA, LV (also see Chap. 3, Fig. 3.23c)

7.8 Tricuspid Atresia

7.8.1 Pathology

Tricuspid atresia is characterized by absence of communication between the right atrium and the right ventricle, which is usually smaller than normal (Fig. 7.24, also see Chap. 3) and the presence of a right–left shunt, which is essential for survival, via an atrial septal defect, usually a patent foramen ovale (the only outlet for blood entering the right atrium). This severe malformation is rare, as it accounts for only 1–3% of all cases of congenital heart disease.

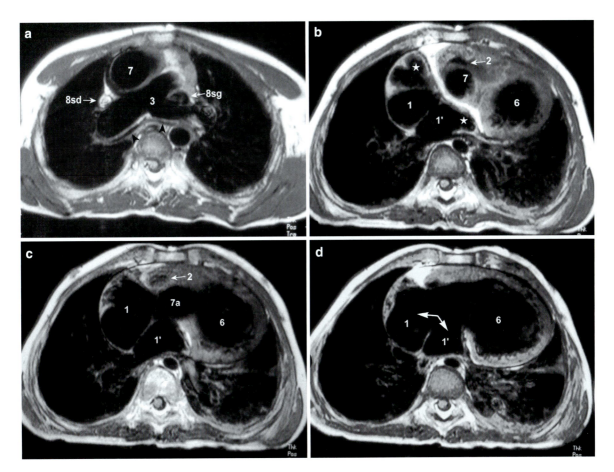

Fig. 7.22 Complex cyanotic heart disease in a 13-year-old child with single LV and tight pulmonary stenosis leading to pulmonary atresia in the context of isomerism (see same patient, Chap. 3, Fig. 3.6). A left Blalock-Taussig shunt was performed as first-line procedure. Assessment before complete correction (see same patient Chap. 8, Fig. 8.9 after complete cavopulmonary shunt). Angiography did not visualize the accessory chamber or the PA branches. The right ventricular outflow tract is not visualized on echocardiography. (**a–d**) Craniocaudad series of axial images: the dilated distal PA trunk is clearly visualized (3) together with its division into right and left branches*. The PA trunk is stenotic at its origin, arising from an almost absent rudimentary RV (2), contrasting with the large single LV (6) (also see Fig. 4.23, Chap. 4). Note the presence of two superior vena cavae, *right* (8sd) and *left* (8sg). The atrium situated on the *right* (1) and on the *left* (1′) has a morphologically right atrial appendage (*stars*)**. There is a large atrial septal defect (*double arrow*). (**e–f**) Front to rear series of axial coronal images: the dilated PA is clearly visualized (3). The right superior vena cava (8sd) drains into the atrium situated

on the *right* (1) and the left superior vena cava (8sg) drains into the atrium situated on the *left* (1′). A palliative Blalock-Taussig shunt (*arrows*) was performed between the left subclavian artery (above) and the left PA (3g below). The liver (L) is in a midline position and the inferior vena cava (*right* – 8id) and abdominal aorta (7i) are juxtaposed on the *right* of the spine*** (also see Chap. 4, Fig. 4.22 and Chap. 5, Fig. 5.23). Note the network of collateral vessels derived from the descending thoracic aorta ensuring proper pulmonary blood supply (*arrows*, **f**) (also see Fig. 7.12)

---

* There are two right pulmonary arteries (right-right symmetry) with an anterior course in the coronal plane and parallel to the respective main bronchi (eparterial); the bronchi are also hypoplastic (*arrowheads*);

** that is, a broad triangular atrial appendage identifies two morphologically right atria (right isomerism), confirming the presence of a morphologically right bronchial division on the *left* (see same case, Chap. 3);

*** right isomerism.

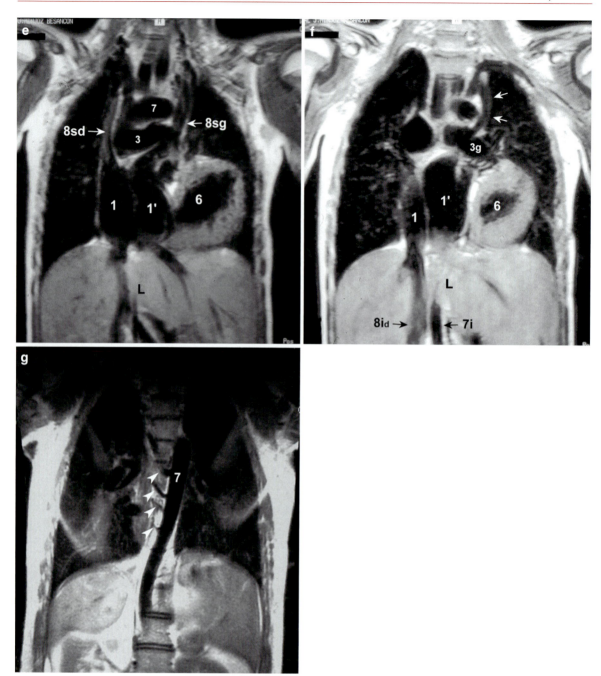

Fig. 7.22 (continued)

7.8.2 Clinicopathological Forms

The clinical presentation varies according to the associated anomalies. This disease is classified according to the type of ventriculoarterial connection, the position of the great vessels (normal, L- or D-malposition), and the PA (normal, stenotic, or hypoplastic) (see Table 7.1, Figs. 7.24–7.26).

Forms without malposition[6] of the great vessels are three times more frequent than forms with malposition, with a predominance of type Ib.

---

[6]The terms malposition and transposition, which concern the respective positions of the great vessels at their origin, were discussed in Chap. 3.

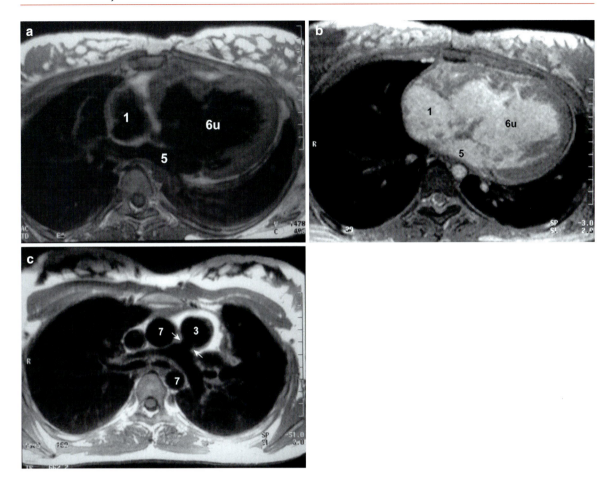

Fig. 7.23 Fourteen-year-old girl with single LV requiring banding at the age of 4 months (postoperative MRI). (**a, b**) Axial spin-echo and cine MRI images through the single LV (6u) showing cardiomegaly; RA (1) and LA (6). (**c**) Axial image through the bifurcation of the PA (3). Banding is well visualized (*arrows*); aorta (7) (also see Chap. 8, Figs. 8.31 and 8.32, Chap. 4, Fig. 4.22 and Chap. 5, Fig. 5.23)

Table 7.1 Tricuspid atresia

Normal position of great vessels
Type Ia with pulmonary atresia (and rudimentary right ventricle)
Type Ib with subvalvular pulmonary stenosis due to small VSD (and presence of right ventricle)
Type Ic pulmonary stenosis due to large VSD (and large right ventricle)
Malposition of great vessels
Type IIa with D-malposition
Type IIb with L-malposition

If the interventricular septum is intact and/or in the presence of pulmonary atresia (type Ia), the patent ductus arteriosus and bronchial vessels must supply all of the pulmonary circulation (severe cyanosis).

In the presence of a large VSD or transposition of the great vessels without pulmonary stenosis, pulmonary blood flow is significantly increased and the clinical presentation is dominated by severe congestive heart failure with no significant cyanosis.

7.9 Ebstein Anomaly

7.9.1 Pathology

Ebstein anomaly accounts for 0.6% of all cases of cyanotic heart disease and is characterized by anomalies of the right (tricuspid) atrioventricular valve and right ventricle (Fig. 7.27).
The malformation of the right tricuspid valve is variable, associating excess valvular tissue and varying

degrees of adherence of the septal and posteroinferior leaflets to the right ventricular wall. In minor forms, only the septal leaflet is inserted more inferiorly than normal. In severe forms, the septal and posteroinferior leaflets are adherent to the septum and right ventricle, making them almost completely nonfunctioning.

The low insertion of the valve leaflets is responsible for incorporation of the right ventricular inlet chamber into the right atrium, which is described as "atrialization" of the right ventricle.

7.9.2 Clinicopathological Forms

The clinical features depend on the severity of the tricuspid valve lesion and especially the associated anomalies.

Ebstein anomaly is associated with obstruction to right ventricular filling due to the decreased volume of the partially atrialized right ventricle. The defective tricuspid valve and decreased compliance of the right ventricle usually induce a significant right–left shunt through the patent foramen ovale or atrioventricular

septal defect. About 50% of cases are symptomatic during infancy with hypoxia, cyanosis, and right heart failure.

The most frequently associated malformation is atrial septal defect (50% of cases), while ventricular septal defect, coarctation, patent ductus arteriosus, and pulmonary stenosis or atresia are observed more rarely.

7.9.2.1 MRI

Once again, MRI is useful to reliably visualize the right ventricular outflow tract. In an with Ebstein anomaly [4], MRI was able to eliminate right ventricular outflow tract obstruction not visualized by echocardiography (Figs. 7.28 and 7.29).

7.10 Treatment

Cyanotic heart disease can be treated medically, surgically, or by interventional catheterization. Medical

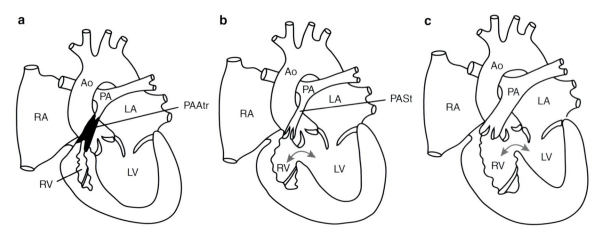

Fig. 7.24 Diagram of variants of tricuspid atresia without malposition of the great vessels (types Ia to Ic): see text and Table 7.1. Aorta (Ao), PA, pulmonary stenosis (PSt), pulmonary atresia (PA Atr), ventricular septal defect (*double arrow*), RA and LA, RV and LV

Fig. 7.25 Ten-year-old child with type Ia tricuspid atresia and pulmonary atresia treated by right Blalock-Taussig shunt followed by central shunt. The stenotic left PA has been dilated by balloon catheter. The distal pulmonary circulation is very poorly visible on echocardiography. Postangioplasty follow-up examination. (**a–c**) Axial images: the atrioventricular groove (*arrowhead*) is prolonged by a white fat signal (in the place of the absent tricuspid valve), which completely separates the large dilated RA (1) and rudimentary RV (2); LV (6). The left PA stenosis (3g) with prestenotic dilatation is clearly visualized. (**d–f**) Anteroposterior series of coronal images. Pulmonary atresia is clearly visible: no PA present (**d**, *arrow*); the left PA is initially dilated (**e**, 3g) and then severely narrowed (**f**, 3g) (also refer to Fig. 7.7)

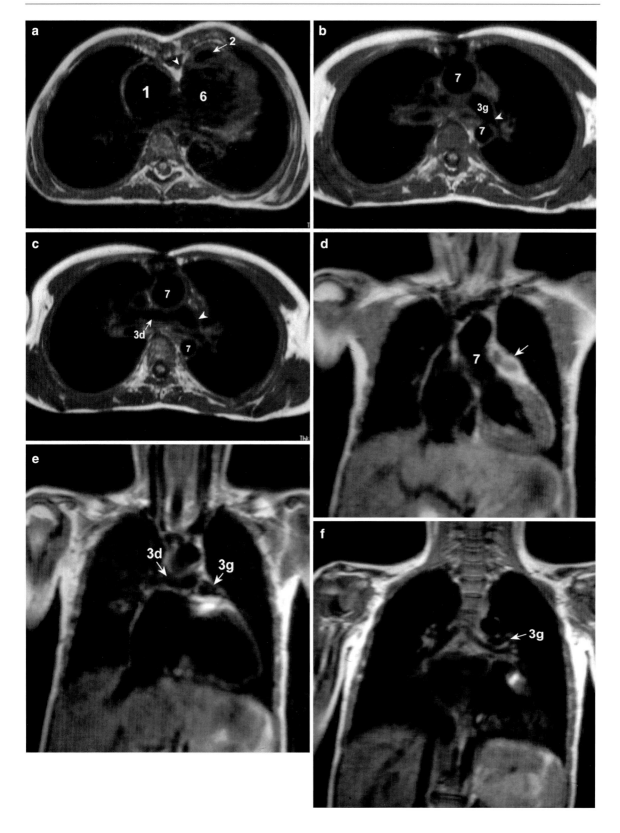

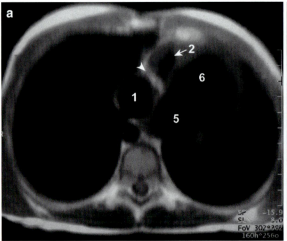

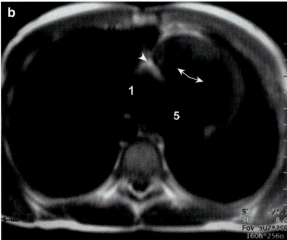

Fig. 7.26 (**a**, **b**) Eleven-year-old child with type Ib tricuspid atresia. (**a**, **b**) Axial fast spin-echo images: the atrioventricular groove (*arrowhead*) is prolonged by a white fat signal (in the place of the absent tricuspid valve) completely separating the dilated RA (1) from the rudimentary RV (2); LA (5), LV (6). This patient was treated by bidirectional cavopulmonary ("hemi-Fontan") shunt (see postoperative appearance in Chap. 8, Fig. 8.10)

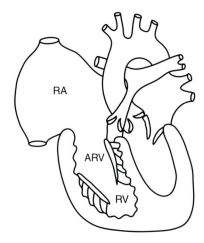

Fig. 7.27 Diagram of Ebstein anomaly of the tricuspid valve. The low insertion of elements of the tricuspid apparatus results in incorporation of part of the RV into the RA, which is enlarged by the atrialized right ventricle (ARV), while the RV is decreased in size

treatment is described only briefly. Surgical treatment has dramatically improved the prognosis of cyanotic heart disease. Palliative surgery or definitive correction usually involves shunting of the PA. The type of procedure determines the modalities of postoperative follow-up by MRI. Surgical management is described in detail and illustrated by diagrams in Chap. 8.

7.10.1 Medical Treatment

Medical treatment essentially consists of oxygen therapy, which does not significantly improve oxygen saturation, but which is useful in the case of severe hypoxia by increasing the proportion of oxygen dissolved in plasma [64]. Phlebotomy may be performed in the case of polycythemia with hematocrit greater than 70%. Acidosis secondary to hypercapnia is corrected by alkalinization. The platelet aggregation inhibitor effects of aspirin are used to prevent thromboembolic complications. Prostaglandin E1 delays closure of the ductus arteriosus in the case of severe hypoxia, as in pulmonary atresia.

7.10.2 Interventional Catheterization

Balloon dilatation of the pulmonary valve in tetralogy of Fallot has been performed by several centers with a certain degree of success. Some teams believe that this procedure can also promote development of the size of the pulmonary arteries [85].

Balloon atrial septostomy (Rashkind procedure) [81] consists of intravenous or umbilical insertion of a guidewire into the right atrium and then into the left atrium via the foramen ovale. The balloon is then

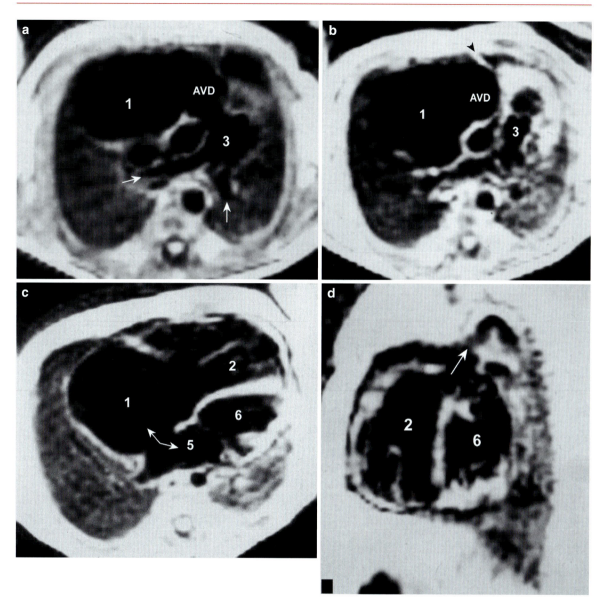

Fig. 7.28 Ebstein anomaly in a 2-day-old hypoxic and cyanotic patient. The right ventricular outflow tract is poorly visualized on echocardiography, especially the infundibular region (obstruction?). (**a–c**) Craniocaudal series of spin-echo axial images demonstrating a dilated RA (1) continuous with the atrialized portion of the right ventricle (ARV) with low anterior insertion of the valves (*arrowhead*). The PA trunk (3) and its left and right branches (R and L) are clearly visualized; note the atrial septal defect (*double arrow*), aorta (7). (**d**) Sagittal image: the right ventricular outflow tract is clearly visualized, with the RV (2) continuous with (*arrow*) the pulmonary infundibulum and PA

inflated and forcibly removed to tear the foramen ovale, resulting in a large ASD in patients with severe cyanosis. This procedure is essentially performed in neonates as first-line treatment of transposition of the great vessels.

Guidewire or radiofrequency perforation of the floor of the pulmonary valve followed by balloon dilatation has been proposed in the case of pulmonary atresia with intact interventricular septum [86].

Balloon dilatation can also be performed to treat postoperative residual PA stenosis. Dilatation of these restenoses may require high pressures [87–89] with a risk of thrombosis and perforation. Stenting of the PA may be performed in the case of failure of balloon

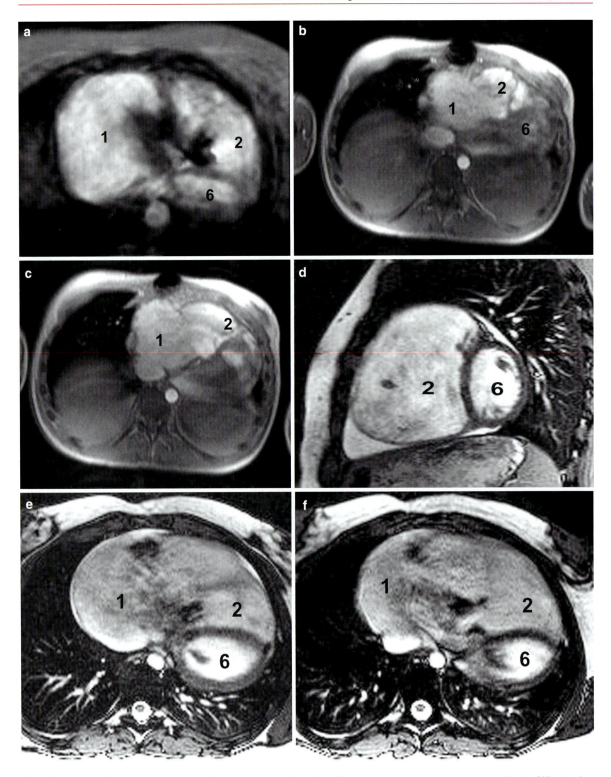

Fig. 7.29 (**a–f**) Ebstein anomaly gradient-echo cine-MR images. Dilated RA (1) continuous with the atrialized portion of the RV with low anterior insertion of the valves is present in these three cases (**a, b–c** and **d–e**). The defective tricuspid valve (insufficiency) and obstruction to right ventricular filling (turbulences) are visible as flow voids (*black areas*) occurring at the level of AV valves

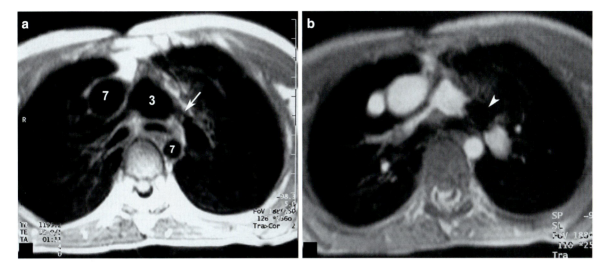

Fig. 7.30 (**a, b**) Pulmonary atresia treated by a conduit and dilatation followed by stenting of the left PA. The stent (*arrow* and *arrowhead*) induces a pronounced signal void artifact on the gradient-echo bright blood image (*arrowhead*). Note the post-stent dilatation of the left PA and hypoplastic right PA; aorta (7)

dilatation. Rigid, self-expanding stents are generally used, as they can subsequently be redilated (Fig. 7.30). Stenting of the right atrium-PA junction can also be performed after Fontan procedure.

7.10.3 Surgery

Complete correction of cyanotic heart diseases is preferable to palliative treatment whenever possible, as only definitive correction can prevent complications such as thrombosis or brain abscess (surgical correction is described in more detail in Chap. 8).

• Palliative surgery

Palliative procedures consist of systemic-pulmonary shunts.

Blalock-Taussig shunt is the oldest procedure (first described in 1945) and consists of end-to-side anastomosis between the subclavian artery and homolateral PA [90, 91] (Figs. 7.6 and 7.22 and see Chap. 8, Fig. 8.2). Modified Blalock-Taussig shunt uses a Gore-Tex® conduit. This operation, performed in pulmonary atresia with VSD, remains the main palliative procedure for tetralogy of Fallot [91, 92] and tricuspid atresia, but is now rarely performed due to the risk of iatrogenic PA stenosis [91, 92].

Potts shunt is a side-to-side anastomosis between the descending aorta and left PA (see Chap. 8, Fig. 8.7).

It is associated with a risk of PA hypertension and is generally performed only when Blalock-Taussig shunt is impossible.

Waterson shunt is a shunt between the ascending aorta and right PA (see Chap. 8, Fig. 8.5), and the central shunt is a shunt between the ascending aorta and PA trunk (see Chap. 8, Fig. 8.4).

The Glenn cavopulmonary shunt is a shunt between the superior vena cava and right PA (see Chap. 8, Fig. 8.10). This procedure, sometimes performed in tricuspid atresia, is now rarely performed, as it can induce superior vena cava syndrome.

Pulmonary artery banding (Fig. 7.23 and Chap. 8, Figs. 8.31 and 8.32) is performed as a palliative procedure to protect the PA in single ventricle and double outlet right ventricle without pulmonary stenosis, multiple ventricular septal defects, and transposition of the great vessels operated by a two-stage procedure.

• Definitive surgery

The type of surgery varies according to the type of cyanotic heart disease and is designed to correct the anomalies of each segment or their anomalous connections.

The Rastelli procedure consists of shunting the PA to the right ventricle via a bioprosthetic valved conduit (homologous graft or porcine xenograft) (see Chap. 8, Fig. 8.12). This procedure is indicated in the case of truncus arteriosus or pulmonary atresia with VSD [93].

The Fontan procedure drains all of the blood from the vena cava to the pulmonary arteries by a shunt from the right atrium to the pulmonary bifurcation (see Chap. 8, Fig. 8.9). It may be performed to treat tricuspid atresia or pulmonary atresia with intact interventricular septum [94]. Other shunt systems are also used, such as complete cavopulmonary shunt between the superior vena cava and right PA (Glenn shunt) plus a connection of the inferior vena cava to the PA via a right intra-atrial conduit.

Arterial switch consists of reimplantation of the aorta onto the left ventricle and the PA onto the right ventricle and is performed to correct transposition of the great vessels (see Chap. 8, Figs. 8.14–8.17).

Another alternative is the Mustard or Senning atrial switch, which reconnects the venous return to the atrium (see Chap. 8, Figs. 8.21 and 8.22). Prior to arterial switch, this procedure was used to treat transposition of the great vessels with pulmonary stenosis and intact interventricular septum.

Carpentier conservative surgery has now replaced the Hunter-Lillehei-Hardy procedure for the treatment of Ebstein anomaly. It consists of remodeling of the right ventricle and repositioning of the tricuspid valves.

7.11 Conclusion

MR imaging has revolutionized the management of congenital heart disease involving the right ventricular outflow tract. It is perfectly complementary to echocardiography and has considerably reduced the indications for more invasive explorations.

References

1. Huhta JC, Piehler JM, Tajik AJ, et al. Two-dimensional echocardiographic detection and measurement of the right pulmonary artery in pulmonary atresia with ventricular septum defect: angiographic and surgical correlation. Am J Cardiol. 1982;49:1235–40.
2. Formanek AG, Witcofski RL, D'souza VJ, Link KM, Karstaedt N. MR imaging of the central pulmonary arterial tree in conotruncal malformation. AJR. 1986;147:1127–31.
3. Link KM, Herrera MA, D'souza VJ, Formanek AG. MR imaging of Ebstein anomaly: results in four cases. AJR. 1988;150:363–7.
4. Kastler B, Livolsi A, Zhu H, Zollner G, Dietemann JL. Potential role of MRI in the diagnostic management of Ebstein anomaly in a newborn. J Comput Assist Tomogr. 1990;14:825–7.
5. Kastler B, Livolsi A, Germain P, Willard D, Wackenheim A. Contribution of MRI in the diagnosis of congenital heart disease in neonates: review of our experience in 65 cases. In: RSNA, 75th assembly and annual meeting, Chicago, Nov. 26–Dec. 1, 1989. Radiology. 1989;173, abstract. p. 484.
6. Soulié P, Binet JP. In: Binet JP, EDITOR. Chirurgie Cardiaque. Paris: Flammarion; 1978. p. 1025–39.
7. Felmlee JP, Ehman RL. Spatial presaturation: a method for suppressing flow artifacts and improving depiction of vascular anatomy in MR imaging. Radiology. 1987;164:559–64.
8. Kastler B. Imagerie du flux. In: Kastler B, editor. Comprendre l'IRM. 6th ed. Masson; 2006. p. 189–213.
9. Atkinson D, Teresi L. Magnetic resonance angiography. Magn Reson Q. 1994;10:149–72.
10. Link KM, Lesko NM. Magnetic resonance imaging in the evaluation of congenital heart disease. Magn Reson Q. 1991;7:173–90.
11. Edelman RR, Chien D, Kim D. Fast selective black blood MR imaging. Radiology. 1991;181(3):655–60.
12. Boiselle PM, White CS. New techniques in cardiothoracic imaging. New York: Informa Healthcare USA, Inc.; 2007. p. 81–2.
13. Wehrli FW, Haacke EM. Principles of MR imaging. In: Potchen EJ, Haacke EM, Siebert JE, Gottschalk A, editors. Magnetic resonance angiography: concepts and applications. St. Louis: Mosby; 1993. p. 9–34.
14. Sechtem U, Pflugfelder PW, White RD, et al. Cine MR imaging: potential for the evaluation of cardiovascular function. AJR. 1987;148:239–46.
15. Sechtem U, Pflugfelder P, Cassidy MC, Holt W, Wolfe C, Higgins CB. Ventricular septal defect: visualization of shunt flow and determination of shunt size by cine MR imaging. AJR. 1987;149:689–92.
16. Weber OM, Higgins CB. MR evaluation of cardiovascular physiology in congenital heart disease: flow and function. J Cardiovasc Magn Reson. 2006;8(4):607–17.
17. Baker EJ, Ayton V, Smith MA, et al. Magnetic resonance imaging at a high field strength of ventricular septal defects in infants. Br Heart J. 1989;62:305–10.
18. Simpson IA, Chung KJ, Glass RF, Sahn DJ, Sherman FS, Hesselink J. Cine magnetic resonance imaging for evaluation of anatomy and flow relations in infants and children with coarctation of the aorta. Circulation. 1988;78:142–8.
19. Mostbeck GH, Caputo GR, Higgins CB. MR measurement of blood flow in the cardiovascular system. AJR. 1992; 159:453–61.
20. Nayler GL, Firmin DN, Longmore DB. Blood flow imaging by cine magnetic resonance. J Comput Assist Tomogr. 1986; 10:715–22.
21. Bogren HG, Klipstein RH, Firmin DN, et al. Quantification of antegrade and retrograde blood flow in the human aorta by magnetic resonance velocity mapping. Am Heart J. 1989;117:1214–22.
22. Rees S, Firmin D, Mohiaddin R, Underwood R, Longmore D. Application of flow measurements by magnetic resonance velocity mapping to congenital heart disease. Am J Cardiol. 1989;64:953–6.

23. Elc NJ, Herfkens RJ, Shimakawa A, Enzmann DR. Phase contrast cine magnetic resonance imaging. Magn Reson Q. 1991;7:229–54.

24. Rebergen SA, Niezen RA, Helbing WA, Van Der Wall EE, De Roos A. Cine gradient-echo MR imaging and MR velocity mapping in the evaluation of congenital heart disease. Radiographics. 1996;16(3):467–81.

25. Geva T, Greil GF, Marshall AC, Landzberg M, Powell AJ. Gadolinium-enhanced 3-dimensional magnetic resonance angiography of pulmonary blood supply in patients with complex pulmonary stenosis or atresia: comparison with x-ray angiography. Circulation. 2002;106(4):473–8.

26. Dorfman AL, Geva T. Magnetic resonance imaging evaluation of congenital heart disease: conotruncal anomalies. J Cardiovasc Magn Reson. 2006;8(4):645–59.

27. Pfefferkorn JR. Absent pulmonary artery. A hint to its embryogenesis. Pediatr Cardiol. 1971;27:737–51.

28. Kucera V, Fiser B, Tuma S, Hucin B. Unilateral absence of pulmonary artery: a report of 19 selected clinical cases. J Thorac Cardiovasc Surg. 1982;30:152–8.

29. Findlay CW, Maier CH. Abnormalities of the pulmonary vessels and their surgical significance. Surgery. 1951;29:604–41.

30. Pool PE, Vogel JHK, Blount SG. Congenital unilateral absence of a pulmonary artery. Am J Cardiol. 1962; 10:706–32.

31. Shakibi JG, Rastan H, Nazarian I, et al. Isolated unilateral absence of the pulmonary artery: review of the world literature and guidelines for surgical repair. Jpn Heart J. 1978; 19:439–51.

32. Cucci C, Doyle E, Lewis JE. Absence of the primary division of the pulmonary trunk: an ontogen theory. Circulation. 1964;29:124–31.

33. Mccartney F, Deverall P, Scott O. Haemodynamic characteristics of systemic arterial blood supply to the lungs. Br Heart J. 1973;35:28–37.

34. La JM. vascularisation systémique non bronchique du poumon. Toulouse: Thèse Méd; 1986.

35. Roujeau J, Morel R. Absence congénitale d'une artère pulmonaire droite. J Fr Méd Chir Thorac. 1962;16:345–59.

36. Boyden EA. Developmental anomalies of the lung. Am J Surg. 1955;89:79–89.

37. Oakler C, Glick G, Mccredie RM. Congenital absence of a pulmonary artery. Am J Med. 1963;34:264–70.

38. Toews WH, Pappas G. Surgical management of absent right pulmonary artery with associated pulmonary hypertension. Chest. 1983;84:497–9.

39. Severinghaus JW, Swenson EW, Finley TN, Lategola MT, Williams J. Unilateral hypoventilation produced in dogs by occluding one pulmonary artery. J Appl Physiol. 1961;16:53.

40. Gill CC, Moodie DS, Mcgoon DC. Staged surgical management of pulmonary atresia with diminutive pulmonary arteries. J Thorac Cardiovasc Surg. 1977;73:436–42.

41. Kleinman PK. Pleural telangiectasia and absence of a pulmonary artery. Radiology. 1979;132:281–4.

42. Rees S. Arterial connection of the lung. Clin Radiol. 1981; 32:1–15.

43. Madoff IM, Gaensler EA, Strieder JW. Congenital absence of the right pulmonary artery. N Engl J Med. 1952;247:149.

44. Newman R, Taradisis G, Chai H. Congenital absence or hypoplasia of pulmonary artery. J Thorac Cardiovasc Surg. 1964;47(6):740–9.

45. Ferguson A, Belbeau R, Gaensler EA. Absence congénitale d'une artère pulmonaire. Respiration. 1969;26:300–12.

46. Morgan P, Foley D, Erickson S. Proximal interruption of a main pulmonary artery with transpleural collateral vessels: CT and MR appearances. J Comput Assist Tomogr. 1991; 15(2):311–3.

47. Seibert R, Quoix E, Burghard G. Mise au point à propos d'un cas d'agénésie unilatérale de l'artère pulmonaire. Rev Pneumol Clin. 1984;40:135–8.

48. Grum CM, Yarnal JR, Cook SA, Cordasco EM, Tomashefski JF. Unilateral hyperlucent lung. Non invasive diagnosis of pulmonary agenesis. Angiology. 1981;32:194–207.

49. Gutgesell HP, Huhta JC, Cohen MH. Twodimensional echographic assessment of pulmonary artery and aortic arch anatomy in cyanotic infants. J Am Coll Cardiol. 1984;4:1242–6.

50. Sondheimer HM, Oliphant M, Schneider B, et al. Computerized axial tomography of the chest for visualization of "absent" pulmonary arteries. Circulation. 1982;65:1020–5.

51. Griffin N, Mansfield L, Redmond KC, Dusmet M, Goldstraw P, Mittal TK, et al. Imaging features of isolated unilateral pulmonary artery agenesis presenting in adulthood: a review of four cases. Clin Radiol. 2007;62(3):238–44.

52. Haworth SG, Rees PG, Taylor JFN, et al. Pulmonary atresia with ventricular septal defect and major aorto-pulmonary collateral arteries. Effect of systemic pulmonary anastomosis. Br Heart J. 1981;45:133–41.

53. Singh SP, Rigby ML, Astley R. Demonstration of pulmonary arteries by contrast injection into pulmonary vein. Br Heart J. 1978;40:55–7.

54. Brocard H, Vannier R, Gallouedec CH. Circulation à contrecourant dans l'artère pulmonaire de poumons non injectés à l'angiocardiopneumographie par voie droite. J Fr Med Chir thorac. 1967;21(3):263–80.

55. Ten Harkel AD, Blom NA, Ottenkamp J. Isolated unilateral absence of a pulmonary artery: a case report and review of the literature. Chest. 2002;122(4):1471–7.

56. Van Praagh A. Classification of truncus arteriosus communis. Am Heart J. 1976;92:129–32.

57. Radeford DJ, Perkins L, Lachman A, Thong YH. Spectrum of DI George syndrome in patients with truncus arteriosus: expanded DI George syndrome. Pediatr Cardiol. 1988; 9:95–101.

58. Li J, Soukias ND, Carvalho J, Ho SY. Coronary arterial anatomy in tetralogy of Fallot: morphological and clinical correlations. Heart. 1998;80(2):174–83.

59. Botnar RM, Stuber M, Kissinger KV, Manning WJ. Freebreathing 3D coronary MRA: the impact of "isotropic" image resolution. J Magn Reson Imaging. 2000;11(4):389–93.

60. Holmqvist C, Hochbergs P, Björkhem G, Brockstedt S, Laurin S. Pre-operative evaluation with MR in tetralogy of fallot and pulmonary atresia with ventricular septal defect. Acta Radiol. 2002;43(3):346.

61. Rees R, Somerville J, Underwood S, Wright J, Firmin D, Klipstein R, et al. Magnetic resonance imaging of the pulmonary arteries and their systemic connections in pulmonary atresia: comparison with angiographic and surgical findings. Br Heart J. 1987;58:621–6.

62. Toussaint M, Guérin F. La cyanose des cardiopathies congénitales. Med Inf. 1980;3:267–76.

63. Hadjo A, Jimenez M, Baudet E, Roques X, Laborde N, Srour S, et al. Review of long-term course of 52 patients with pulmo-

nary atresia an ventricular septal defect. Anatomical and surgical considerations. Eur Heart J. 1995;16:1668–74.

64. Dupuis C, et al. Cardiologie pédiatrique. In: Classification et terminologie des cardiopathies congénitales. Paris: Flammarion 1991.

65. Gaudeau S, Corone P. Approche clinique du diagnostic des cardiopathies congénitales. Rev Prat. 1980;30(19):1195–275.

66. Fallot A. Contribution à l'anatomie pathologique de la maladie bleue (cyanose cardiaque). Mars Med. 1988;25:418–20.

67. Iselin M. Cardiopathies cyanogènes. E.M.C., Radiodiagnostic; Cœur Poumon, 32-015-B-10; 1999. p. 24.

68. Van Praagh R, Van Praagh S, Nebesar RA, et al. Tetralogy of Fallot: underdevelopment of the pulmonary infundibulum and its sequelae. Am J Cardiol. 1970;26:25–33.

69. Geva T, Ayres NA, Pac FA, Pignatelli R. Quantitative morphometric analysis of progressive infundibular obstruction in tetralogy of Fallot. Circulation. 1995;92:886–92.

70. Soulie P, Binet JP. In: Soulie P, editor. Cardiopathies congénitales. Paris: Flammarion; 1978. p. 94–129.

71. Rao BNS, Anderson RC, Edwards JE. Anatomic variations in the tetralogy of Fallot. Am Heart J. 1971;81(3):361–371.

72. Dabizzi RP, Teodori G, Barletta GA, Caprioli G, Baldrighi G, Baldrighi V. Associated coronary and cardiac anomalies in the tetralogy of Fallot. An angiographic study. Eur Heart J. 1990;11:692–704.

73. Halt M, Kastler B, Livolsi A, Mardini M, Willard D, Wackenheim A. Fallotsche tetralogie: studie mit Hilfe der Kernspintomographie. Röfo (Forschrite im Gebiet der Röntgenstrahlung). 1991;54:111–4.

74. Geva T, Sandweiss BM, Gauvreau K, Lock JE, Powell AJ. Factors associated with impaired clinical status in long-term survivors of tetralogy of Fallot repair evaluated by magnetic resonance imaging. J Am Coll Cardiol. 2004;43(6):1068–74.

75. Liao PK, Edwards EF, Julsrud PR, et al. Pulmonary blood supply in patients with pulmonary atresia and ventricular septal defect. J Am Coll Cardiol. 1985;6:1343–50.

76. Somerville J, Saravelli O, Ross D. Complex pulmonary atresia with congenital systemic collaterals. Classification and management. Arch Mal Coeur. 1978;71:322–8.

77. Choi YH, Seo JW, Yun YS, Kim SH, Lee HJ. Morphology of the tricuspid valve in pulmonary atresia with intact. Ventricular septum. Pediatr Cardiol. 1998;19:381–9.

78. Anderson RH, Henry CN, Becker AE. Morphologic aspects of complete transposition. Cardiol Young. 1991;1:141–53.

79. Kurosawa H, Imai Y, Kawada M. Coronary arterial anatomy in regard to the arterial switch procedure. Cardiol Young. 1991;1:54–62.

80. Berry LM, Padbury J, Novoa-Tark L, Emmanoilides GC. Premature "closing" of the foramen ovale in transposition of the great arteries with intact ventricular septum: rare cause of sudden neonatal death. Pediatr Cardiol. 1998;19:246–8.

81. Waldhausen JA, Boruchow I, Miller WW, Rashkind WJ. Transposition of the great arteries with ventricular septal defect. Palliation by atrial septostomy and pulmonary artery banding. Circulation. 1969;39(5 Suppl 1):I215–21.

82. Hoyer MM, Zuberbuhler JR, Anderson RH, Del Nido P. Morphology of ventricular septal defect in complete transposition. J Thorac Cardiovasc Surg. 1992;104:1203–11.

83. Robertson DA, Silverman NH. Malaligned outlet septum with subpulmonary ventricular septal defect. Defined echocardiographically. Cardiology. 1990;16:459–68.

84. Schiebler GL, Edwards JE, Burchell HB, Duschane JW, Ongley PA, Wood EH. Congenital corrected transposition of the great vessels: a study of 33 cases. Pediatrics. 1961;27(Part II):851.

85. Guerin P, Jimenez M, Dos Santos P, Choussat A. Percutaneus dilatation of the pulmonary tract in tetralogy of Fallot. Arch Mal Coeur. 1996;89:541–5.

86. Piechaud JF, Ladeia AM, Da Cruz E, et al. Perforation des atrésies pulmonaires à septum interventriculaire intact chez le nouveau-né et le nourrisson. Arch Mal Cœur. 1993;86:581–6.

87. Gentles TL, Lock JE, Perry SB. High pressure balloon angioplasty of branch pulmonary artery stenosis: early experience. J Am Coll Cardiol. 1993;22:867–72.

88. Nakanishi T, Matsumoto Y, Seguchi M, Nakasawa M, Imai Y, Momma K. Balloon angioplasty for postoperative pulmonary artery stenosis in transplantation of the great arteries. J Am Coll Cardiol. 1993;22:859–66.

89. Worms AM, Marcon F, Chehab G, Michalski H. Angioplastie percutanée de sténose de branches artérielles pulmonaires. Etude coopératives. Arch Mal Cœur Vaiss. 1992;85:527–31.

90. Blalock A, Taussig HB. The surgical treatment of malformations of the heart in which there is pulmonary stenosis or pulmonary atresia. JAMA. 1945;128(3):189–202.

91. Moulton AL, Brenner JI, Ringel R, Nordenberg A, Berman MA, Ali S, et al. Classic versus modified Blalock-Taussig shunts in neonates and infants. Circulation. 1985;72:1135–44.

92. Gladman G, Mc Crindle BW, Williams WG, Freedom RM, Benson LM. The modified Blalock-Taussig shunt: clinical impact and morbidity in Fallot's tetralogy in the current era. J Thorac Cardiovasc Surg. 1997;114:25–30.

93. Pearl JM, Laks H, Drinkwater Jr DC, Loo DK, George BL, Williams RG. Repair of conotruncal abnormalities with the use of the valved conduit: improved early and midterm results with the cryopreserved homograft. J Am Coll Cardiol. 1992;20:191–6.

94. Muster AJ, Zales VA, Ilbawi MN, Backer CL, Duffy CE, Mavroudis C. Biventricular repair of hypoplastic right ventricle assisted by pulsatile bidirectional cavopulmonary anastomosis. J Thorac Cardiovasc Surg. 1993;105:112–9.

95. Lynch D, Higgins C. MR Imaging of unilateral pulmonary artery anomalies. J Comput Assist Tomogr. 1990;14(2):187–91.

96. Catala F, Marti-Bonmati L, Morales-Marin P. Proximal absence of the right pulmonary artery in the adult: computed tomography and magnetic resonance findings. J Thorac Imaging. 1993;8(3):244–7.

97. Debatin J, Moon R, Spritzer C, Macfall J, Sostman H. MRI of absent left pulmonary artery. J Comput Assist Tomogr. 1992;16(4):641–5.

98. Gomes A. MR imaging of congenital anomalies of the thoracic aorta and pulmonary arteries. Radiol Clin North Am. 1989;27(6):1171–80.

Although the incidence of congenital heart disease is quite low [1], rapid diagnosis is essential to allow early management. Spectacular progress in cardiovascular surgery over the last three decades has transformed the prognosis of these malformations., A dramatic increase has occurred in the population of the so-called "grown up congenital heart" or "GUCH" patients in the past years, and now, the population of GUCH patients is larger than the population of children with congenital malformations in western countries. This new population has to contend with new problems, and needs a specialized long-term follow-up. In these patients who often have to undergo multiple complex surgical correction, the use of echocardiography is often limited due to the poor acoustic window. Hence other techniques, such as MRI or CT-scan are required for visualization of these complex surgical montages.

For decades, MRI has played an essential role in the assessment of congenital anomalies. Preoperatively, MRI appears complementary to echocardiography [2–6], and has proven to be essential especially for the evaluation of the right ventricular outflow tract and the caliber of the pulmonary artery [6–8, 10]. Postoperatively also, MRI has proven to be very useful for evaluation of the surgical corrections, which sometimes require very complex procedures [9–21]. The spectacular progress that has been made in MRI in the last few years with respect to imaging speed, MRA, and flow analysis has strongly reinforced its contribution. For anatomical imaging, MRI results are comparable to CT, which has also made significant technical advances in this field. However, MRI has an edge over multidetector CT in that it offers the advantage of depicting complex cardiac anatomy measuring cardiac function and flow in one examination. Furthermore, it is nonionizing, which should be a concern in this population where postoperative long-term imaging is

required, particularly when follow-up begins in a pediatric population.

8.1 Examination Technique

The investigation starts with acquisition of a first series of ECG-Gated black blood anatomical images (fast spin-echo or double IR sequences) (see Chap. 1). The choice of other imaging planes (other axial, coronal, oblique, and/or sagittal series) cannot be standardized, but is determined case by case as a function of the patient's medical file (procedures performed, current clinical data, problems not resolved by echocardiography, etc.) (Table 8.1). In order to optimize the yield of MRI (with the shortest possible imaging protocol), this approach must integrate the information obtained as one goes along the course of the examination (sequences in the various planes).

Small vascular structures and surgical procedures can be best visualized by acquiring stacks of overlapping 3–5 mm thick images (i.e., 2–3 mm overlap) (see Chap. 2, Examination technique).

The patency of rapid flow cardiovascular structures and surgical procedures (aorta, pulmonary artery, systemic–pulmonary shunt) is relatively easy to confirm on spin-echo sequences, as they are classically visualized as zones of signal void (black low signal intensity, see Chap. 1). However, low-flow cardiovascular structures and surgical procedures (dilated chambers and vessels, veins and cavopulmonary shunts, etc.), particularly when using spin-echo type sequences (see Chap. 1), may give signals suggestive of thrombus, as slowly circulating blood (some types of venous flow and/or even diastolic arterial flow) may have an intermediate intravascular signal, or even a high signal intensity, sometimes simulating thrombus or arterial obstruction [22]. This situation was clarified by applying sequences with saturation bands outside the Fov of interest [23–26] (which restore the usual contrast between black circulating blood and gray thrombus), adding a double inversion pulse at the beginning of the sequence for blood pool signal suppression, and optimizing black blood imaging [27]. Single slice or better multislice double IR T2-weighted sequences allowing excellent image quality during one breath-hold [28] are now becoming the gold standard for black blood imaging and are used routinely in replacement of fast spin-echo sequences. Bright-blood imaging [29–34], velocity mapping [35–43], and various MR angiography techniques [24, 25, 44, 45] are also particularly useful in this setting (see Chap. 1). Black blood sequences should however be performed before gadolinium injection as the latter impairs proper blood suppression by the IR pulse.

8.2 Corrective and Palliative Pulmonary Artery Revascularization Surgery

8.2.1 Palliative Shunts

In patients with cyanotic heart disease and right ventricular outflow obstruction, patent ductus arteriosus and foramen ovale initially help to maintain adequate pulmonary blood flow. At birth, ductus arteriosus closes and the foramen ovale becomes insufficient creating a life-threatening situation. When definitive surgical correction cannot be performed immediately, a temporizing palliative procedure connecting the systemic arterial or venous and pulmonary circulation is usually required before a more complete procedure (which will subsequently restore the connection between the atrium or right ventricle and the pulmonary circulation, see below).

Palliative shunts create anastomotic connections between the systemic circulation (venous or arterial) and the pulmonary circulation. The oldest procedure, the Blalock–Taussig shunt, comprises end-to-side anastomosis between the subclavian artery and the homolateral pulmonary artery (see Chap. 7; [46]). A modified Blalock–Taussig shunt (side-to-side anastomosis) using a Gore-Tex® and other types of shunts have been

subsequently proposed: central shunt between the ascending aorta and the pulmonary trunk, Waterston shunt between the ascending aorta and the right pulmonary artery, Potts shunt between the descending aorta and the left pulmonary artery, and Glenn low pressure shunt between the superior vena cava and the right pulmonary artery.

Echocardiography is not always reliable to assess the patency of a palliative shunt. Even when combined with Doppler, it is sometimes limited for the evaluation of these small extracardiac vascular shunts, often masked by lung or the sternum, which form a screen to echocardiography.

8.2.1.1 Blalock–Taussig Shunts

This procedure is exceptionally performed in Tetralogy of Fallot, but remains the main palliative procedure for pulmonary atresia and VSD and tricuspid atresia or complex congenital disease not amenable to early definitive repair [47] (see Chap. 7). It consists of realizing a surgical end-to-side anastomosis of the native amputated subclavian artery to the homolateral pulmonary artery, and was first performed with success in November 1944 by Drs. Alfred Blalock and Helen Taussig in a cyanotic child [46]. The "classic" Blalock–Taussig shunt has been for the most part replaced by the "modified" Blalock–Taussig using a prosthetic material to connect the corresponding subclavian and pulmonary arteries [47, 48].

Right or left Blalock–Taussig shunts performed between the subclavian artery and the homolateral pulmonary artery are difficult to visualize on echocardiography, but their patency can be confirmed indirectly by the presence of flow on the Doppler study. Confirmation of the patency and display of these shunts when echocardiography is inconclusive requires further imaging investigations.

MRI is a reliable noninvasive method to evaluate Blalock–Taussig shunts. A pioneer study using spin-echo sequences confirmed the efficacy of MRI in 11 out of a series of 17 angiographically controlled palliative shunts [12]. Although black blood SE sequences MRI can easily distinguish between shunt occlusion and patency, it is more difficult to demonstrate narrowing [13]. However, MRI clearly visualizes the patency and course of the shunt [14, 15, 49]. We believe that adequate assessment of the shunt requires complete visualization of the shunt on at least two imaging planes with over-lapped serial images [14, 15]. This multiplanar approach provides more reliable evaluation of these small vascular structures. Axial images are performed first, as they help to guide coronal oblique images in the axis of the pulmonary artery. Systemic–pulmonary shunts are visualized over their entire course including the subclavian and pulmonary insertions (Figs. 8.1 and 8.2 and see Chap. 7, Figs. 7.6 and 7.22). In a personal series [15], the patency and absence of stenosis of the shunt were confirmed in ten patients based on the absence of narrowing of the shunt on spin-echo sequences observed on axial and coronal oblique images. Shunt patency should also be confirmed by performing a third sequence of sagittal images, cine-MRI, and contrast-enhanced MRA offering luminal imaging on a large field of view [10].

Two other points should be stressed:

- The lung homolateral to the other lung to the shunt is often hypertrophied compared (due to preferential perfusion to the side of the shunt)
- In classical Blalock–Taussig shunts (without interposition of Gore-Tex®), the anastomosed subclavian artery has a horizontal or even downwardly angled course, and sometimes presents narrowing of its pulmonary insertion.

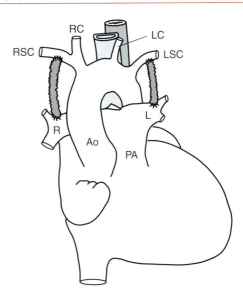

Fig. 8.1 Diagram of Blalock–Taussig shunt. The anastomosis between the subclavian artery and the homolateral pulmonary artery is usually performed on the opposite side to the aortic arch* (on the *right*, R), but can also be performed on the same side** (on the *left*, L). Right and left subclavian arteries (RSC and LSC), right and left pulmonary arteries (R and L PA), aorta (Ao), left and right carotid arteries (RC and LC). * As the right subclavian artery, arising from the brachiocephalic trunk, is more easily mobilized than the left subclavian artery, ** particularly in the case of right arch associated with tetralogy of Fallot, Blalock–Taussig shunt, when it is indicated, is performed on the left side to avoid kinking of the subclavian artery

8.2.1.2 Other Palliative Shunts

MRI can also be used for postoperative assessment of other palliative procedures, especially central shunts (between ascending aorta and pulmonary trunk, Figs. 8.3 and 8.4), the Waterston shunt (anastomosis between ascending aorta and right pulmonary artery), and the Potts shunt (direct side-to-side anastomosis between descending aorta and usually the left pulmonary artery, Figs. 8.5 and 8.6), which are now performed less frequently. These procedures expose the patient to the risk of pulmonary artery hypertension. They were introduced decades ago and are generally performed only when the Blalock–Taussig shunt is impossible [50–54].

The last type of shunt, the Glenn low pressure shunt (anastomosis between superior vena cava and right pulmonary artery) or bidirectional Glenn shunts (see Sect. 8.2.2, Fig. 8.7b–d) are performed to palliate tricuspid atresia or pulmonary atresia with an intact interventricular septum [51] (see Chap. 7), as the first step of total cavo-pulmonary derivation.

The direction of these shunts varies according to the type of procedure performed and the underlying congenital heart disease (position and relations between aorta and pulmonary artery). They are generally visualized on axial and coronal images (preferably serial "intertwined and overlapping" series, see Table 8.1), which must cover the zone of interest comprising the shunts (Figs. 8.3, 8.4, 8.6 and 8.8):

- Central shunt (Fig. 8.4): axial images of the ascending aorta and pulmonary trunk
- Waterston shunt (Fig. 8.8): axial images of the ascending aorta and right pulmonary artery and images in the axis of the shunt
- Potts shunt (Fig. 8.5): posterior coronal images of the descending aorta and left pulmonary artery
- Glenn shunt or bidirectional Glenn shunt (Fig. 8.10): anterior coronal (and sagittal) images of the superior vena cava and right pulmonary artery

8.2.1.3   Complications

The most frequent complication of these palliative procedures is shunt occlusion and/or stenosis of the related pulmonary artery (Fig. 8.2d, e). Anastomotic pseudoaneurysm or periprosthetic hematoma may also occur [55–58].

Evaluation of these shunts is also facilitated by velocity mapping techniques, which assess flow in the shunt and separately in the right and left pulmonary arteries (stenoses, preferential flow) [24–40]. Lung volumes must also be evaluated (unilateral hypertrophy).

8.2.2   Definitive Corrections

"Definitive" surgical correction consists of reconnecting the right atrium or right ventricle to the pulmonary artery. In the case of a nonfunctioning right ventricle (single ventricle), or an obstacle such as tricuspid atresia, this revascularization procedure used to be classically performed from the right atrium (directly onto the right atrial appendage or with interposition of a conduit – classical Fontan procedure [59], Fig. 8.7a) or from the vena cava, particularly the superior vena cava, modified Fontan or cavopulmonary shunt (Figs. 8.7b–e, 8.9 and 8.10). Conversely, when there is a discontinuity between the right ventricle and the pulmonary vessels (transposition of the great vessels with pulmonary stenosis and VSD, truncus arteriosus or severe tetralogy of Fallot), revascularization is performed from the right ventricle (via a Rastelli conduit [18], Figs. 8.11, 8.12 and 8.17). These conduits sometimes include a valve (nonferromagnetic and therefore avoiding any interfering artifacts).

MRI must be performed with coronal and axial images for the Fontan procedure and sagittal and axial images for the Rastelli procedures (see Table 8.1). MRI

is useful to detect thrombosis or narrowing of the conduit (RA-PA or RV-PA, respectively) in these procedures, which are difficult to assess by echocardiography because of their retrosternal situation [19]. MRI also assesses the caliber of pulmonary vessels. The other complications observed in this type of procedure are pseudoaneurysm, hematomas (and abscesses) at zones of anastomosis, and, in the Fontan procedure, right atrial dilatation and frequent intraatrial thrombosis (due to excess pressure).

As indicated above, MRI is also very useful for the preoperative assessment and follow-up of cavopulmonary shunts (low pressure, Glenn and Fontan variants) which have superseded classical Fontan corrections and which are also very difficult to visualize by echocardiography. Cavopulmonary shunts can be assessed on anterior coronal and sagittal images of the superior vena cava and right pulmonary artery (Figs. 8.9 and 8.10; Table 8.1).

8.3   Surgical Correction of Transposition of the Great Vessels

Complete transposition (D-transposition) of the great vessels consists of atrioventricular concordance (normal position) and ventriculoarterial discordance (see Chap. 3, Transposition): the aorta (situated anteriorly and to the right – D-transposition) arises from the morphologically right ventricle situated to the right of the left ventricle (D-loop) and the pulmonary artery (situated posteriorly and centrally) arises from the morphologically left ventricle (Figs. 8.14a and 8.15a).[1] D-transposition of the great vessels can also

---

[1] Corrected D-transposition of the great vessels is a distinct entity with double atrioventricular and ventriculoarterial discordance (see Chap. 3, Segmental analysis).

Fig. 8.2 Blalock–Taussig shunt performed in a newborn [13] with tetralogy of Fallot and severe hypoplasia of the pulmonary artery trunk and branches (also see Chap. 7, Figs. 7.6 and 7.22f). (**a**) Coronal oblique image in the axis of the right pulmonary artery (*3d*); the size, course, and patency of the shunt (*black arrow*); and its subclavian (*25d, above*) and pulmonary (*below*) insertions (*white arrows*) are fully visualized on a single image (coronal oblique); left atrium (*5*), left ventricle (*6*), aorta (*7*), trachea (*T*). (**b**) Sagittal image showing the shunt (*arrow*) situated immediately posteriorly to and along the superior vena cava (*8s*), which drains into the right atrium (*1*). The shunt is inserted between the subclavian artery superiorly and the right pulmonary artery (seen in cross-section on this image) inferiorly. (**c, d**) Axial spin-echo (**c**) and gradient-echo (**d**) images with flow compensation showing the patent shunt (*arrows*), that is, circulating blood is black on the spin-echo sequence (**c**) and white on the gradient-echo flow sequence (**d**). In (**d**), the shunt is inserted inferiorly on the right pulmonary artery (*3d*). (**e, f**) Axial images performed during subsequent follow-up, showing narrowing and stenosis (*arrow*) of the inferior insertion on the right with pulmonary artery and consequently upstream pulmonary trunk and left pulmonary artery dilatation (*3*). This patient subsequently underwent a Rastelli procedure (Fig. 8.12)

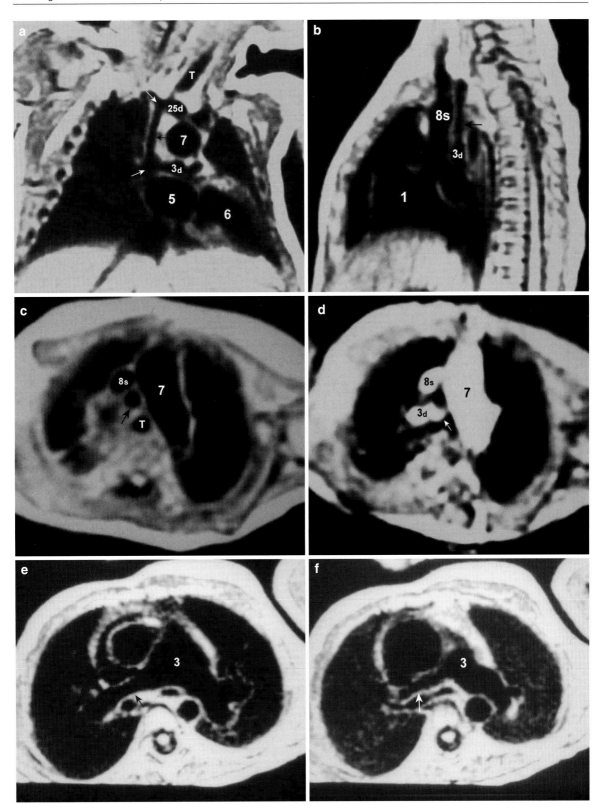

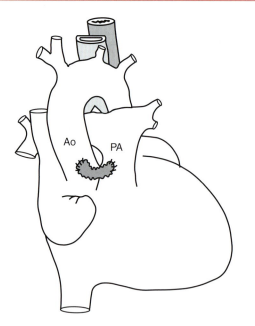

Fig. 8.3 Diagram of the central shunt performed between the ascending aorta (Ao) and pulmonary artery (PA)

be associated with other congenital cardiac anomalies. Hemodynamically therefore, there are two parallel systemic and pulmonary circulatory systems (Fig. 8.13a).[2]

In this type of anomaly, mixing of the two circulations (supplying the pulmonary trunk) is ensured by ductus arteriosus as long as it remains patent (Fig. 8.14a) and/or by a ventricular septal defect when present. Surgical correction must therefore be performed rapidly. Two variants have been proposed: arterial switch and atrial switch.

8.3.1 Arterial Switch (Jatene Procedure)

Introduced in the late 1970s, the arterial switch procedure [60] consists of detachment of the aorta and pulmonary artery and reattachment to the contralateral

ventricles[3]: the pulmonary artery is reconnected to the right ventricle and the aorta to the left ventricle (with reimplantation of the coronary arteries) (Fig. 8.13). This correction, now performed routinely [61, 62], is described as "anatomical": right ventricle → pulmonary artery and left ventricle → aorta (Figs. 8.15 and 8.16). In the absence of VSD, performance of a Raskind procedure [63] and perfusion of prostaglandine to maintain the ductus arteriosus are mandatory. Arterial switch must follow rapidly, while the left ventricle is still able to cope with the high pressure systemic circulation (sufficiently "muscular" ventricle), that is, in practice, before the second to third week of life.

Restoration of ventriculopulmonary continuity may require insertion of a valved conduit (Rastelli procedure, Fig. 8.17). In the case of perimembranous VSD, restoration of the left ventricular outflow tract may require a left ventricle–aorta patch baffle through the VSD (Figs. 8.18 and 8.19).

The most frequent complications of this type of procedure are stenoses at the site of anastomotic sutures. They are more frequent at the supravalvular segment of the right ventricular outflow tract at the site of removal of the coronary arteries[4] and are more clearly visualized on cine-MRI sequences (Figs. 8.16 and 8.17). More rarely, pseudoaneurysm can also occur at the site of anastomotic sutures.

MRI clearly visualizes the zones of anastomosis of the aorta and particularly the pulmonary artery (short-axis sagittal images, Figs. 8.15–8.17; Table 8.1) [9, 16, 17].

Compared to the atrial switch described in the following paragraph, an arterial switch restores the left ventricle as the systemic ventricle. However, it cannot be proposed in patients with pulmonary stenosis, an unresectable right ventricular outflow obstruction, or a coronary artery anomaly.

---

[2]Superior and inferior venae cavae → morphologically right atrium → morphologically right ventricle → aorta → systemic circulation → superior and inferior venae cavae. Pulmonary veins → morphologically left atrium → morphologically left ventricle → pulmonary artery → pulmonary circulation – lung → pulmonary veins.

[3]So-called "anatomical" correction: restoration of normal circulation: right ventricle – pulmonary artery and left ventricle – aorta: Superior and inferior venae cavae → morphologically right atrium → morphologically right ventricle → pulmonary artery (in the place of the aorta) → pulmonary circulation – lung → pulmonary veins → morphologically left atrium → morphologically left ventricle → aorta (in the place of the pulmonary artery) → systemic circulation → superior and inferior venae cavae.

[4]The coronary arteries are harvested from the supravalvular segment of the right side and reimplanted with the aorta on the left side.

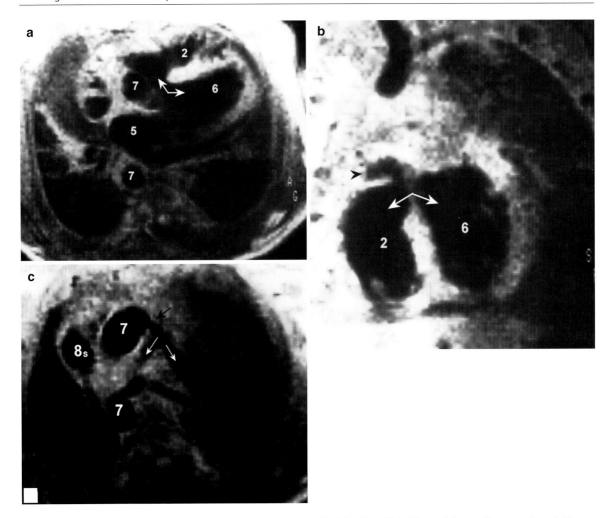

Fig. 8.4 Central shunt [14] in a newborn with pulmonary atresia and VSD. (**a**) Preoperative MRI demonstrating the VSD (*double arrow*) between the right (*2*) and left (*6*) ventricles; right-sided ascending and descending aorta (*7*); left atrium (*5*). (**b**) Preoperative short-axis image demonstrating pulmonary atresia (*arrowhead*) and confirming the VSD (*double arrow*) between the right (*2*) and left (*6*) ventricles. (**c**) Postoperative axial image visualizing the shunt (*black arrow*) between the ascending aorta (*7*) and pulmonary artery. Note that the aortic arch is on the *right*, as frequently observed in this type of anomaly. The pulmonary artery and its branches are hypoplastic (*white arrows*); superior vena cava (*8s*)

8.3.2 *Atrial Switch*

The introduction in 1958 of the atrial switch by Senning has dramatically changed the prognosis of patients born with transposition of the great vessel, offering them a possibility of reaching adulthood [64]. The Senning procedure consists of inverting venous connections to the atrium [65]. Systemic venous return is redirected (via a systemic venous pathway – baffle (or "neocavity") created within the left atrium) to the left ventricle and pulmonary artery, and the pulmonary venous return is redirected (pulmonary venous pathway – baffle) to the right ventricle and aorta. The right ventricle then

definitively functions as a "systemic" ventricle. The systemic venous baffle is created with interatrial septum and part of the wall of the right atrium (Figs. 8.20 and 8.21). Some years later Mustard [66] described an alternative in which the atrial septum is excised and or synthetic baffle is used to redirect the venous return [66] (Figs. 8.20 and 8.22). This type of surgery was performed in the early era of transposition of the great vessels surgical treatment. Because of late complications, namely arrhythmias with risks of sudden death and right ventricular dysfunction [67–70], it has largely been replaced since the mid 1980s by the arterial switch. In the 1990s, it had been proposed in some patients with

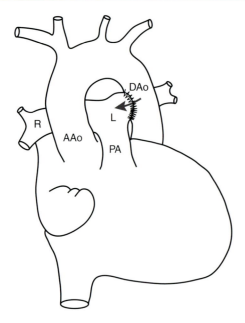

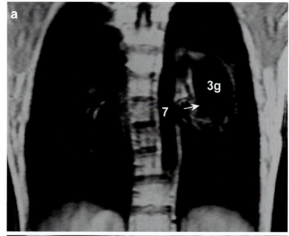

Fig. 8.5 Diagram of Potts shunt: direct side-to-side shunt (*arrow*) between the descending aorta (DAo) and left (L) pulmonary artery (PA). Right pulmonary artery (R), ascending aorta (AAo)

transposition of the great vessels and pulmonary artery obstruction (and intact interventricular septum) or when arterial switch was not performed in time. Owing to the large number of survivors, there is still a great interest in long-term follow-up [70].

Multiplanar MRI is particularly useful for the follow-up of these corrections. Vascular complications observed with these procedures include systemic and pulmonary vein obstructions baffle leak (extensive atrial suture lines). Detection of venous pathway obstruction was already possible in the early times of MRI [19]. Short-axis axial images clearly visualize the neocavity in the Senning procedure (Fig. 8.21), but coronal images are also useful to visualize superior and inferior venae cavae particularly in the Mustard procedure (Fig. 8.22; Table 8.1). Mainly performed decades ago, atrial switches leave, as mentioned, the right ventricle as the systemic ventricle with a potential on the long term of tricuspid and right ventricular insufficiency,[5] atrial arrhythmias, and cardiac arrest [67–70]. Assessment of right ventricular function and the right atrioventricular valve (tricuspid) is based on gradient-echo cine-MRI sequences [17, 21, 30, 71]. A

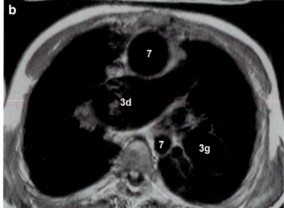

Fig. 8.6 Potts shunt in a patient with tricuspid atresia already treated by Blalock–Taussig shunt. Posterior coronal image (**a**) clearly showing the direct side-to-side anastomosis (*arrow*) between the descending aorta (*7*) and significantly dilated left pulmonary artery (*3g*). This enlargement is also seen on the axial image (**b**)

recent study showed that the extent of late gadolinium right ventricular enhancement is correlated to ventricular alterations and clinical outcome [72].

8.4 Surgical Correction of Coarctation of the Aorta

The poor outcome of nonoperated coarctations of the aorta reported in older series is the main argument in favor of surgical correction [73]. The indication for surgery takes into account, the patient's age, and the site, severity, and extent of coarctation. It is essentially based on demonstration of significant coarctation

---

[5]The tricuspid valve and right ventricle are not "designed" to support on the long term, the load of the systemic circulation.

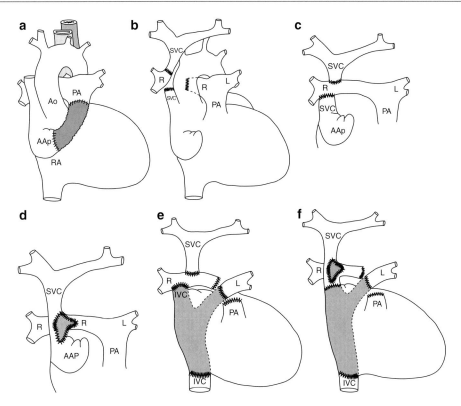

Fig. 8.7 Diagram of Fontan procedures and cavopulmonary variants. (**a**) Classical Fontan: revascularization of the pulmonary artery (PA) from the right atrium (RA), on the right atrial appendage (AAp) either directly or via a conduit, aorta (Ao). (**b**) Classical Glenn (low pressure) cavopulmonary shunt between superior vena cava (SVC) and right pulmonary artery (R). Left pulmonary artery (PA L), ascending Aorta (AAo). These two operations are now performed less frequently, as they have been replaced by cavopulmonary shunts. (**c**) End-to-side bidirectional cavopulmonary shunt of the two inferior and superior stumps of the SVC onto the right pulmonary artery. (**d**) Side-to-side bidirectional cavopulmonary shunt with interposition of a Gore-Tex® patch between the superior vena cava and right pulmonary artery. This variant, called "hemi-Fontan," represents an alternative to the previous procedure (**c**) in the case of stenotic or hypoplastic pulmonary arteries. These two operations are performed prior to definitive complete cavopulmonary correction. (**e**, **f**) Complete cavopulmonary shunt: Formation of a right intraatrial conduit between the inferior vena cava (IVC) and left pulmonary artery (L). This conduit is also connected to the SVC. This procedure has superseded the classical Fontan procedure. It is performed following a bidirectional cavopulmonary shunt (**c**, **d**). In the absence of preliminary bidirectional cavopulmonary shunt, this procedure and the conduit are performed at the same operation

corresponding to a significant systolic transisthmic pressure gradient reduction of the aortic lumen by more than 50%, demonstration of a collateral circulation, hypoplasia of the horizontal segment, and hypoplasia of the proximal segment of the descending aorta (see Chap. 6) [74].

Apart from severe neonatal forms, in which surgery must be performed as an emergency, the optimal timing of the procedure is still controversial. Excessively early surgery increases the operative risks, residual stenoses, and recoarctations. Excessively late repair leads to residual hypertension and increases the cardiovascular risks. While an operation between the ages of 2 months and 4 years appeared to be sufficient in the recent past [74, 75], the longer survival and the low incidence of residual hypertension in patients operated before the age of 1 year now justify operation between the ages of 6 months and 1 year [76, 77]. Combining anatomical and functional information, as compared to CT-scan, MRI has proven to be the best suited for both diagnosis of coarctation and postsurgical follow-up [78, 79].

8.4.1 Types of Procedures

The Crafoord procedure is the reference technique for the treatment of isolated coarctation (Fig. 8.23b). It

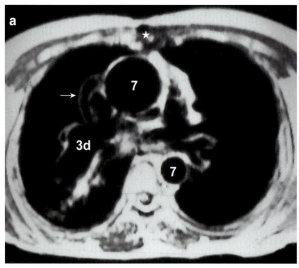 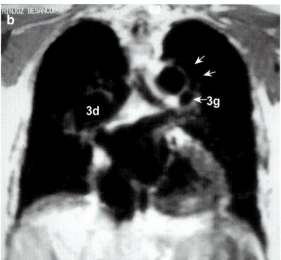

Fig. 8.8 Waterston shunt. Axial image in a patient with pulmonary atresia and VSD, and interrupted pulmonary artery. The shunt (*arrow*) connects the ascending aorta (*7*) and right pulmonary artery (*3d*). Note the marked dilatation of the pulmonary artery (**a**). Absence of confluence of the right (*3d*) and left (*3g*) pulmonary arteries is clearly visible on these two views, particularly on the axial image (also see the same patient, Chap. 7, Fig. 7.11). Nonconfluent branch pulmonary arteries require bilateral palliative shunts. A Blalock–Taussig shunt was thus also performed on the left side (*arrows*, **b**), between the left subclavian artery and left pulmonary artery (*3g*); sternotomy wire artifact (*star*)

consists of sufficiently large resection of the stenosis to eliminate all ductal tissue, followed by end-to-end anastomosis of the two aortic segments [80]. In the case of late diagnosis of coarctation in adolescents or adults, the more fragile and less mobile resected aortic margins may sometimes be too far apart to allow direct anastomosis, and interposition of a prosthetic conduit may be necessary (Fig. 8.23). A conduit may also be required in very long coarctations with a hypoplastic aortic isthmus or in the presence of associated aneurysm (Fig. 8.23c, f).

In serious neonatal forms, progress in intensive care now allows surgery to be performed on a hemodynamically stable neonate [76], an essential factor for the success of surgery. In these difficult cases, simple resection-anastomosis is often impossible due to the length of the stenotic segment and/or associated hypoplasia of the horizontal aorta. Alternative techniques have been proposed that can be encountered in surgical follow-up [74, 77].

The widely used modified Crafoord procedure consists of anastomosis of the descending aorta in the concavity of the arch, which simultaneously reduces hypoplasia of the arch (see Chap. 6, Fig. 6.18).

The technique described by Waldhausen uses a left subclavian artery flap to enlarge the narrowed segment (Fig. 8.23d) [81]. The prime advantage of this technique was that it limited the risk of restenosis (as it uses living tissue, which continues to grow). However, it has been abandoned, because sacrifice of the left

Fig. 8.9 Complex cyanotic heart disease with tight pulmonary stenosis and single ventricle, in a context of right isomerism (see preoperative images, Chap. 3, Fig. 3.6 and Chap. 7, Fig. 7.22). A left Blalock–Taussig shunt was performed as first-line procedure. Correction by complete cavopulmonary shunt. Postoperative follow-up at the age of 13 years. (**a**) Anterior coronal spin-echo image through the conduit (*C*) continuous (*arrow*) with the left pulmonary artery (*3g*) (see Fig. 8.7e); right superior vena cava (*8sd*), thoracic aorta (*7*), hepatic vein (*hv*). (**b**) Coronal image through the left superior vena cava (*8sg*) also anastomosed onto the right pulmonary artery (*3g*) (see Fig. 8.7e), right atrium (*1*), single left ventricle (*6*). (**c**) More posterior coronal image through the right superior vena cava (*8sd*) anastomosed end-to-side to the right pulmonary artery (*3d*). The conduit (c) is connected to a right (*8id*) and left (*8ig*) inferior vena cava, which receives an HV: this left inferior vena cava and hepatic vein initially drained into the left-sided right atrium (see Chap. 3, Fig. 3.6d); abdominal aorta (*7i*). (**d**) Axial spin-echo image through the conduit (C) in the atria

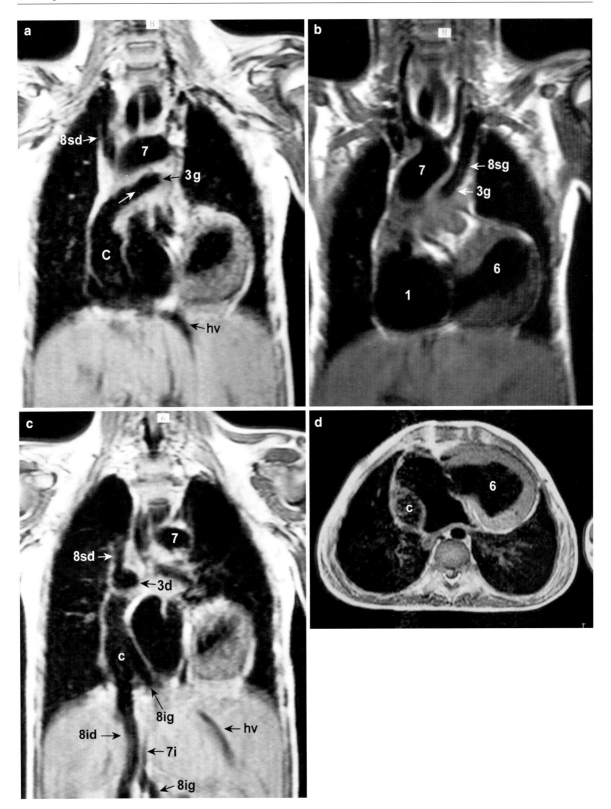

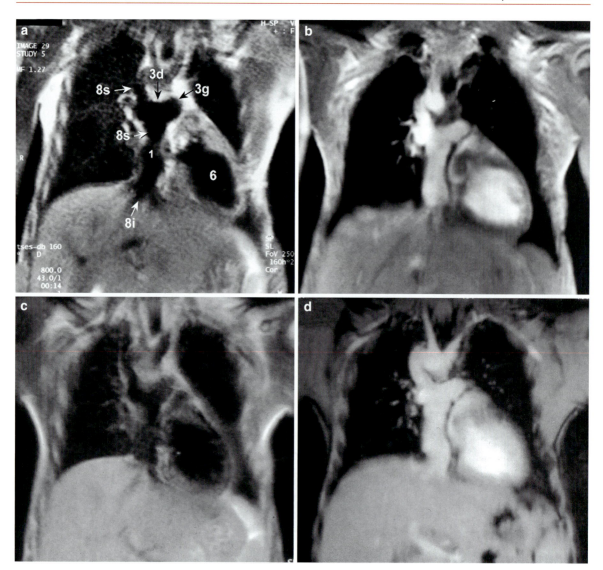

Fig. 8.10 Bidirectional cavopulmonary shunt ("hemi-Fontan") in a case of type 3b tricuspid atresia. Postoperative MRI: a first MRI was performed at the age of 7 years (**a, b** – December 1997) and a second MRI was performed at the age of 11 years (**c, d, e** – May 2001) (see preoperative images, Chap. 7, Fig. 7.26). (**a**) Anterior coronal fast spin-echo (Haste) image through the two superior vena cava stumps (*8s*) connected to the right pulmonary artery (*3d*) (see Fig. 8.7e). The shunt is patent (circulating black flow); inferior vena cava (*8i*); left pulmonary artery (*3g*), right atrium (*1*), left ventricle (*6*). (**b**) Anterior coronal cine-MRI at the same level, more clearly confirming patency of the shunt (circulating white flow). (**c, d**) Same views as in (**a**) and (**b**): the shunt is still functional 3 years later. (**e**) Gadolinium-enhanced MR angiography (Dota-Gd, Guerbet, France) and MIP reconstruction: all of the procedure is visualized together with the venous drainage and drainage of the brachiocephalic veins into the superior vena cava and all of the inferior vena cava and right atrium (*1*). This patient also had a right-sided aortic arch (see Chap. 5, Fig. 5.11d, e). (**f–h**) Classical Fontan procedure in a patient presenting tricuspid atresia: revascularization of the pulmonary artery (*3*) from the right atrium (*1*), on the right atrial appendage (*1d*) via a conduit (*arrows*). Note the dilated ascending aorta (*7a*) and left ventricle (*6*); descending aorta (*7d*), left atrium (*5*). Compare this rather simple surgical correction to the more complex bidirectional cavopulmonary shunts (Figs. 8.9 and 8.10a–d)

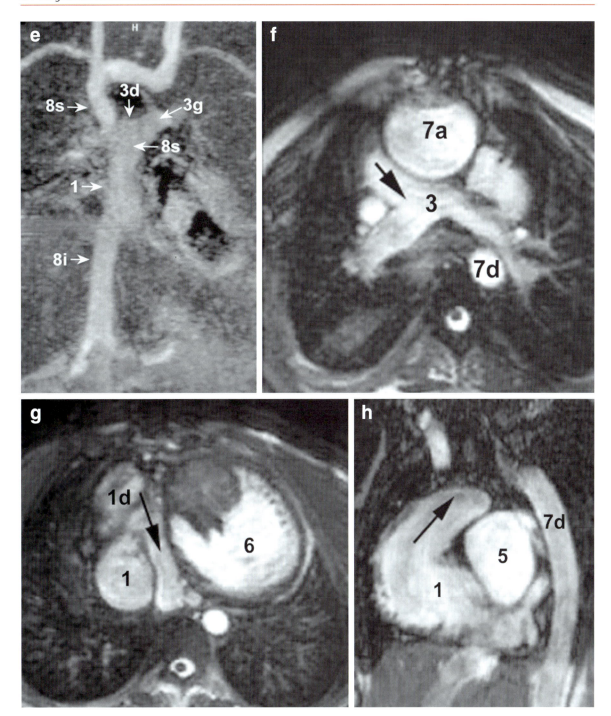

Fig. 8.10 (continued)

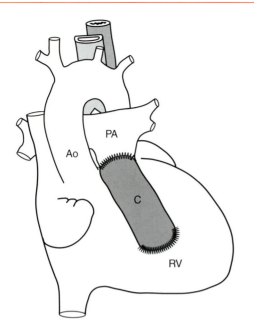

Fig. 8.11 Diagram of Rastelli procedure. Pulmonary artery (PA) revascularization is performed from the right ventricle (RV) by insertion of a Dacron® conduit (C), aorta (Ao)

subclavian artery can lead to complications ranging from minor functional disorders to shortening of the left arm.

Dacron® prosthetic patch aortoplasty (Fig. 8.23e) has also gone out of favor, as it can predispose to aneurysm formation.

In infantile coarctation syndromes, ligation of ductus arteriosus is performed during the same procedure, but the treatment of associated malformations, particularly closure of a VSD, may require a second operation.

As a less invasive method, percutaneous transluminal angioplasty with dilatation of the coarctation by balloon catheter has been proposed. It has not been largely diffused because of its rate of recoarctation. It is rarely performed as a first-line procedure in Europe, where it is mainly reserved for recoarctations [82]. This technique is sometimes used in the USA to treat relatively minor coarctation. To overcome recoarctation problems, stenting has been proposed [83, 84]. Stenting has also been useful in complications such as pseudoaneurysm. However, surgical treatment still has the best long-term results [85].

8.4.2 Complications

Radiologists and Cardiologists must be familiar with the complications of these interventions [76, 77, 79, 86, 87].

8.4.2.1 Early Complications

Early postoperative complications are rare but serious. Hemorrhages occur more frequently on neglected coarctations and require emergency reoperation.

The postcoarctectomy syndrome is related to paradoxical hypertension following the operation. Hypertensive crises are accompanied by abdominal pain due to vasomotor disorders that can be responsible for intestinal bleeding and mesenteric infarction and can be treated by antihypertensives.

Paraplegia due to spinal cord ischemia is an exceptional complication (0.4% cases) [88] that can be prevented by preserving the collateral circulation, particularly intercostal, during the operation which requires identification of these vessels by preoperative imaging (see Chap. 6, Figs. 6.12, 6.13, and 6.18).

8.4.2.2 Late Complications

Restenosis should be suspected clinically by a reduction of femoral pulses and a blood pressure gradient between upper and lower limbs. Doppler echocardiography is used to measure the transisthmic gradient, which is greater than 20 mmHg. MRI visualizes the stenosis. Percutaneous angioplasty is the preferred first-line procedure, as it is relatively simple to perform and is particularly effective in the case of a tight and localized stenosis [82]. There is a potential risk of rupture of the aortic wall, although it has been rarely reported. Regular MRI follow-up is justified by the late risks of restenosis (Fig. 8.24), aneurysm, dissection, fistulas, and rupture [89, 90].

Aortic aneurysms at the operated zone (Fig. 8.25) are more frequently observed after prosthetic patch aortoplasty.

Nearly half of the operated patients develop late hypertension, which is more frequent in the case of delayed surgery. Recurrent hypertension some time

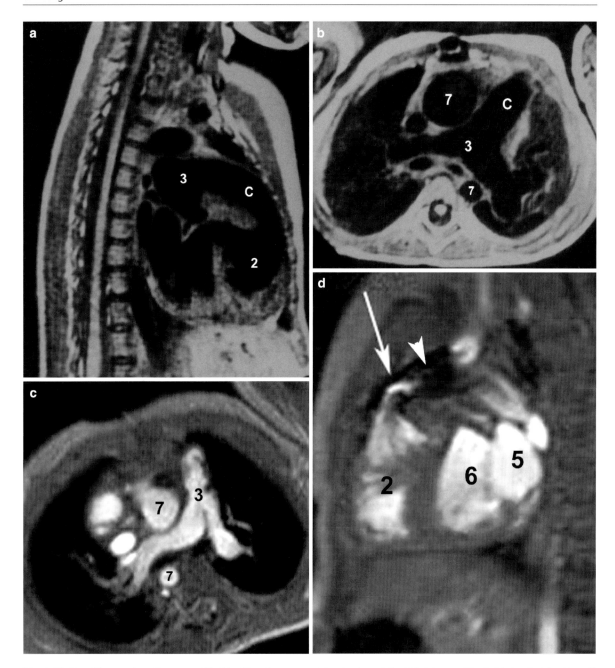

Fig. 8.12 Rastelli procedure. Two-year-old girl with pulmonary atresia and intact interventricular septum (severe tetralogy of Fallot). Restoration of ventriculopulmonary continuity by a valved conduit (*C*) containing a bioprosthesis (Rastelli procedure) clearly visible on the sagittal fast spin-echo image (**a**) and also on the axial image (**b**). This patient had already undergone a right Blalock–Taussig shunt (Fig. 8.2) (also see Fig. 8.17). (**c, d**) Other Rastelli procedure. Truncus arteriosus in a 10-month infant. Postoperative assessment. Axial and LAO cine-MR images. Note the significant narrowing (*arrow*) and poststenotic systolic flow void jet (signal void – *arrowhead*); right ventricle (*2*), pulmonary artery (*3*), left atrium (*5*), left ventricle (*6*) aorta (*7*) (also see Fig. 8.17)

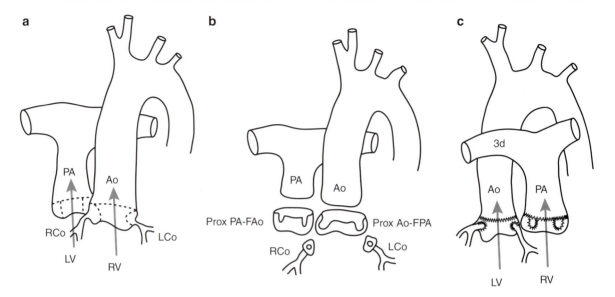

Fig. 8.13 Diagram of arterial switch. (**a**) Preoperative view showing transposition of the vessels: the aorta (Ao) emerges from the right ventricle (RV) and the pulmonary artery (PA) emerges from the left ventricle (LV). Right and left coronary arteries (RCo and LCo). (**b**) Image showing the vessels at their origin and removal of the coronary arteries with a cuff of arterial wall on the proximal aortic segment, the future pulmonary artery (Prox Ao-FPA). The proximal pulmonary artery segment is the future aorta (Prox PA-FAo). (**c**) Arterial switch with coronary artery reimplantation. Filling of the defect at the zone of resection of the coronary arteries by small pericardial patches (zone at risk of postoperative stenosis, see Figs. 8.16 and 8.17). Note that the right branch of the pulmonary artery (*3d*) now crosses in front of and to the right of the aorta (and not posteriorly as in the normal situation, see Figs. 8.15 and 8.16)

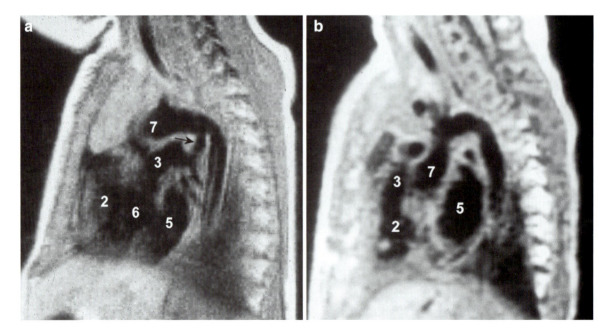

Fig. 8.14 Complete transposition of the great vessels (D-transposition) in a neonate: correction by arterial switch. (**a**) Preoperative sagittal image: the aorta (*7*), situated anteriorly and to the right, and the pulmonary artery (*3*), situated posteriorly and on the left, run parallel without crossing ("gun barrel image"). The aorta emerges from the right ventricle (*2*) and the pulmonary artery emerges from the left ventricle (*6*). The patent ductus arteriosus (*arrow*) is clearly visualized; left atrium (*5*). (**b**) Postoperative sagittal image showing the switch. In contrast with the preoperative image (**a**), the pulmonary artery (*3*) is situated anteriorly and emerges from the right ventricle (*2*) and the aorta (*7*) is situated posteriorly (also see Chap. 1, Fig. 1.8, Chap. 3, Figs. 3.17–3.20 and Chap. 7, Figs. 7.14 and 7.15)

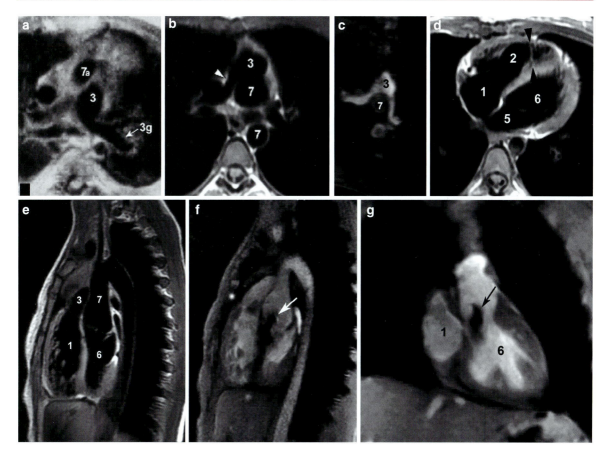

Fig. 8.15 Complete transposition of the great vessels (D-transposition), correction by arterial switch follow-up at the age of 9 years. (**a**) Preoperative axial image: the aorta (*7a*), situated anteriorly and to the right (D-transposition), emerges from the right ventricle and the pulmonary artery (*3*), situated posteriorly and to the left in a central position, emerges from the left ventricle; left pulmonary artery (*3g*). Correction was realized in the neonatal period. Follow-up at the age of 9 years (GEMS 3T images). Postoperative axial images (**b–g**): The aorta (*7a*), situated posteriorly and to the right in a central position, emerges from the left ventricle and the pulmonary artery (*3*), situated anteriorly and to the right, emerges from the right ventricle. The right pulmonary artery (*white arrow heads*) crosses in front of and to the right of the aorta (and not posteriorly as in the normal arrangement); also note (**d**) that the morphologically right ventricle (*2*) is on the right (right loop); it is identified by the presence of a moderator band (between the *two black arrowheads*); left ventricle – *6*). Sagittal oblique (LAO) images in the plane of the aorta (**e**, **f**) and coronal (**g**) image through the aorta (*7*) and left ventricle (*6*), display a dilated aortic root. Gradient-echo cine-MR images (**f, g**) demonstrate an aortic regurgitation (jet of signal void – *arrow*, whose summit or conus is situated at the site of coaptation of the aortic valves); right atrium (*2*), left atrium (*5*), (also see Chap. 1, Fig. 1.8, Chap. 3, Figs. 3.17–3.20, Chap. 7, Figs. 7.14, 7.15, and Fig. 7.28, Chap. 6 for the aortic root dilatation)

after the operation is suggestive of restenosis. The geometry of the aortic arch, particularly gothic-shaped arches, has also been incriminated in residual or recurrence of hypertension and developing left ventricular hypertrophy [91–94].

Scoliosis after left thoracotomy is another possible complication.

8.5 Extensive Coarctation and Interrupted Aortic Arch

In these forms, the extent of the interrupted or hypoplastic segment and the size of the patent ductus arteriosus are useful features to be taken into account by the surgeon.

In the presence of extensive hypoplasia (Fig. 8.23f) interposition of a Dacron® conduit is indicated. In more localized forms, curative treatment consists of suture of ductus arteriosus and aorta allowing proximal mobiliza-

tion of the distal aortic segment with end-to-side anastomosis to the ascending aorta (Fig. 8.26).

In severe, extensive coarctations (transitional forms with interrupted aortic arch), many techniques have

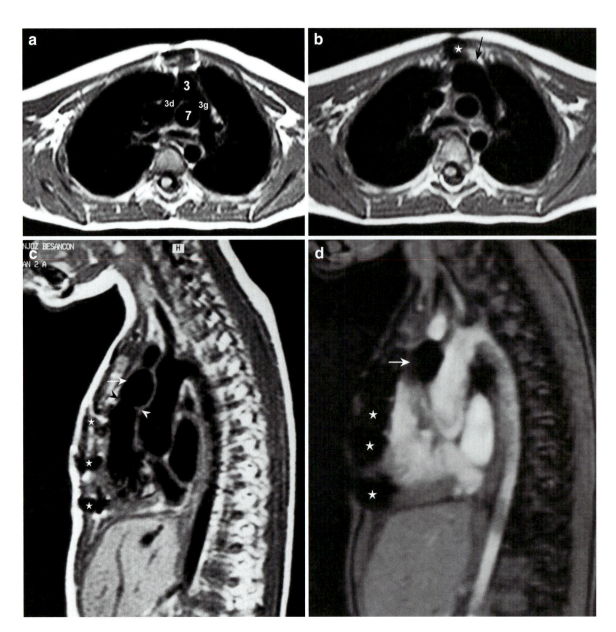

Fig. 8.16 Complete transposition of the great vessels (D-transposition): correction by arterial switch. Follow-up at the age of 2 years. (**a**, **b**) Axial spin-echo sequences: the right branch (*3d*) of the pulmonary artery (*3*) crosses the aorta (*7*) anteriorly and to the right (and not posteriorly as in the normal arrangement). The pulmonary artery is dilated (*arrow*) above a stenosis (see (**d**)); left branch of the pulmonary artery (*3g*). Sagittal spin-echo (**c**) and cine-MRI images (systole – (**d**), diastole – (**e**)). On the

black blood image (**c**), the flow obstruction (*arrowheads*) on the anastomotic zone is clearly demonstrated by the downstream suprastenotic dilatation (*arrow*). The white blood image (**d**) confirms the obstacle by showing a large signal-void zone above the stenosis (turbulence – *arrow*): The flow void artifact is more marked during systole (**d**) compared to diastole (**e**). Also note the sternotomy wire artifacts (*stars*) in front of the pulmonary artery (more marked on the gradient-echo sequence)

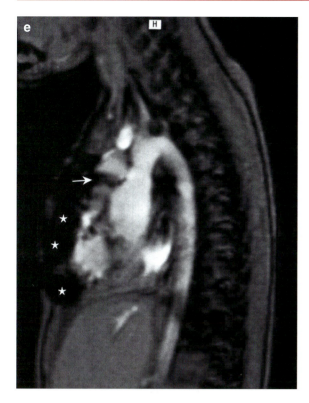

Fig. 8.16 (continued)

been proposed, particularly a palliative procedure that is performed first when many other anomalies are also present. They consist of creating a Dacron® shunt between the proximal segment of the aorta (ascending aorta or horizontal segment) and the descending aorta (Fig. 8.23f). In very long thoracoabdominal coarctations, sometimes very long Dacron® conduits are required, which can be easily visualized by MRI (Fig. 8.28).

8.6 Other Types of Surgery

8.6.1 Tetralogy of Fallot

Tetralogy of Fallot is the most frequent form of cyanotic congenital heart disease (0.25–0.8% prevalence). Proper surgical management has drastically improved the 20-year survival rate (up to 90%) [95–97].

Temporary procedures (essentially Blalock–Taussig shunt) are still performed in patients with a very narrow or atretic pulmonary artery. MRI, as mentioned above,

allows assessment of size and patency of the shunts [49, 78]. Surgical correction of tetralogy of Fallot, designed to repair the infundibular stenosis, consists of incising the right ventricular outflow tract with excision of the hypertrophied parietal and septal muscle bands. The conoventricular septal defect is closed by a patch. The right ventricular (infundibular or transannular) outflow tract obstruction is usually treated by infundibular and pulmonary incision and enlarged by a pericardial or Dacron® tract patch (Figs. 8.29b and 8.30). Common postoperative complications include residual pulmonary outflow tract stenosis, branch pulmonary arterial stenosis or occlusion, and shunt stenosis or occlusion. Pulmonary valve regurgitation resulting in right ventricular dilatation and dysfunction was almost universal, particularly in patients operated before recent surgical progress began to focus on efforts to preserve pulmonary valve integrity. Patients are exposed to heart failure, atrial and ventricular arrhythmias, and cardiac arrest in the long run [95, 97–99]. In repaired tetralogy of Fallot, MRI is aimed at quantifying right ventricular enlargement and dysfunction, pulmonary valve regurgitation (see Fig. 1.17b, Chap. 1), tricuspid valve insufficiency, and residual narrowing or stenosis on right ventricular outflow tract (see Fig. 1.17a, Chap. 1), pulmonary arterial tree, and aorto-pulmonary collateral circulation [95, 97–99].

Note that as seen in Chap. 7, proximal branches of coronary arteries must be visualized during preoperative assessment of tetralogy of Fallot to detect an abnormal major coronary branch (5% of cases – [100]) crossing the pulmonary infundibulum anteriorly over the ventriculotomy zone (Fig. 8.29a) (particularly abnormal origin of the left anterior descending artery from the right coronary artery) [101]. Visualization of coronary arteries is becoming available with MRI [102, 103] (see Chap. 1, Fig. 1.10).

8.6.2 Pulmonary Artery Banding

Preoperative and postoperative assessment of the quality of the pulmonary arterial supply, for which MRI is an excellent imaging modality, was discussed in Chap. 7.

Pulmonary artery banding (Figs. 8.31 and 8.32) is designed to reduce pulmonary blood flow and prevent secondary pulmonary artery hypertension. Now that one-stage definitive corrections of congenital heart

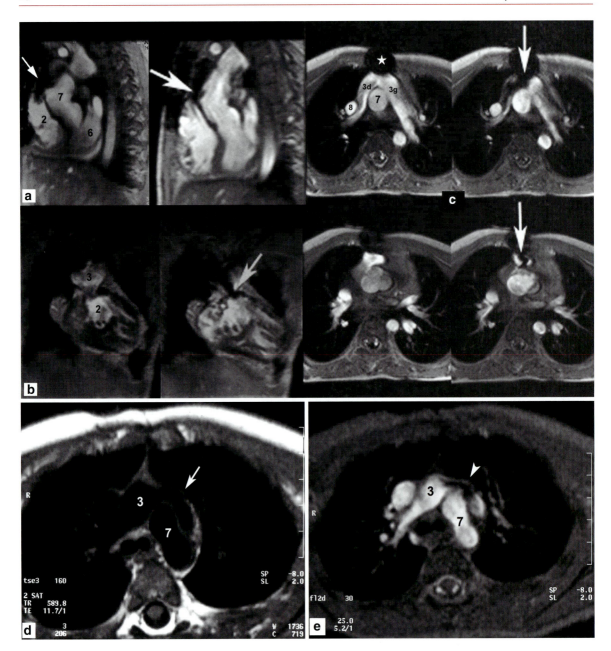

Fig. 8.17 Complete transposition of the great vessels (D-transposition) with pulmonary stenosis: correction by arterial switch and restoration of continuity by a valved conduit (Rastelli procedure). Postoperative cine-MRI sequences: (**a**) Sagittal, (**b**) coronal, and (**c**) axial cine-MR images. On the sagittal (**a**), coronal, (**b**) and also the axial (**c**) images in systole, the stenosis of the valved conduit is seen as a signal-void turbulent jet (*arrows*) located above the site of pulmonary anastomosis (zone of coronary artery resection). Note that on the axial images, the right branch (*3d*) of the pulmonary artery (*3*) crosses the aorta (*7*) anteriorly and to the right; left pulmo-

nary artery (*3g*), superior vena cava (*8*). Also note the marked artifact related to sternotomy wires (*star*); pulmonary artery (*3*), right ventricle (*2*), left ventricle (*6*). Other case of complete transposition of the great vessels (D-transposition) corrected by arterial switch. (**d, e**) Axial fast-spin echo and cine-MR images at the level of the pulmonary artery (*3*) bifurcation. On both images, note the significant stenosis of the left pulmonary artery (*arrow* and *arrowhead*) appearing as a signal-void turbulent jet on the white blood image (*arrowhead*); aorta (*7*) (also see Fig. 8.12a–d)

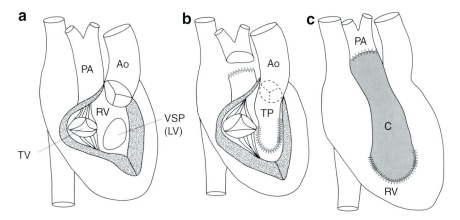

Fig. 8.18 Complete transposition (D-transposition) with per-imembranous ventricular septal defect (VSD). Diagram of the switch with Rastelli procedure and left ventricle-to-aorta tunnel through the VSD (modified from [18]). (**a**) Open view of the right ventricle (RV) from which the aorta (Ao) emerges. The patent perimembranous VSD in the left ventricle (LV) and the right atrioventricular valve (tricuspid, TV) can be seen. (**b**) Restoration of continuity on the left ventricular outflow tract by creation of a tunneling patch (TP) between the left ventricle and the aorta through the VSD. (**c**) Restoration of ventriculopulmonary continuity by Rastelli procedure with insertion of a valved conduit (C) between the pulmonary artery (PA) and the right ventricle (RV)

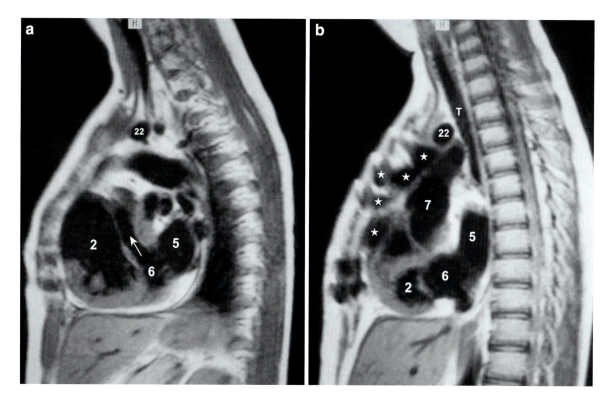

Fig. 8.19 Rastelli procedure with left ventricle-to-aorta tunnel. Eight-year-old boy with transposition of the great vessels and VSD with severe subpulmonary obstruction. Complete correction was performed 3 years previously with arterial switch, separation of the pulmonary artery from the left ventricle and restoration of ventriculopulmonary continuity by a valved conduit containing a bioprosthesis (Rastelli procedure). A left ventricle-to-aorta tunnel was created with a patch through the perimembranous VSD. Left and right sagittal spin-echo images (**a**, **b**). Tunneling patch (*arrow*) emerging from the left ventricle (6) to the aorta (7). The Rastelli procedure on the right ventricular outflow tract is difficult to evaluate because of sternotomy wire artifacts (*stars*); right ventricle (2), left atrium (5), trachea (T), brachiocephalic vein (22). This patient also had a right-sided aortic arch (see Chap. 5, Fig. 5.11a–c)

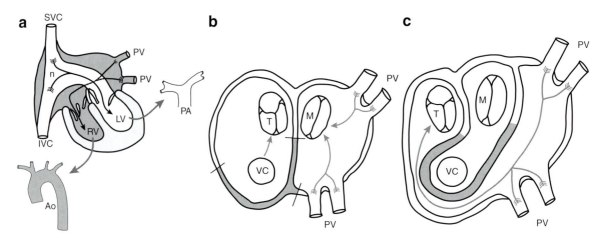

Fig. 8.20 Diagram of the Senning (and/or Mustard) procedure: atrial switch. (**a**) Coronal view: the superior vena cava (SVC) and inferior vena cava (IVC) enter the baffle ("neocavity") (systemic venous pathway), which is connected to the left ventricle (LV) and pulmonary artery (PA), while the pulmonary veins are connected (pulmonary venous pathway) to the right ventricle (RV) and aorta (Ao). (**b, c**) Preoperative and postoperative axial images of the atria: the neocavity is formed from interatrial septum and part of the wall of the right atrium (*shaded zone*). Merging SVC and IVC ti baffle (VC) right atrioventricular valve (tricuspid T), pulmonary veins (PV), left atrioventricular valve (mitral M)

disease can be successfully performed in much younger subjects, this procedure is at present indicated only in a limited number of selected patients.

It is performed as a palliative procedure to protect the pulmonary artery, in the absence of pulmonary stenosis, in single ventricles, double outlet right ventricle, and tricuspid atresia with increased blood flow [104]. Banding is also indicated for the same reason in multiple ventricular septal defects and two-stage operations for transposition of the great vessels. It has been evaluated as a first-step technique for later second-stage more complete repair by a bidirectional cavopulmonary shunt by Fontan or Damus procedure [105–107].

Fig. 8.21 (**a–m**) Complete transposition of the great vessels (D-transposition) in a 7-year-old infant corrected by a Senning procedure (atrial switch). (**a–d**) Postoperative axial fast spin-echo images through the ventricular chambers; the right ventricle (*2* – moderator band: *arrowheads*) is on the right (right loop) and is hypertrophied as it is connected to the aorta and the systemic circulation (the right ventricle acts as the systemic ventricle). Good visualization of the systemic venous pathway – baffle ("neocavity" – *n*). The "neocavity" drains blood from both venae cavae: The vena cavae (*stars* – inferior vena cava – (**a–d**)) merge into the "neocavity" (*n*) (systemic venous pathway – baffle) connected (*arrow* on the right – image (**d**)) to the left ventricle (*6*) (and pulmonary artery – transposition). The pulmonary venous pathway is also well displayed: Blood entering the left atrium (*5* – derived from pulmonary veins! pulmonary venous pathway) travels (*arrow* on the left – image (**d**)) around the neocavity (*n*) and drains into the right atrium (*1*), which is connected to the right ventricle (*2*). These findings of systemic and venous rerouted blood pathways are confirmed on the postoperative coronal images (Fast spin-echo – (**e**), (**f**) and cine-MR – (**g**)) and CE-MRA native axial reconstructions (**h**, **i**); pulmonary veins (*white arrows*): the superior and inferior vena cavae (*stars*) do not connect with the right atrium (*1*), but with the "neocavity" situated between the right atrium (*1*) and the left atrium (*5*). (**j–m**) Postoperative axial (**j**) and sagittal oblique (**k–m**) CE-MRA (**j–l**) and cine-MR (**m**) images through the great vessels which remain transposed (as an atrial switch was performed): the aorta (*7*), situated anteriorly (and to the *right*), and the pulmonary artery (*3*), situated posteriorly (and on the *left*), run parallel ("gun barrel image")

8.6.3 Damus Procedure

End-to-side shunt between the pulmonary artery trunk and the ascending aorta (Damus procedure [108]) is sometimes proposed in severe left ventricular outflow tract obstruction. The pulmonary artery is supplied by a second distal shunt on the pulmonary artery trunk or its branches. A review of the experience in 38 patients including 9 double outlet right ventricle and 38 uni-ventricular heart and subaortic stenosis showed that the 5-year survival rate is 72% [109]. MRI has not been extensively evaluated in this type of operation [110]. Sagittal, LAO, and coronal images centered on the pulmonary artery and aorta must be performed.

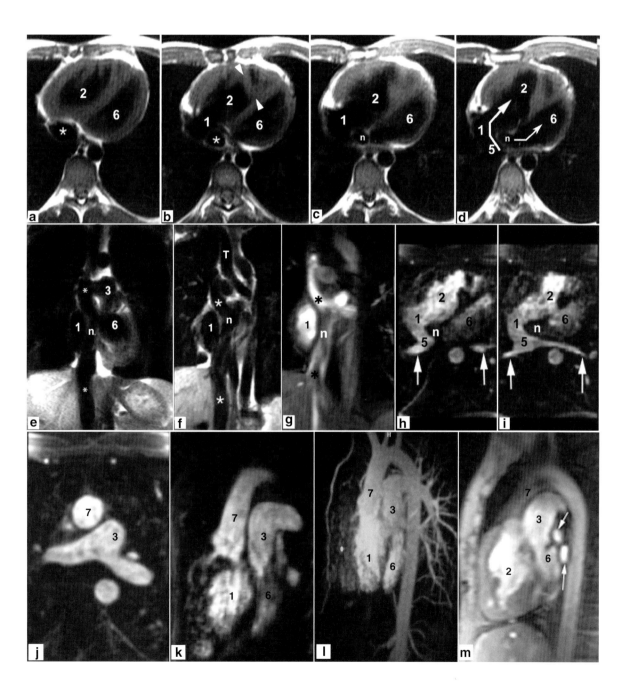

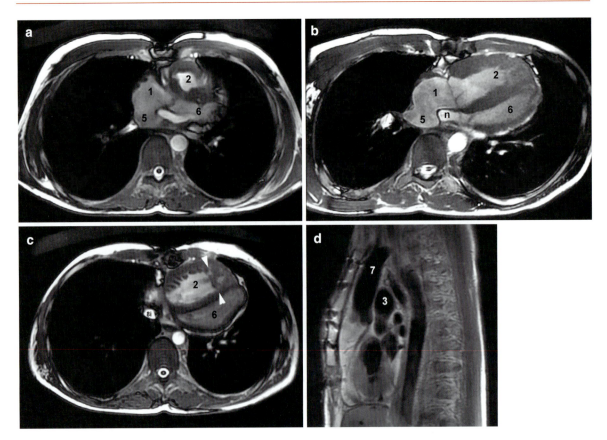

Fig. 8.22 (**a–c**) Complete transposition of the great vessels (D-transposition) in a female patient corrected by a Mustard procedure in the neonatal period (atrial switch). Follow-up MRI at the age of 25 years. 3T (GEMS) Postoperative axial balanced-SSFP (Fiesta) images through the ventricular chambers; the right ventricle (*2* – moderator band: *arrowheads*) is on the right (right loop) and is hypertrophied as it is connected to the aorta and the systemic circulation (the right ventricle acts as the systemic ventricle). The vena cava (here the inferior vena cava – *8i*) merges into the "neocavity" (*n*) (systemic venous pathway – baffle) connected to the left ventricle (*6*) (and pulmonary artery – transposition). Blood entering the left atrium (*5* – derived from pulmonary veins! pulmonary venous pathway) around the neocavity (*n*) drains into the right atrium (*1*), which is connected to the right ventricle (*2*). (**d**) Postoperative sagittal oblique double IR black blood image through the great vessels which remain transposed (as an atrial switch was performed): the aorta (*7*), situated anteriorly (and to the *right*), and the pulmonary artery (*3*), situated posteriorly (and on the *left*), run parallel without crossing ("gun barrel image"). (**e–j**) Other case of complete transposition of the great vessels (D-transposition): Young man treated by Mustard procedure at the age of 1 year (atrial switch).

A second procedure on the systemic aspect (SVC) was performed at the age of 4 years for obstruction on venous pathway. The patient now presents with conduction disorders constituting an indication for pacemaker. MRI is performed to verify patency of the superior vena cava for pacemaker placement. (**e**) Coronal spin-echo image: MRI demonstrates superior vena cava obstruction (*arrow*). (**f**) Coronal oblique gradient-echo image according to the line shown on image (**a**): the superior vena cava is blind (*arrow*) with countercurrent shunting of blood to the inferior vena cava via the azygos vein (*AzV*) and internal mammary vein (*arrowheads*). (**g**) Coronal oblique spin-echo image: note dilatation of the azygos vein, which acts as a shunt (*arrows*). (**h**) Axial spin-echo image through the root of the aorta and pulmonary artery: the great vessels remain transposed (an atrial switch was performed); at its origin, the ascending aorta (*7a*) is situated anteriorly and to the right (D-transposition) of the pulmonary artery (*3*). (**i**) Axial spin-echo image through the termination of the superior vena cava; the superior vena cava is filled by complex scar tissue. (**j**) Axial spin-echo image through the ventricular chambers: the right ventricle (*2*) is on the right (right loop) and is hypertrophied as it is connected to the aorta and the systemic circulation (the right ventricle acts as the systemic ventricle)

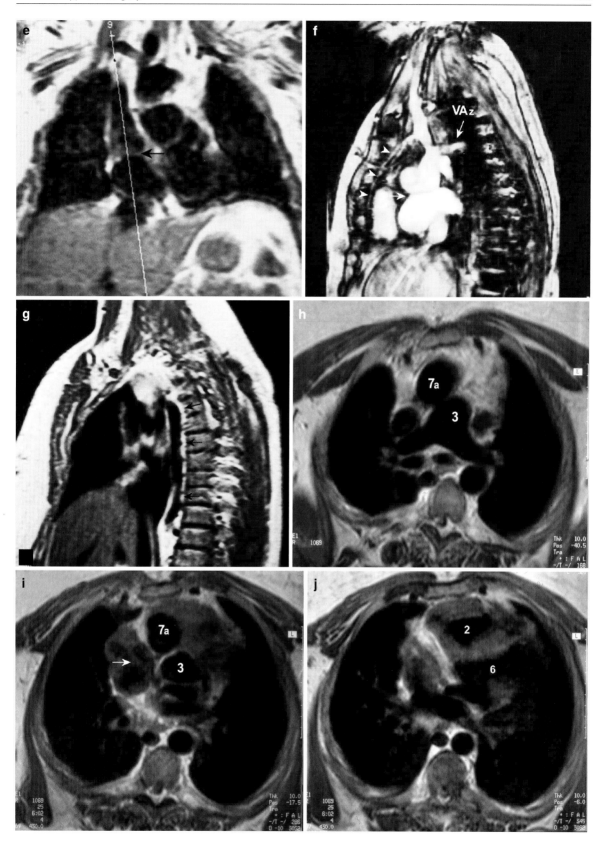

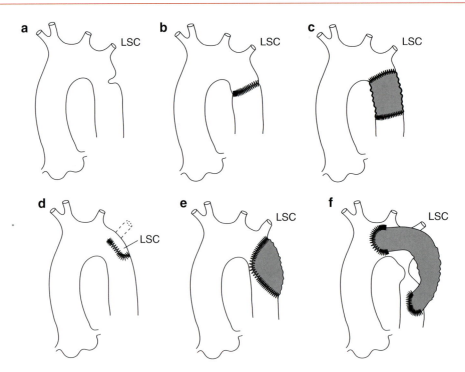

Fig. 8.23 Coarctation surgery. (**a**) Coarctation of the aorta (Ao). Left subclavian artery (LSC). (**b**) Crawford procedure: sufficiently large resection of the stenosis to eliminate all ductal tissue, followed by end-to-end anastomosis of the two aortic segments. (**c**) End-to-end interposition of a Dacron® conduit is sometimes necessary, if the ends of the aorta are too fragile or too far apart to allow direct anastomosis. (**d**) Waldhausen procedure uses a left subclavian artery wall flap to enlarge the stenosis. (**e**) Patch aortoplasty: repair by Dacron® patch. (**f**) Interposition of a Dacron® conduit to act as a palliative shunt in severe forms of coarctation associated with other anomalies or in very extensive forms of coarctation

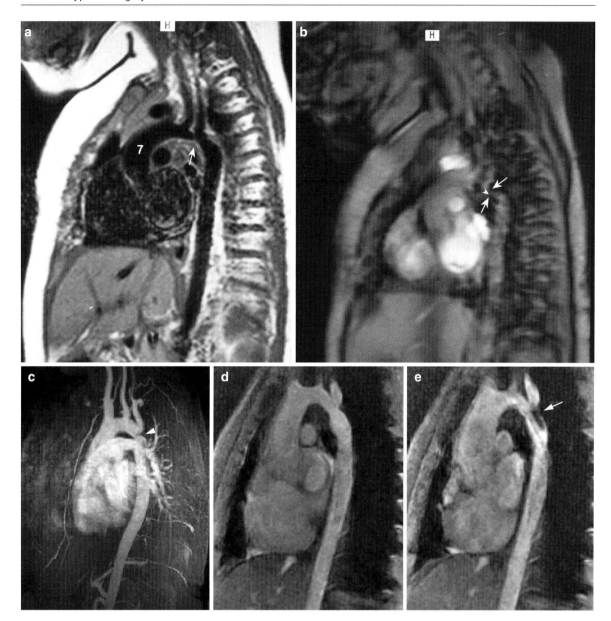

Fig. 8.24 Preductal coarctation corrected by Crawford procedure during the neonatal period. Follow-up at 6 months. (**a**) Spin-echo image: persistent coarctation with a small diaphragm (*arrow*) over the left subclavian artery (suspected on Doppler echocardiography with a gradient of 42 mmHg) aorta (*7*). (**b**) Cine-MRI image: the signal void jet, arising (*arrowhead*) downstream at the site of stenosis (*arrows*), confirms the narrow lumen. (**c–e**) Other example of Crawford procedure in an adolescent female patient. Postoperative assessment. LAO cine-MR images of the aorta. Note the slight narrowing (*arrowhead*) at the suture site on the aorta followed by subtle signal void (*arrows*) present on cine-MRI during systole (image on the *right*) and not during diastole (image in the *middle*) (also see Chap. 5, Figs. 5.8e and 5.18d, e; Chap. 6, Fig. 6.18d, e and Chap. 8, Figs.8.23b for the Crawford procedure)

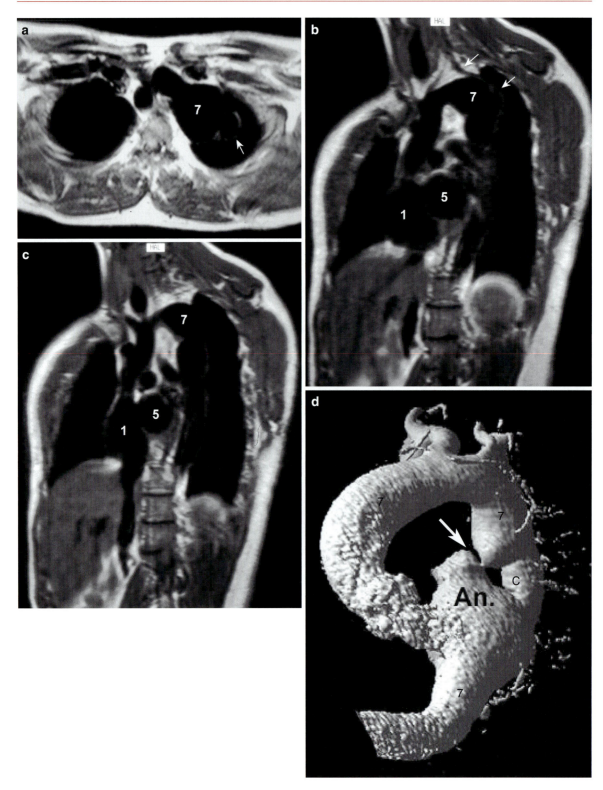

Fig. 8.25 (**a–c**) Preductal coarctation operated at the age of 13 years with sacrifice of the left subclavian artery (Waldhausen procedure). Note the postoperative aneurysmal dilatation of the aorta (7) visible on axial and LAO spin-echo images. The dilatation involves the origin of the retro-esophageal right subclavian artery (arteria lusoria – *arrows*); right atrium (*1*) and left atrium (*5*). (**d**) A Dacron® conduit (*C*) was inserted 15 years ago in this patient with severe coarctation (*arrow*) of the aorta (7). The aneurysm (*An*) at the distal anastomosis is depicted on this CE-MRA 3D MIP reconstruction (Dota-Gd, Guerbet, France)

Fig. 8.26 Surgical correction of type B interrupted aortic arch (**a**): suture of the ductus arteriosus (DA) and left subclavian artery (LSC) allowing mobilization of the distal aortic segment (DAo) which is advanced proximally and sutured end-to-side to the ascending aorta (AAo) (**b**); right and left common carotid arteries (RC and LC), right subclavian artery (RSC) (also see Chap. 6, Fig. 6.20 and 6.21)

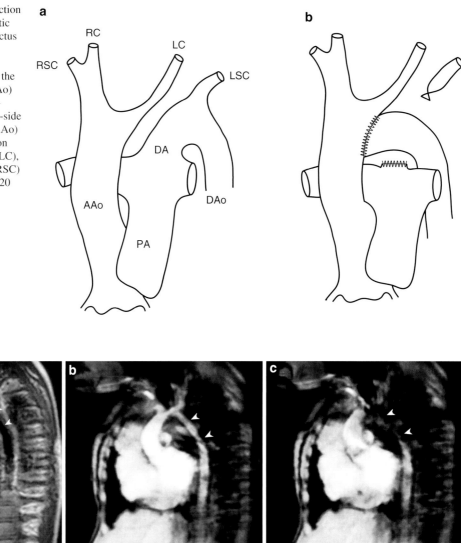

Fig. 8.27 Surgical correction of interrupted aortic arch with interposition of a Dacron® conduit. Interrupted aortic arch with extensive hypoplasia and VSD operated during the neonatal period. Follow-up at 16 months. The Dacron® conduit (straight segment – *arrowhead*) is clearly visible on the two LAO spin-echo (**a**) and cine-MRI images ((**b**), diastole and (**c**), systole). It is patent, but appears to be slightly narrowed compared to the native ascending and descending aorta, as reflected by the significant turbulent flow during systole (signal void – *arrowheads* – in (**c**) compared to (**b**)) (also see Chap. 6, Figs. 6.20 and 6. 21)

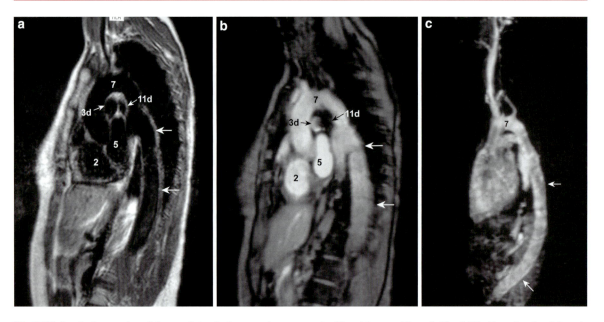

Fig. 8.28 Surgical correction of thoracoabdominal coarctation: a Dacron® conduit shunt was performed between the descending thoracic aorta (aorta – 7) and the abdominal aorta. LAO spin-echo (**a**), cine-MRI (**b**), and gadolinium-enhanced MR angiography (**c**) images show that the shunt (*arrows*) is patent and presents a nor- mal caliber (also see Chap. 6, Fig. 6.10). Note that the right pul- monary artery (*3d*) is black on the spin-echo sequence and white on the gradient-echo sequence (flow) and the right main bronchus is black on the spin-echo and gradient-echo sequences (air); right ventricle (*2*); left atrium (*5*) right main bronchus (*11d*)

Fig. 8.29 Diagram of the procedure designed to enlarge the right ventricular outflow tract in tetralogy of Fallot. (**a**) Incision (*fine dotted line*) performed on the infundibulum and pulmonary artery (PA). A major coronary branch (6% of cases) crossing in front of the pulmonary infundibulum may be situated on the zone of the ventriculotomy incision. For example, the left anterior descending artery (LAD) can arise abnormally (*large dots*) from the right coronary artery (RCo); left coronary and circumflex arteries (LCo and Cx), aorta (Ao). (**b**) Enlargement of the right ventricular outflow tract by a pericardial or synthetic patch

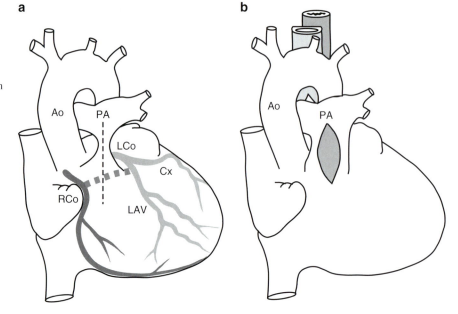

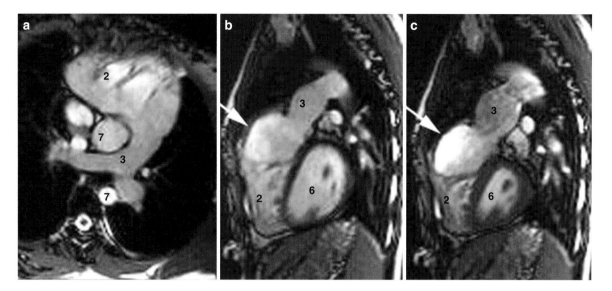

Fig. 8.30 Enlargement of the right ventricular outflow tract by a pericardial patch in a patient with tetralogy of Fallot. Axial (**a**) and sagittal (**b, c**) cine-MR images. Note the dilatation (*arrow*) at the site of the patch. Aorta (*7*), right ventricle (*2*), pulmonary artery (*3*) left ventricle (*6*)

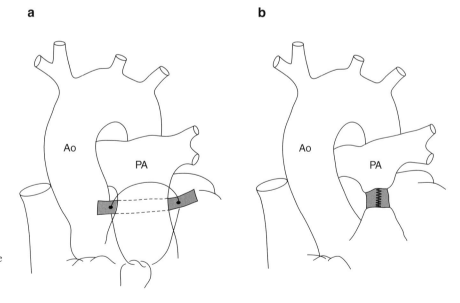

Fig. 8.31 Diagram of pulmonary artery banding. (**a**) The synthetic band is placed around the origin of the pulmonary artery (PA). (**b**) The diameter of banding is adjusted so that the pulmonary artery systolic pressure is equal to 1/3 of the systemic blood pressure. Aorta (Ao)

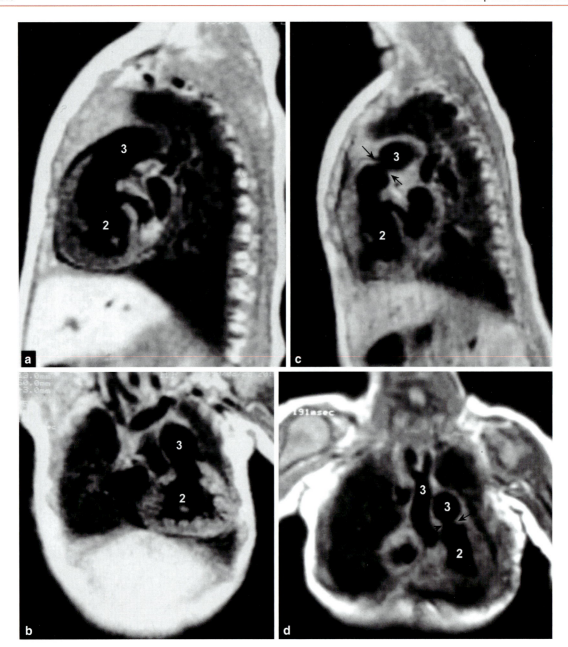

Fig. 8.32 Double outlet right ventricle; pulmonary artery banding. Coronal and sagittal spin-echo images. Preoperative (**a**, **b**) and postoperative (**c**, **d**) images demonstrating the efficacy of banding on the pulmonary artery diameter (*arrows*); right ventricle (*2*), pulmonary artery (*3*) (also see preoperative images of the same patient, Chap. 3, Fig. 3.24 and Chap. 7, Fig. 7.19)

Table 8.1 Postoperative MRI assessment

Palliative procedures and surgical correction of pulmonary revascularization			
Palliative shunts	*Anastomosis*	*Complications*	*Slices centered on shunt (always axial)*
Blalock–Taussig	SCA – homolateral PA	Stenosis, occlusion	Axial – coronal oblique
Central shunt	Asc Ao – PA trunk	Preferential flow and lung	Axial (Asc Ao – PA trunk)
Waterston	Asc Ao – RPA	hypertrophy	– LAO in axis of shunt
Potts	Desc Ao – LPA	Homolateral/anastomosis	Axial – sagittal oblique
Glenn (and bidirectional	SVC – RPA	Stenosis, thrombosis of SVC	(Asc Ao – RPA)
cavopulmonary)		and site of anastomosis	Posterior coronal
			(Asc Ao – LPA)
			Anterior coronal
			(SVC – RPA)
Complete Fontan corrections and variants	*Anastomosis*	*Complications*	*Slices centered on conduit (always axial)*
Classical Fontan (Glenn,	LA – PA	Thrombosis – narrowing of	Axial – Coronal
see above)	SVC – RPA	conduit, pseudoaneurysms	Axial – Coronal
Bidirectional cavopulmonary	SVC – RPA and	RA dilatation (Fontan)	Axial – Coronal
Complete cavopulmonary	IVC – LPA conduit	Thrombosis – narrowing of	Axial – Sagittal
Rastelli	RV – PA	conduit, pseudoaneurysms	
		Narrowing of conduit,	
		pseudoaneurysms	
Correction of transposition of great vessels			
Type	*Technique*	*Complications*	*Slices (always axial)*
Arterial switch	Ao-PA arterial switch	Stenosis at anastomotic	Axial – Sagittal –
Atrial switch	Atrial switch	sutures (RV outflow +++),	short-axis
Senning	SVC and IVC to	pseudoaneurysms	
Mustard	neocavity	Obstructions – systemic and	Axial – short-axis – coronal
	IAS and RA patch	pulmonary venous stenoses	
	Pericardial patch	tricuspid and RV insufficiency	
Coarctation surgery			
Type	*Technique*	*Complications*	*Slices (always axial)*
Crafoord	Resection – anastomosis	Restenosis, pseudoaneurysms,	Axial – LAO – coronal
Dacron® conduit		HT	Axial – LAO – coronal
Waldhausen	Resection – Dacron®		Axial – LAO – coronal
Patch aortoplasty	conduit – anastomosis		
	Flap derived from left		
	subclavian vein		
	Resection – Dacron®		
	enlargement patch		

8.7 Conclusion

Since the first, already very promising reports on the potential of MRI for postoperative assessment of congenital heart disease, considerable technological progress has transformed the follow-up of these patients. MRI is perfectly complementary to echocardiography (difficult in this field), making the Doppler echocardiography-MRI combination extremely efficient noninvasive and nonionizing imaging combination.

References

1. Hoffman JIE, Christhianson R. Congenital heart disease in a cohort of 19.502 births with long term follow up. Am J Cardiol. 1978;42:641–7.
2. Fletcher BD, Jacobstein MD, Nelson DA, et al. Gated magnetic resonance imaging of congenital cardiac malformations. Radiology. 1984;150:137–40.
3. Higgins CB, Byrd III BF, Farmer DW, et al. Magnetic resonance imaging in patients with congenital heart disease. Circulation. 1984;70:851–60.

4. Jacobstein MD, Fletcher BD, Nelson AD, et al. ECG-gated nuclear magnetic resonance imaging: appearance of the congenitally malformed heart. Am Heart J. 1984;107:1014–20.

5. Didier D, Higgins CB, Fisher MR, et al. Congenital heart disease: gated MR imaging in 72 patients. Pediatr Radiol. 1986;158:227–35.

6. Kastler B, Livolsi A, Germain P, et al. MRI in congenital heart disease of newborns. Preliminary results in 23 patients. Eur J Radiol. 1990;10:109–17.

7. Kersting-Sommerhoff BA, Sechtem UP, Higgins CB. Evaluation of pulmonary blood supply by nuclear magnetic resonance imaging in patients with pulmonary atresia. J Am Coll Cardiol. 1988;11:66–71.

8. Formanck AG, Witeofski RI, Souza VJ, et al. MR imaging of the central pulmonary arterial tree in conotroncus malformation. Am J Roentgenol. 1986;147:1127–31.

9. Julsrud PR. Magnetic resonance imaging of the pulmonary arteries and veins. Semin Ultrasound CT MR. 1990;11:184–205.

10. Dorfman AL, Geva T. Magnetic resonance imaging evaluation of congenital heart disease: conotruncal anomalies. J Cardiovasc Magn Reson. 2006;8(4):645–59.

11. Soulen RL, Dooner RM. Magnetic resonance imaging of rerouted pulmonary blood flow. Radiol Clin North Am. 1985;23:737–44.

12. Jacobstein MD, Fletcher BD, Nelson AD, Riemenchneider TA, Alfidi RJ. MRI: evaluation of palliative systemic pulmonary shunts. Circulation. 1984;70:650–6.

13. Katz ME, Glazer HS, Siegel MJ, Gutierrez F, Levill RG, Lee JK. Mediastinal vessels: post-operative evaluation with MRI. Radiology. 1986;161:647–51.

14. Kastler B, Livolsi A, Willard D, Wackenheim A. MRI in the pre- and post-surgical evaluation of congenital heart disease in newborns. RSNA, 75th Assembly and Annual Meeting, Chicago, Nov 26–Dec 1, 1989. Radiology. 1989;173:Abstract 35.

15. Kastler B, Livolsi A, Germain P, et al. Evaluation of Blalock-Taussig shunts in newborns: value of oblique MRI planes. Int J Card Imaging. 1991;7:1–5.

16. Kastler B, Livolsi A, Tajamady T, Willard D, Wackenheim A. Intérêt de l'IRM dans le diagnostic et le suivi postopératoire des cardiopathies congénitales en période néonatale. Radiologie. 1989;9:331–6.

17. Chung KJ, Simpson IA, Glass RF, et al. Cine MRI after surgical repair in patients with transposition of the great arteries. Circulation. 1988;77:104–9.

18. Rastelli GC, McGoon DC, Wallace RB. A new approach to "anatomic" transposition of the great arteries with ventricular sptum defect and subpulmonary stenosis. J Thorac Cardiovasc Surg. 1969;58:545–52.

19. Campbell RM, Moreau GA, Johns JA, et al. Detection of caval obstruction by MRI after intraatrial repair of transposition of the great arteries. Am J Cardiol. 1987;60:688–91.

20. Julsrud PR, Ehman RL, Hagler DJ, Ilstrup DM. Extracardiac vasculature in candidates for Fontan surgery: MR imaging. Radiology. 1989;173:503–6.

21. Higgins CB. MRI of congenital heart disease. In: Higgins CB, editor. Essentials of cardiac radiology and imaging. Philadelphia, PA: Lippincott; 1992. p. 283–331.

22. von Schulthess GK, Fisher S, Crooks LE, et al. Gated MR imaging of the heart: Intracardiac signals in patients and healthy subjects cardiac. Radiology. 1985;156(1):12532.

23. Felmlee JP, Ehman RL. Spatial presaturation: a method for suppressing flow artifacts and improving depiction of vascular anatomy in MR imaging. Radiology. 1987;164:559–64.

24. Kastler B. Dans: Comprendre l'IRM: Imagerie du flux; B Kastler. 6th ed. Paris: Masson; 2006. p. 189–213.

25. Atkinson D, Teresi L. Magnetic resonance angiography. Magn Reson Q. 1994;10:149–72.

26. Link KM, Lesko NM. Magnetic resonance imaging in the evaluation of congenital heart disease. Magn Reson Q. 1991;7:173–90.

27. Edelman RR, Chien D, Kim D. Fast selective black blood MR imaging. Radiology. 1991;181(3):655–60.

28. Boiselle PM, White CS. New techniques in cardiothoracic imaging. New York, NY: Informa Healthcare; 2007. p. 81–2.

29. Wehrli FW, Haacke EM. Principles of MR imaging. In: Potchen EJ, Haacke EM, Siebert JE, Gottschalk A, editors. Magnetic resonance angiography: concepts and applications. St Louis, MO: Mosby-Year Book; 1993. p. 9–34.

30. Sechtem U, Pflugfelder PW, White RD, et al. Cine MR imaging: potential for the evaluation of cardiovascular function. AJR Am J Roentgenol. 1987;148:239–46.

31. Sechtem U, Pflugfelder P, Cassidy MC, Holt W, Wolfe C, Higgins CB. Ventricular septal defect: visualization of shunt flow and determination of shunt size by cine MR imaging. AJR Am J Roentgenol. 1987;149:689–92.

32. Baker EJ, Ayton V, Smith MA, et al. Magnetic resonance imaging at a high field strength of ventricular septal defects in infants. Br Heart J. 1989;62:305–10.

33. Simpson IA, Chung KJ, Glass RF, Sahn DJ, Sherman FS, Hesselink J. Cine magnetic resonance imaging for evaluation of anatomy and flow relations in infants and children with coarctation of the aorta. Circulation. 1988;78:142–8.

34. Weber OM, Higgins CB. MR evaluation of cardiovascular physiology in congenital heart disease: flow and function. J Cardiovasc Magn Reson. 2006;8(4):607–17.

35. Mostbeck GH, Caputo GR, Higgins CB. MR measurement of blood flow in the cardiovascular system. AJR Am J Roentgenol. 1992;159:453–61.

36. Nayler GL, Firmin DN, Longmore DB. Blood flow imaging by cine magnetic resonance. J Comput Assist Tomogr. 1986;10:715–22.

37. Bogren HG, Klipstein RH, Firmin DN, et al. Quantification of antegrade and retrograde blood flow in the human aorta by magnetic resonance velocity mapping. Am Heart J. 1989;117:1214–22.

38. Rees S, Firmin D, Mohiaddin R, Underwood R, Longmore D. Application of flow measurements by magnetic resonance velocity mapping to congenital heart disease. Am J Cardiol. 1989;64:953–6.

39. Elc NJ, Herfkens RJ, Shimakawa A, Enzmann DR. Phase contrast cine magnetic resonance imaging. Magn Reson Q. 1991;7:229–54.

40. Ilner PJ, Firmin DN, Rees RSO, et al. Valve and great vessel stenosis: assesment with MR jet velocity mapping. Radiology. 1991;178:229–35.

41. Rebergen SA, Van Der Wall EE, Doornbos J, De Roos A. Magnetic resonance measurement of velocity and flow: technique, validation, and cardiovascular applications. Am Heart J. 1993;126:1439–56.

42. Pelc NJ, Sommer G, Li KCP, Brosnan TJ, Herfkens RJ, Enzmann DR. Quantitative magnetic resonance flow imaging. Magn Reson Q. 1994;10:125–47.

43. Rebergen SA, Niezen RA, Helbing WA, Van Der Wall EE, De Roos A. Cine gradient-echo MR imaging and MR velocity mapping in the evaluation of congenital heart disease. Radiographics. 1996;16(3):467–81.

44. Kastler B, IRM des malformations cardiovasculaires. Edition. Paris: Elsevier; 2001.

45. Lohan DG, Krishnam M, Saleh R, Tomasian A, Finn JP. Time-resolved MR angiography of the thorax. Magn Reson Imaging Clin N Am. 2008;16(2):235–48.

46. Blalock A, Taussig HB. The surgical treatment of malformations of the heart in which there is pulmonary stenosis or pulmonary atresia. JAMA. 1945;128(3):189–202.

47. Gladman G, Mc Crindle BW, Williams WG, Freedom RM, Benson LM. The modified Blalock-Taussig shunt: clinical impact and morbidity in Fallot's tetralogy in the current era. J Thorac Cardiovasc Surg. 1997;114:25–30.

48. Moulton AL, Brenner JI, Ringel R, Nordenberg A, Berman MA, Ali S, et al. Classic versus modified Blalock-Taussig shunts in neonates and infants. Circulation. 1985;72:1135–44.

49. Ichida F, Hashimoto I, Miyazaki A, et al. Magnetic resonance imaging: evaluation of the Blalock-Taussig shunts and anatomy of the pulmonary artery. J Cardiol. 1992;22(4):669–78.

50. Potts WJ. Congenital heart disease in cyanotic children. Calif Med. 1953;785:101–3.

51. Fenn JE, Glenn WW, Guilfoil PH, Hume M, Patino JF. Circulatory bypass of the right heart. II. Further observations on vena caval-pulmonary artery shunts. Surg Forum. 1956;6:189–93.

52. Waterston DJ, Stark J, Ashcraft KW. Ascending aorta-to-right pulmonary artery shunts: experience with 100 patients. Surgery. 1972;72(6):897–904.

53. Williams WG, Rubis L, Trulser GA, Mustard WT. Palliation of tricuspid atresia. Potts-Smith, Glenn, and Blalock-Taussig shunts. Arch Surg. 1975;110(11):1383–6.

54. Barragry TP, Ring WS, Blatchford JW, Foker JE. Central aorta-pulmonary artery shunts in neonates with complex cyanotic congenital heart disease. J Thorac Cardiovasc Surg. 1987;93(5):767–74.

55. Trusler GA, Miyamura H, Culham JA, Fowler RS, Freedom RM, Williams WG. Pulmonary artery stenosis following aortopulmonary anastomose. Br Heart J. 1976;38(9): 957–60.

56. Nwaneri NJ, Fortune RL. Aneurysm of the pulmonary artery. Rare long term complication of central aorto-pulmonary shunts for congenital heart disease. Report of two cases with review of the literature. J Cardiovasc Surg (Torino). 1986;27(1):94–9.

57. Schmaltz AA, Neudorf U, Sack S, Galal O. Interventions in congenital heart disease and their sequelae in adults. Herz. 1999;24(4):293–306.

58. Hull DA, Shinebourne E, Gerlis L, Nicholson AG, Sheppard MN. Rupture of pulmonary aneurysms in association with long-standing Waterston shunts. Cardiol Young. 2001;11(1):123–7.

59. Fontan F, Baudet E. Surgical repair of tricuspide atresia. Thorax. 1971;26(3):240–8.

60. Jatene AD, Fontes VF, Paulista PP, Souza LC, Neger F, Galantier M, et al. Anatomic correction of transposition of the great vessels. J Thorac Cardiovasc Surg. 1976;72(3):364–70.

61. Wernovsky G, Jonas RA, Colan SD, Sanders SP, Wessel DL, Castanñeda AR, et al. Results of the arterial switch operation in patients with transposition of the great arteries and abnormalities of the mitral valve or left ventricular outflow tract. J Am Coll Cardiol. 1990;16(6):1446–54.

62. Wernovsky G, Mayer JE Jr, Jonas RA, Hanley FL, Blackstone EH, Kirklin JW, et al. Factors influencing early and late outcome of the arterial switch operation for transposition of the great arteries. J Thorac Cardiovasc Surg. 1995;109(2):289–301; discussion 301–2.

63. Waldhausen JA, Boruchow I, Miller WW, Rashkind WJ. Transposition of the great arteries with ventricular septal defect. Palliation by atrial septostomy and pulmonary artery banding. Circulation. 1969;39(5 Suppl 1):I215–21.

64. Senning A. Surgical correction of transposition of the great vessels. Surgery. 1959;45:966–80.

65. Corno AF, Parisi F, Marino B, Ballerini L, Marcelletti C. Palliative Mustard operation: an expanded horizon. Eur J Cardiothorac Surg. 1987;1(3):144–7.

66. Mustard WT. Successful two-stage correction of transposition of the great vessels. Surgery. 1964;55:469–72.

67. Deanfield J, Camm J, Macartney F, et al. Arrhythmia and late mortality after Mustard and Senning operation for transposition of the great arteries: an eight-year prospective study. J Thorac Cardiovasc Surg. 1988;96:569–76.

68. Wong KY, Venables AW, Kelly MJ, et al. Longitudinal studies of ventricular function after the Mustard operation of transposition of the great arteries: a long term follow up. Br Heart J. 1988;60:316–22.

69. Ebenroth ES, Hurwitz RA. Functional outcome of patients operated for d-transposition of the great arteries with the Mustard procedure. Am J Cardiol. 2002;89(3):353–6.

70. Dos L, Teruel L, Ferreira IJ, Rodriguez-Larrea J, Miro L, Girona J, et al. Late outcome of Senning and Mustard procedures for correction of transposition of the great arteries. Heart. 2005;91(5):652–6.

71. Lorenz CH, Walker ES, Graham Jr TP, Powers TA. Right ventricular performance and mass by use of cine MRI late after atrial repair of transposition of the great arteries. Circulation. 1995;92(9 Suppl):II233–9.

72. Babu-Narayan SV, Goktekin O, Moon JC, Broberg CS, Pantely GA, Pennell DJ, et al. Late gadolinium enhancement cardiovascular magnetic resonance of the systemic right ventricle in adults with previous atrial redirection surgery for transposition of the great arteries. Circulation. 2005; 111(16):2091–8.

73. Campbell M. Natural history of coarctation of the aorta. Br Heart J. 1970;32:633–40.

74. Fixler DE. Coarctation of the aorta. Cardiol Clin. 1988;6(4): 561–71.

75. Dupuis C, Kachaner J, Freedom RM, Payot M, Davignon A. Coarctation de l'aorte. In: Cardiologie pédiatrique. Paris: Flammarion Médecine Sciences; 1991. p. 265–84.

76. Tronc F, Curtil A, Robin J, Ninet J, Champsaur G. Coarctation et son traitement chirurgical. Arch Mal Coeur Vaiss. 1997;90:1729–36.

77. Di Filippo S, Sassolas F, Bozio A. Résultats à long terme après chirurgie de coarctation aortique chez le nouveau-né et l'enfant. Arch Mal Coeur Vaiss. 1997;90:1723–8.

78. Didier D, Saint-Martin C, Lapierre C, Trindade PT, Lahlaidi N, Vallee JP, et al. Coarctation of the aorta: pre and postoperative evaluation with MRI and MR angiography; correlation with echocardiography and surgery. Int J Cardiovasc Imaging. 2006;22(3–4):457–75.

79. Shih MC, Tholpady A, Kramer CM, Sydnor MK, Hagspiel KD. Surgical and endovascular repair of aortic coarctation: normal findings and appearance of complications on CT angiography and MR angiography. AJR Am J Roentgenol. 2006;187(3):W302–12.

80. Crafoord C. Classics in thoracic surgery. Correction of aortic coarctation. Ann Thorac Surg. 1980;30(3):300–2.

81. Waldhausen JA, Nahrwold DL. Repair of coarctation of the aorta with a subclavian flap. J Thorac Cardiovasc Surg. 1966;51(4):532–3.

82. Worms AM, Marcon F, Michalski H, Chehab G. Angioplastie percutanée de recoarctation de l'aorte: résultats dans 18 cas à court et moyen terme. Arch Mal Coeur Vaiss. 1993; 86: 573–9.

83. Diethrich EB, Heuser RR, Cardenas JR, Eckert J, Tarlian H. Endovascular techniques in adult aortic coarctation: the use of stents for native and recurrent coarctation repair. J Endovasc Surg. 1995;2(2):183–8.

84. Pilla CB, Fontes VF, Pedra CA. Endovascular stenting for aortic coarctation. Expert Rev Cardiovasc Ther. 2005;3(5): 879–90.

85. Karl TR. Surgery is the best treatment for primary coarctation in the majority of cases. J Cardiovasc Med. 2007;8(1): 50–6. Review

86. Brouuwer RM, Erasmus ME, Ebols T, Eijgelaar A. Influence of age on survival, late hypertension and recoarctation in elective coarctation repair. Including long term results after elective aortic coarctation repair with a follow up from 25 to 44 years. J Thorac Cardiovasc Surg. 1994;108(3):525–31.

87. Conte S, Lacour-Gayet F, Serraf A. Surgical management of neonatal coarctation. J Thorac Cardiovasc Surg. 1995;109(4): 663–74.

88. Vanhulle C, Durand I, Tron P. Paraplégie par ischémie médullaire après cure chirurgicale d'une coarctation de l'aorte. Arch Pédiatric. 1998;5:633–6.

89. Bogaert J, Kuzo R, Dymarkowski S, Janssen L, Celis I, Budts W, et al. Follow-up of patients with previous treatment for coarctation of the thoracic aorta: comparison between contrast-enhanced MR angiography and fast spin-echo MR imaging. Eur Radiol. 2000;10(12):1847–54.

90. Oliver JM, Gallego P, Gonzalez A, Aroca A, Bret M, Mesa JM. Risk factors for aortic complications in adults with coarctation of the aorta. J Am Coll Cardiol. 2004;44(8): 1641–7.

91. Ou P, Bonnet D, Auriacombe L, Pedroni E, Balleux F, Sidi D, et al. Late systemic hypertension and aortic arch geometry after successful repair of coarctation of the aorta. Eur Heart J. 2004;25(20):1853–9.

92. Ou P, Mousseaux E, Celermajer DS, Pedroni E, Vouhe P, Sidi D, et al. Aortic arch shape deformation after coarctation surgery: effect on blood pressure response. J Thorac Cardiovasc Surg. 2006;132(5):1105–11.

93. Ou P, Celermajer DS, Mousseaux E, Giron A, Aggoun Y, Szezepanski I, et al. Vascular remodeling after "successful" repair of coarctation: impact of aortic arch geometry. J Am Coll Cardiol. 2007;49(8):883–90.

94. Ou P, Celermajer DS, Raisky O, Jolivet O, Buyens F, Herment A, et al. Angular (Gothic) aortic arch leads to enhanced systolic wave reflection, central aortic stiffness, and increased left ventricular mass late after aortic coarctation repair: evaluation with magnetic resonance flow mapping. J Thorac Cardiovasc Surg. 2008;135(1):62–8.

95. Geva T, Sandweiss BM, Gauvreau K, Lock JE, Powell AJ. Factors associated with impaired clinical status in long-term survivors of tetralogy of Fallot repair evaluated by magnetic resonance imaging. J Am Coll Cardiol. 2004; 43(6):1068–74.

96. Murphy JG, Gersh BJ, Mair DD, Fuster V, Mcgoon MD, Ilstrup DM, et al. Long-term outcome in patients undergoing surgical repair of tetralogy of Fallot. N Engl J Med. 1993;329(9):593–9.

97. Nollert G, Fischlein T, Bouterwek S, Böhmer C, Klinner W, Reichart B. Long-term survival in patients with repair of tetralogy of Fallot: 36-year follow-up of 490 survivors of the first year after surgical repair. J Am Coll Cardiol. 1997;30(5):1374–83.

98. Vliegen HW, Van Straten A, De Roos A, Roest AA, Schoof PH, Zwinderman AH, et al. Magnetic resonance imaging to assess the hemodynamic effects of pulmonary valve replacement in adults late after repair of tetralogy of Fallot. Circulation. 2002;106(13):1703–7.

99. Li W, Davlouros PA, Kilner PJ, Pennell DJ, Gibson D, Henein MY, et al. Doppler-echocardiographic assessment of pulmonary regurgitation in adults with repaired tetralogy of Fallot: comparison with cardiovascular magnetic resonance imaging. Am Heart J. 2004;147(1):165–72.

100. Li J, Soukias ND, Carvalho J, Ho SY. Coronary arterial anatomy in tetralogy of Fallot: morphological and clinical correlations. Heart. 1998;80(2):174–83.

101. Dabizzi RP, Teodori G, Barletta GA, Caprioli G, Baldrighi G, Baldrighi V. Associated coronary and cardiac anomalies in the tetralogy of Fallot. An angiographic study. Eur Heart J. 1990;11:692–704.

102. Botnar RM, Stuber M, Kissinger KV, Manning WJ. Free-breathing 3D coronary MRA: the impact of "isotropic" image resolution. J Magn Reson Imaging. 2000;11(4):389–93.

103. Holmqvist C, Hochbergs P, Björkhem G, Brockstedt S, Laurin S. Pre-operative evaluation with MR in tetralogy of Fallot and pulmonary atresia with ventricular septal defect. Acta Radiol. 2002;43(3):346.

104. Freedom RM, Beson LN, Smallhorn JF, Williams WG, Trusler GA, Rowe RD. Subaortic stenosis, the univentricular heart and banding the pulmonary artery: an analysis of the course of 43 patients with univentricular heart pallated by pulmonary banding. Circulation. 1985;73:758–64.

105. Daenen W, Eyskens B, Meyns B, Gewillig M. Neonatal pulmonary artery banding does not compromise the short-term function of a Damus-Kaye-Stansel connection. Eur J Cardiothorac Surg. 2000;17(6):655–7.

106. Cerillo AG, Murzi B, Giusti S, Crucean A, Redaelli S, Vanini V. Pulmonary artery banding and ventricular septal defect enlargement in patients with univentricular atrioventricular connection and the aorta originating from an incomplete ventricle. Eur J Cardiothorac Surg. 2002; 22(2):192–9.

107. Chang YH, Kim WH, Lee JY, Kim SJ, Lee C, Hwang SW, et al. Pulmonary artery banding before the Damus-Kaye-Stansel procedure. Pediatr Cardiol. 2006;27(5): 594–9.

108. Damus PS. Correspondence. Ann Thorac Surg. 1975; 20:724–5.

109. Lui RC, Williams WG, Trusler GA, Freedom RM, Coles JG, Rebeyka IM, et al. Experience with the Damus-Kaye-Stansel procedure for children with Taussig-Bing hearts or univentricular hearts with subaortic stenosis. Circulation. 1993;88(5 Pt 2):II170–6.

110. Dos L, Pen V, Silversides C, Provost Y, Oeschlin E, Horlick E, et al. Images in cardiovascular medicine. Cardiac magnetic resonance imaging and multidetector computed tomography scan illustrating Damus-Kaye-Stansel operation. Circulation. 2007;115:e440–2.

Adams FH, Emmanouilides GC, Riemenshneider TA. Heart disease in infants, children, and adolescent. Baltimore: Williams and Wilkins; 1987.

Elliot LP. Cardiac imaging in infants, children, and adults. Philadelphia: JB Lippincott; 1991.

Heim de Balsac R, Métianu C, Durand M, Dubost Ch. Traite des cardiopathies congenitales. Paris: Masson; 1954.

Higgins CB, Silvermann NH, Kerting-Sommerhoff B, Schmidt KG. Congenital heart disease, echocardiography and magnetic resonance imaging. New York: Raven; 1990.

Khonsiari S. Cardiac surgery: safeguards and pittfalls in operative techniques. Philadelphia: Lippincott Williams and Wilkins; 1996.

Yen Ho S, Baker EJ, Rigby ML, Anderson RH. Color atlas of congenital heart disease morphologic and clinical correlations. London: Mosby-Wolfe; 1995.

B. Kastler, *MRI of Cardiovascular Malformations*,
DOI: 10.1007/978-3-540-30702-0, © Springer-Verlag Berlin Heidelberg 2011

Index

B. Kastler, *MRI of Cardiovascular Malformations*,
DOI: 10.1007/978-3-540-30702-0, © Springer-Verlag Berlin Heidelberg 2011

Printing and Binding: Stürtz GmbH, Würzburg